Recent Advances in
CLINICAL PHARMACOLOGY

PAUL TURNER MD BSc FRCP
Professor of Clinical Pharmacology, the University of London;
Consultant Physician, St Bartholomew's Hospital, London

DAVID G. SHAND PhD MRCP
Professor of Pharmacology and Medicine,
Duke University,
Durham, North Carolina

Recent Advances in
CLINICAL PHARMACOLOGY

EDITED BY

PAUL TURNER

DAVID G. SHAND

NUMBER ONE

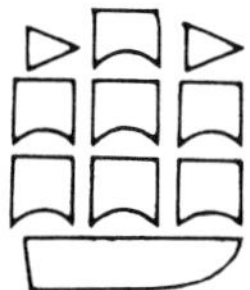

CHURCHILL LIVINGSTONE
EDINBURGH LONDON AND NEW YORK   1978

CHURCHILL LIVINGSTONE
Medical Division of Longman Group Limited

Distributed in the United States of America by Longman
Inc., 19 West 44th Street, New York, N.Y. 10036, and by
associated companies, branches and representatives
throughout the world.

First published 1978

ISBN 0 443 01572 4

British Library Cataloguing in Publication Data

Recent advances in clinical pharmacology.
  No.1.
  1. Pharmacology
  I. Turner, Paul, b.1933   II. Shand, David G
  615'.7   RM300   78-40710

Printed in Great Britain by Bell and Bain Ltd, Glasgow

Preface

While we felt honoured by the invitation to edit this first volume of a new series of Recent Advances, we hesitated to accept for several reasons. Firstly, clinical pharmacology is a young discipline and rapid changes are taking place in our understanding of the pharmacological basis of normal human body function, of diseases and of its treatment. It was, therefore, inevitable that the delay between the writing of chapters for this volume and their publication would mean that some material would already be out-of-date, and that other subjects, important at the time of publication, would be omitted because their importance had grown since the book's planning stage. This explains, for example, the absence of a chapter devoted to human H_2 receptor activity and blockade. Secondly, we were reluctant to ask colleagues who are already heavily committed to research to give up their time to yet more writing, for we know only too well, the heavy pressures from many sides to contribute to books and symposia. We thank them most sincerely for their willingness to collaborate with us.

Nevertheless, we were attracted by the thought of an on-going series of volumes devoted to advances in clinical pharmacology, for we are convinced that a better use of drugs in the prevention and treatment of disease depends upon a deeper understanding of the scientific principles underlying drug action. We hope, therefore, that this volume will prove of interest and value not only to students of clinical pharmacology, but to prescribing doctors in all clinical disciplines.

David G. Shand
Paul Turner

Contributors

ALAN BENNETT PhD DSc
Professor of Pharmacology, King's College Hospital, London

D. G. GRAHAME-SMITH MA MB BS PhD FRCP
Rhodes Professor of Clinical Pharmacology, University of Oxford; Honorary Consultant Physician, Oxford Area Health Authority; Honorary Director, MRC Unit of Clinical Pharmacology, Oxford

CYRUS R. KUMANA BSc MB BS MRCP
Clinical Pharmacologist/Cardiologist and Assistant Professor of Medicine, McMaster University, Hamilton, Ontario

GRAHAM E. MARLIN MB BS FRACP
Specialist, Respiratory Unit, Repatriation General Hospital, Concord, New South Wales

ALAN S. NIES MD
Professor of Medicine and Pharmacology, Division of Clinical Pharmacology, University of Colorado School of Medicine, Denver

M. W. ORR MD MA BSc MRCPsych
Lecturer in Psychiatry, Department of Psychiatry, University of Oxford (Warneford Hospital)

L. F. PRESCOTT MD FRCP
Consultant Physician, Royal Infirmary, and Reader in Clinical Pharmacology, University Department of Therapeutics, Edinburgh

ALAN RICHENS PhD MRCP
Reader in Clinical Pharmacology, St Bartholomew's Hospital and Institute of Neurology, London

DAVID ROBERTSON MD
Assistant Professor of Medicine and Pharmacology, Vanderbilt University, Nashville

T. ZVONKO RUMBOLDT MD
Chief, Clinical Pharmacology Unit, General Hospital, 5800 Split, Yugoslavia

DAVID G. SHAND PhD MRCP
Professor of Pharmacology and Medicine, Duke University, Durham, North Carolina

W. LEIGH THOMPSON PhD MD FACP
Director, Clinical Pharmacology Program, University Hospitals of Cleveland; Associate Professor of Medicine and Pharmacology, Case Western Reserve University, Cleveland

PAUL TURNER MD BSc FRCP
Professor of Clinical Pharmacology in the University of London; Consultant Physician to St Bartholomew's Hospital, London

RAYMOND L. WOOSLEY MD PhD
Associate Professor of Medicine and Pharmacology, Vanderbilt University School of Medicine, Nashville

Contents

1. Clinical pharmacokinetics—Recent advances in pharmacokinetics *David Shand* Some aspects of the relationship between plasma drug levels and their pharmacological effects *Paul Turner*   1

2. Prostaglandins *Alan Bennett*   17

3. Selectivity of beta-adrenoceptor agonists and antagonists *Cyrus R. Kumana Graham E. Marlin*   31

4. Antihypertensive drugs *David Robertson   Alan S. Nies*   55

5. Antiarrhythmic drugs *Raymond L. Woosley   T. Zvonko Rumboldt*   93

6. Drug therapy of shock *W. Leigh Thompson*   123

7. Antiepileptic drugs *Alan Richens*   147

8. Clinical psychopharmacology *D. G. Grahame-Smith   M. W. Orr*   163

9. Drug toxicity *L. F. Prescott*   189

Index   205

1. Clinical pharmacokinetics

David Shand   Paul Turner

RECENT ADVANCES IN PHARMACOKINETICS

David Shand

Considerable advances have been made in the last decade which have changed pharmacokinetics from a purely descriptive, mathematical science, albeit at a very sophisticated level, to one in which the biology of the system has received increasing attention. This more physiological approach arose out of the need to understand and quantify the factors that determine drug concentrations to better predict what might happen in patients whose disease or drug therapy can lead to quite profound alterations in drug disposition. The intense interest of clinical pharmacology in such matters is therefore not surprising. While overemphasis on pharmacokinetics has been criticised, perhaps with some justification, the fundamental principle that a drug's effects are related to its concentration at the receptor which, in turn, is often reflected by circulating drug levels has been amply confirmed. It has also been repeatedly shown that differences in drug disposition resulting from normal variation, disease and the coadministration of other drugs may profoundly alter drug effectiveness and toxicity. Indeed, routine plasma level monitoring for some drugs with a narrow therapeutic index has become an integral part of medical practice.

This chapter will not attempt an exhaustive review of the literature, but will focus on the development of 'physiological' pharmacokinetics. As most of the studies have been performed on drugs that are metabolised by the liver, we shall confine discussion to that area, though the concepts have equal validity for other eliminating organs.

Historically, the earliest drugs investigated, such as antipyrine, the oral anticoagulants and phenylbutazone, were very poorly extracted by the liver, so that their clearance was rate-limited by the activity of the drug metabolising enzymes and tended to be slowed by drug binding in blood. Furthermore, alterations in drug metabolism were reflected by changes in the elimination rate constant, or its more familiar expression drug half-life ($T\frac{1}{2}$). It was on the basis of the disposition of this type of compound that our classical concepts of pharmacokinetics were developed. A major impetus to the development of a more physiological approach was the introduction of several important drugs, such as lignocaine, propranolol and the tricyclic antidepressants, which differed dramatically from those previously investigated in that they were very efficiently extracted by the liver. Drawing on the experience of the 1950s with compounds used as indicators to measure liver blood flow, it was clear that the elimination of highly extracted compounds would be affected by changes in liver blood flow. Unlike these indicators, however, it was desirable that the drugs be given by mouth and it became evident that the anatomical arrangement of the hepatic portal circulation was an extremely important factor in their disposition. It became clear that after their absorption across the gut into the portal vein, drug would be exposed to elimination by the liver before it could reach the systemic circulation and thence the site of action (Harris and Riegelman, 1969). Such presystemic or 'first pass' metabolism was an obvious cause of reduced systemic availability, despite the fact that the drug might be completely absorbed across the intestinal mucosa. There followed a series of publications that sought to define and quantify the effects of route of administration on drug disposition (Gibaldi, Boyes and Feldman, 1971; Rowland, 1972). At about that time Rowland and his co-workers (1973) published an important paper describing a kinetic model of hepatic elimination which incorporated blood flow as well as enzyme activity. While this was not the only perfusion-limited model available, it was simple and came at just the time when the effect of organ blood flow on elimination were being reinvestigated. It has since undergone minor modifications to incorporate the effects of drug binding in the blood (Shand, Cotham and Wilkinson, 1976). In addition, a more physiological approach to volume of distribution had been suggested by Gillette (1971) who expressed this somewhat vague parameter in terms of real body volumes and the avidity of drug binding in blood and tissue. Thus within the span of a decade the biological determinants of drug disposition had become sufficiently focused to allow a classification of hepatic drug elimination on the basis of extraction ratio that helped predict the effects of disease and drug interactions on circulating drug concentrations (Wilkinson and Shand, 1975).

Clearance concepts

A most critical development has been the fuller application of the clearance concept of drug elimination. The value of using drug clearance rather than $T_{\frac{1}{2}}$ as an index of the elimination process cannot be overemphasised. This is not to say that drug half-life is not a most useful parameter, but only that it is a poor index of the efficiency of the elimination process, because it is determined just as much by volume of distribution as by elimination due to clearance. Furthermore, changes in the elimination process are, in the case of some drugs, not well reflected by altered drug half-life. By contrast, knowledge of a drug's clearance can tell us much more, because it can be used to gauge the efficiency of elimination, which, in turn can tell us which biological factors are likely to be important to the drug's disposition. Several clearance terms are now in common use.

Intrinsic clearance

The activity of the drug metabolising enzymes can be expressed as a clearance term, the intrinsic clearance (Branch, Nies and Shand, 1973). Hepatic intrinsic clearance is defined as the volume of liver water cleared of drug in unit time and is therefore independent of liver blood flow. It can be measured in vitro by rearrangement of the Michalis–Menten equation (Gillette, 1971)

$$Cl_i' = \frac{v}{s} = \frac{V_{max}}{Km + S}$$

Under first order conditions, this reduces to

$$Cl_i' = \frac{V_{max}}{Km} \tag{1}$$

Intrinsic clearance is one of the factors that determines the ability of the whole organ to eliminate drug: the others are blood flow and drug binding in blood. If we wish to relate enzyme activity, which is dependent on free drug concentration, to the elimination of total drug from the blood which is in both bound and free forms, intrinsic clearance must be computed as

$$Cl_i = Cl_i' \, fB \qquad (2)$$

where fB is the fraction of drug in blood. Let us now see how the various factors determine hepatic clearance.

Hepatic clearance
The amount of total drug removed in the Liver (R) under first order conditions is by definition given by the concentration of free drug in liver (C_L) multiplied by the intrinsic clearance:

$$R = C_L \times Cl_i' \qquad (3)$$

Now the basic postulate of the model of Rowland et al (1973) is that drug in the liver is in equilibrium with that in the emergent venous blood so that C_L is equal to the free drug concentration in hepatic venous blood. If C_{HV} is the concentration of total drug then,

$$C_L = C_{HV} \cdot fB \qquad (4)$$

so that

$$R = C_{HV} \cdot fBCl_i' \qquad (5)$$

Removal rate at steady state is also given by the Fick principle as

$$R = Q(C_A - C_{HV}) \qquad (6)$$

where Q is liver blood flow and C_A the drug concentration in arterial blood. Combining the two equations for R and rearranging gives

$$\frac{C_{HV}}{C_A} = \frac{Q}{Q + Cl_i' \, fB} \qquad (7)$$

But organ clearance (Cl_h) is given by:

$$Cl_h = Q \cdot E = \frac{Q(C_A - C_{HV})}{C_A} = Q\left[1 - \frac{C_{HV}}{C_A}\right]$$

where E is the extraction ratio. Substituting for C_{HV}/C_A from equation (7) gives

$$Cl_h = Q \cdot E = Q\left[\frac{Cl_i' \, fB}{Q + Cl_i' \, fB}\right] \qquad (8)$$

This 'well-stirred' or 'venous equilibration' model allows us to predict the effects altering the biological determinants. From the equation, two intrinsic clearance terms are evident. Cl_i' is calculated in terms of free drug which is available to the enzymes and represents enzyme activity alone (intrinsic free drug clearance.) The term $Cl_i' \, fB$ is calculated in terms of total drug concentrations and is clearly dependent on drug binding in blood (intrinsic total drug clearance.) It represents the clearance of total drug in blood that would result from enzyme activity in the absence of any flow consideration. Several experiments under controlled conditions in the perfused rat liver suggest that this model adequately described the effects of altered blood flow on the elimination of propranolol (Branch et al, 1973) and lidocaine (Shand, Kornhauser and Wilkinson, 1975; Pang and Rowland, 1977b). It also predicts the effects of altered drug binding in blood (Shand et al, 1976) and route of administration (Shand et al, 1975) on drug disposition. The model has also been used to predict whole organ extraction ratio from in vitro measurements of the Michaelis–Menten constants using equations (1) and (8) (Rane, Wilkinson and Shand, 1977).

The 'venous equilibration' model is not the only one available. Indeed, a pharmacokinetic model was fully developed by Brauer (1963) based on the assumption that the liver comprised a set of parallel tubes, from which drug was eliminated as a first order process. Thus drug concentration was visualised as declining exponentially along the length of the sinusoid. This 'sinusoidal' model has its proponents (Winkler, Keiding and Tygstrup, 1973; Keiding et al, 1976). In this case the description of hepatic clearance takes the form of a cumulative exponential:

$$Cl_h = Q \left[1 - \exp^{-\left(\frac{-Cl_i' \, fB}{Q}\right)} \right] \qquad (9)$$

While the 'venous equilibration' and 'sinusoidal' models have very different critical assumptions, it should be emphasised that in practice the differences in hepatic clearance and extraction that each predicts is not very large (Wilkinson, 1976; Pang and Rowland, 1977a). What is more important is that the broad principles involved are not critically dependent on the model chosen. In particular, it is evident that the effects of altered intrinsic clearance, blood flow and binding in blood depends very much on the drug in question.

Determinants of hepatic drug clearance
When intrinsic clearance is very low compared to blood flow, then the hepatic extraction is low and both kinetic models reduce to

$$Cl_h \simeq Cl_i' \, fB \qquad (10)$$

and elimination is dependent only on enzyme activity and drug binding. Antipyrine is a poorly extracted drug as it is non-protein bound so that its clearance is dependent only on enzyme activity and unaffected by blood flow changes (Branch et al, 1974). This accounts for its popularity as a model drug to investigate the many factors that may alter hepatic enzyme activity.

At the other extreme, drugs with very high intrinsic clearances have high extraction ratios and demonstrate flow dependent kinetics as the equations reduce to:

$$Cl_h \simeq Q \qquad (11)$$

Notable examples of flow-dependent compounds are propranolol (Branch et al, 1973) and lignocaine (Stenson, Constantino and Harrison, 1971). The effects of liver blood flow on hepatic drug clearance has been fully reviewed recently (Wilkinson 1976; Nies, Shand and Wilkinson, 1976). It is only in the intermediate range of extraction ratios where both intrinsic clearance and flow can affect organ clearance that the models differ in their predictions, but as mentioned these differences are quite small.

The effects of altered drug binding in blood are also dependent on the intrinsic clearance. Thus with poorly extracted compounds, hepatic clearance is essentially proportional to the free fraction in blood, so that increased binding will reduce clearance and reduced binding increase it. This type of elimination has been termed restrictive and occurs with such drugs as warfarin (Levy and Yacobi, 1974) and phenytoin (Gugler et al, 1975). On the other hand, when intrinsic clearance is very high, altered binding has little effect on organ clearance as drug can be functionally stripped from its binding sites during its passage through the liver. Such non-restricted elimination has been shown to apply to the kinetics of propranolol (Evans, Nies and Shand, 1973). While the restrictive/non-restrictive classification is somewhat naive, as even the elimination of highly extracted drugs can be reduced by a very high degree of binding (Shand et al, 1976), it does have the merit of emphasising that not all drugs are affected in the same way by altered binding in the blood.

Systemic clearance

Systemic clearance is defined as the volume of blood cleared of drug from the systemic circulation in unit time. It is calculated from the amount of drug reaching the systemic circulation and the resultant area under the blood concentration/time curve (AUC). For example, after i.v. administration of a dose, D, systemic clearance is given by

$$\mathrm{Cls} = \frac{D_{i.v.}}{AUC_{i.v.}} \tag{12}$$

Clearance from the systemic circulation is made up of the sum of all of the clearances due to individual organs. If only one organ is involved, say the liver, then systemic clearance is equal to hepatic clearance and can be related to the blood flow to the organ of elimination (Q) to give a measure of the efficiency of elimination, the extraction ratio (E) because

$$\mathrm{Cls} = Q \times E$$

Once clearance and extraction have been established, then a great deal can be deduced about which factors will be most important to the disposition of the drug. In addition to intrinsic clearance, drug binding and organ blood flow, the anatomical arrangement of the portal circulation is also important.

Oral drug clearance

Considerable amounts of certain drugs can be eliminated by the liver before reaching the systemic circulation. This process has been called presystemic (or 'first pass') elimination and is simple to quantify as it is determined by the hepatic extraction ratio of the drug. Thus the fraction of the dose removed is equal to the hepatic extraction ratio (E) and that fraction entering the systemic circulation is simply the remainder $(1 - E)$. For example, if the hepatic extraction ratio is 0.7, then 70 per cent of the dose will be eliminated presystemically and only 30 per cent will be available to exert its effects in the systemic circulation. It is clear that significant presystemic elimination will occur only with relatively well extracted drugs like lignocaine (Boyes et al, 1970) and propranolol (Shand and Rangno, 1972) but not with poorly extracted drugs like antipyrine, tolbutamide and warfarin (Andreason and Vesell, 1974).

The apparent oral clearance of a drug is simply given by

$$\mathrm{Cl}_o = \frac{D_o}{AUC_o} \tag{13}$$

As this represents systemic clearance of $(1 - E)$ of the dose,

$$\mathrm{Cl}_o = \frac{(1 - E)D_o}{QE} \tag{14}$$

One important consequence of the first pass effect seems paradoxical at first: that the apparent clearance of an oral dose is equal to the intrinsic clearance of total drug provided the drug is fully absorbed and eliminated only by the liver. This can be seen by solving equation (8) of the 'venous equilibration' model for intrinsic total drug clearance when

$$Cl_i' \, fB \;=\; \frac{QE}{(1 - E)} \tag{15}$$

substitution from equation (14) then gives

$$Cl_i' fB \;=\; Cl_o \;=\; \frac{D_o}{AUC_o} \tag{16}$$

Thus the average steady state concentrations (or AUC) of all drugs after oral administration depends only on intrinsic clearance and not on blood flow irrespective of the hepatic extraction ratio. In simple terms the flow independence of oral drug clearance occurs because alterations in hepatic blood flow change presystemic elimination and hepatic clearance equally and in opposite directions. For example, reducing blood flow will increase hepatic extraction and presystemic elimination, so that less drug is available presystemically. At the same time, however, the fall in flow reduces hepatic clearance so that the reduced amount of drug that enters the circulation is cleared more slowly, and average concentration (or AUC) is unchanged. It should be emphasised that while AUC is unaltered, the shape of the plasma concentration/time curve will change. Taking the case of reduced flow, the reduced systemic availability leads to low peak levels, while the fall in systemic clearance will prolong the $T_{1/2}$ leading to higher trough concentrations.

The effects of altered intrinsic clearance also depend on the extraction ratio of the drug in question. With poorly extracted compounds, drug clearance is enzyme-dependent and unaffected by the route of elimination. In this case systemic oral and intrinsic clearances are for all intents and purposes the same, so that changes in intrinsic clearance produce equal changes in drug clearance after both routes of administration. Further, because there is no presystemic effect, the change in enzyme activity is seen largely as an alteration in $T_{1/2}$. Highly extracted drugs are not so obviously affected by changes in intrinsic clearance because their elimination is more flow dependent. However, systemic availability is altered quite markedly. For example if hepatic extraction is changed only from 0.9 to 0.95, a much bigger change in availability $(1 - E)$ from 0.1 to 0.05 occurs. For this reason, differences in intrinsic clearance of highly extracted drugs are seen more dramatically after oral administration and result in changes in peak levels with little alteration in drug $T_{1/2}$ (Kornhauser et al, 1978). These considerations have also received support from the study of Alvan et al (1977) on the effects of enzyme induction with pentobarbital on the disposition of the highly extracted drug alprenolol. They showed quite clearly that enzyme induction lowered drug concentration (AUC) largely after oral administration and that the systemic clearance and $T_{1/2}$ was little affected. Similar results were obtained by Meikle et al (1969) for induction of metyrapone elimination by diphenylhydantoin.

Another important development stemming from the investigation of highly extracted drugs has been the ability to estimate liver blood flow from pharmacokinetic data (Wilkinson and Shand, 1975). Provided the drug used is fully absorbed across the gut and is eliminated only by the liver, the blood flow can be estimated from a knowledge of the AUC's after oral (AUC_o) and i.v. ($AUC_{i.v.}$) administration as rearrangement of equation (8) for flow gives

$$Q = \frac{Cls \times Cl_i'\ fB}{Cl_i'\ fB - Cls} \qquad (17)$$

Substituting for Cls (equation (12)) and $Cl_i'\ fB$ (equation (16)) gives

$$Q = \frac{D_{i.v.} \cdot D_o}{AUC_{i.v.}\ D_o - AUC_o \cdot D_{i.v.}} \qquad (18)$$

This approach has been used to estimate liver blood flow using impramine (Gram and Christiansen, 1975), alprenolol (Alvan et al, 1977) and propranolol (Kornhauser et al, 1978). In the latter study, a most powerful pharmacokinetic technique was used. An i.v. tracer dose of propranolol was given at the same time as the unlabelled drug was administered orally. By measuring the labelled and native drug, the kinetics following i.v. and oral administration can be measured simultaneously, thus avoiding two studies. As shown by Houghton and Richens (1974) this technique was particularly useful in determining the non-linear kinetics of phenytoin. In the case of propranolol all of the biological determinants of disposition, including intrinsic clearance and blood flow, could be quantified (Kornhauser et al, 1978). In addition to measuring the kinetics of the parent compound, this approach can be most useful in determining the kinetics of metabolite generation and elimination, when a labelled metabolite is administered together with the parent drug as in the case of procainamide and its N-acetylated metabolite (Dutcher et al, 1977).

Volume of distribution

Volume of distribution has traditionally been a difficult parameter as its value seldom conforms to known physiological spaces. Furthermore, it cannot be determined directly but must be computed from drug clearance and a rate constant of elimination. In the case of the two compartmental models, those values can be obtained, the volume of the central compartment (Vc), that of the peripheral compartment (Vp) and a steady state volume of distribution (Vd_{ss}) which is the sum of Vc and Vp. Vd_{ss} only applies when there is no net flux of drug between the compartment and therefore is only attained at one instant of time after a single injection and during steady state infusion when it becomes a somewhat meaningless parameter as drug concentration under these circumstances is determined by clearance alone. The most widely used volume term is Vd_{beta} which is calculated on the basis of the terminal phase of elimination. Although in strict kinetic sense this is not the most satisfactory parameter, it does have the merit of describing the drug's kinetics during the dominant, terminal phase.

While one can define volume of distribution as a constant which relates drug clearance and a given rate constant of elimination, it does have biological meaning as it is determined by the relative degrees of drug binding in blood (or plasma) and the tissues of the rest of the body. Gillette (1971) was the first to visualise volume of distribution in terms of real body spaces and the degree of binding within them. The relationship described takes the form:

$$Vd_{total} = V_B + V_T \cdot \frac{f_B}{f_T}$$

in which V_B is blood volume, V_T the volume of extravascular water, and f_B and f_T the fractions of free drug in blood and tissues, respectively. Thus $V_B + V_T$ becomes total body water and real values can be inserted into the equation and calculate the average value for tissue binding. The utility of this approach has been to highlight the quantitative aspects of altering binding in blood or plasma on volume of distribution, and emphasise that changes in the degree of plasma binding do not always produce proportional changes in Vd. For example, let us take two drugs whose binding in blood is reduced from 95 to 90 per cent (f_B increases from 0.05 to 0.10). With the first drug, assume that there is not tissue binding ($f_T = 1.0$), that blood volume is 5 litres and V_T is 35 litres. Using the Gillette equation, Vd will increase from an initial value of $5 + 35 \times 0.05 = 6.75$ litres to $5 + 35 \times 0.1 = 8.5$ litres, a relatively small change. On the other hand, if tissue binding is very high $V_T = 0.1$ the with this drug Vd will increase from $5 + 35 \times 0.05/0.1 = 22.5$ litres to $5 + 35 \times 0.1/0.1 = 40$ litres, a much larger change. These examples illustrate (1) that in vitro changes in binding are dampened in vivo and (2) that the percentage changes in Vd produced are greater the larger the initial Vd.

It should be emphasised that the above changes apply to *total* drug concentration, but it is *free* drug concentration that determines effect. If we use the Gillette approach to measure Vd_{free} and thus to simulate free drug concentration, the relationship becomes:

$$Vd_{free} = \frac{V_B}{f_B} + \frac{V_T}{f_T}$$

as $Vd_{total} = Vd_{free} \cdot f_B$

If we work through the previous example, we see that Vd_{free} for the first drug with poor tissue binding falls from $5/0.05 + 35 = 135$ litres to $5/0.1 + 35 = 85$ litres, a large change, while for the highly tissue bound drug, Vd_{free} falls from $5/0.05 + 35/0.1 = 450$ litres to $5/0.1 + 35/0.1 = 400$ litres, a very much smaller change. Thus when we consider Vd_{free} we come to the opposite and more important conclusion that changing drug binding in blood produces much larger changes in Vd_{free} (and free drug concentration) when initial Vd is small than when it is large. Thus we have demonstrated that the immediate effect of altered binding (for example by another drug) is greatest when drug are poorly concentrated in tissues. As pointed out by Wardell's (1974) excellent article, this is simply because a greater proportion of these drugs is available in the circulation for redistribution into the tissues.

The situation with altered drug binding is still more difficult, because after redistribution occurs, drug clearance is also affected, again dependent on the drug in question. For example, if elimination is restrictive, drug clearance is enhanced by reduced binding, such that it compensates for the altered binding. When a new steady state is reached total plasma concentrations are halved, but free fraction was doubled, so that steady state free drug concentration returns to control values. This explains why redistribution interaction with this type of compound are transient. Such appears to be the case for the interaction between chloral hydrate and warfarin (Boston Collaborative Drug Surveillance Program, 1972). On the other hand, if elimination is non-restrictive, no such compensation occurs and total concentrations rise to reach their initial level. As free drug fraction has been increased, free drug concentrations should remain permanently elevated. No such interaction with non-restrictive drugs has yet been described but the theoretical argument is a compelling one.

It will have been noted that in describing the effect of altered binding we have not mentioned elimination rate of half-life, but have implied that it changes in opposite directions with our two examples. We can assess the biological determinants of T½ by combining Rowland's and Gillette's equations to give

$$T_{\frac{1}{2}} = 0.693 \left[\frac{Vd_{total}}{Q} + \frac{Vd_{total}}{\cdot \; ClfB} \right]$$

From this rather imposing relationship it can be seen that T½ will depend not only on drug binding but also on the magnitude of intrinsic clearance. Several simulations have been presented (Wilkinson and Shand, 1975) so that two examples will suffice. Take a drug with a low Vd which is eliminated restrictively, like warfarin. In this case reducing binding in blood will increase total drug clearance almost proportionally. However, Vd total will increase, but not to the same extent, so that T½ is shortened and elimination is accelerated (Levy and Yacobi, 1974). Conversely, if elimination is non-restrictive as with propranolol, reduced binding has no effect on total drug clearance but Vd total increases so that T½ is prolonged by reduced binding (Evans et al, 1973).

From the previous discussion, it is evident that the effects of drug binding are the most complex that we have to deal with. However, by applying a more physiological approach, the complexities can be rationalised and even quantified. In dealing with such data, it will be found most useful to calculate the pharmacokinetic parameters in terms of free drug as these reflect the active moeity.

A classification
The proposed classification of drug elimination on the basis of extraction ratio is a useful way to summarise the physiological approach to kinetics. If a drug has a *low* extraction ratio, due to a small intrinsic clearance relative to flow, hepatic clearance will be low and independent of flow changes but highly sensitive to alterations in enzyme activity. This may be caused by interindividual differences, alterations by enzyme induction and inhibition, or disease states. In addition, there will be only a small first-pass effect after oral administration and most of the administered dose will reach the systemic circulation intact. Variations in the intrinsic clearance will be seen largely as changes in T½ with both routes of administration. On the other hand, for a drug with a *high* extraction ratio hepatic clearance will predominantly reflect liver blood flow rather than drug-metabolising activity. Consequently, the clearance and half-life will be sensitive to changes in flow and insensitive to alterations in metabolic activity. Such a drug will exhibit significant presystemic hepatic elimination after an oral dose, and the availability will be readily affected by changes in intrinsic clearance. Unlike the i.v. route, altered enzyme activity will change drug concentrations after oral adminis-tration, but changes in peak levels, rather than T½ will predominate. Although altered blood flow will not change average steady state levels, T½ will change so that differ-ences in peak and trough levels will be evident. Between these two extremes, corres-ponding to an extraction of about 30 to 70 per cent, there will be an intermediate mixture of properties, clearance being partly dependent on liver blood flow and hepatic metabolism, and to an extent that can be predicted only by a precise knowledge of the extraction ratio.

In the case of altered drug binding, the elimination of poorly extracted drugs will tend to be restricted, such that total drug clearance is proportional to free drug. Decreased binding will accelerate elimination and tend to compensate for the binding change, so that free drug concentrations are little changed, even though total drug levels fall. Thus the effects of altered binding will be transient. With avidly extracted compounds, however, altered binding in blood has much less effect on total drug clearance so that free drug levels will reflect the change in binding. Furthermore, because volume of distribution depends on binding in blood, reduced binding will prolong $T_{1/2}$ because distribution is increased with little change in clearance. Thus altered binding in blood tends to change the $T_{1/2}$ for drugs with high and low extraction in opposite directions.

In conclusion, our understanding of the roles played by blood flow, intrinsic clearance, drug binding and route of administration in drug disposition has increased considerably in the last decade. The realisation that these factors do not affect all drugs to the same extent has introduced a degree of complexity, but the newer approaches that have developed provide a basis for rationalising and predicting their effects on both free and total drug concentration in many clinical situations.

REFERENCES

Alvan, G., Piafsky, K., Lind, M. & Von Bahr, C. (1977) Effect of pentobarbital on the disposition of alprenolol. *Clinical Pharmacology and Therapeutics*, **22**, 316–321.

Andreason, D. B. & Vesell, E. S. (1974) Comparison of plasma levels of antipyrine, tolbutamide and warfarin after oral and intravenous administration. *Clinical Pharmacology and Therapeutics*, **16**, 1059–1065.

Boston Collaborative Drug Surveillance Program (1972) Interaction between chloral hydrate and warfarin. *New England Journal of Medicine*, **286**, 53–55.

Boyes, R. N., Scott, D. B., Jebson, P. J., Godman, M. J. & Julian, D. G. (1971) Pharmacokinetics of lignocaine in man. *Clinical Pharmacology and Therapeutics*, **12**, 105–116.

Branch, R. A., Nies, A. S. & Shand, D. G. (1973) The disposition of propranolol. VIII. General implications of the effects of liver blood flow on elimination from the perfused rat liver. *Drug Metabolism and Disposition*, **1**, 687–690.

Brauer, R. W. (1963) Liver circulation and function. *Physiolical Reviews*, **43**, 115–213.

Dutcher, J. S., Strong, J. M., Lucas, S. V., Lee, W.-K. & Atkinson, A. J. (1977) Procainamide and N-acetylprocainamide kinetics investigated simultaneously with stable isotope methodology. *Clinical Pharmacology and Therapeutics*, **22**, 447–457.

Evans, G. H., Nies, A. S. & Shand, D. G. (1973) The disposition of propranolol. III. Decreased half-life and volume of distribution as a result of plasma binding in man, monkey, dog and rat. *Journal of Pharmacology and Experimental Therapeutics*, **186**, 114–122.

Gibaldi, M., Boyes, R. N. & Feldman, S. (1971) Influence of first-pass effect on availability of drugs on oral administration. *Journal of Pharmaceutical Sciences*, **60**, 1338–1340.

Gillette, J. R. (1971) Factors affecting drug metabolism. *Annals of the New York Academy of Sciences*, **179**, 43–66.

Gram, L. F. & Christiansen (1975) First-pass metabolism of imipramine in man. *Clinical Pharmacology and Therapeutics*, **17**, 555–563.

Gugler, R., Shoeman, D. W., Huffman, D. H., Cohlmia, J. B. & Azarnoff, D. L. (1975) Pharmacokinetics of drugs in patients with the nephrotic syndrome. *Journal of Clinical Investigation*, **55**, 1182–1189.

Harris, P. A. & Riegelman, S. (1969) Influence of the route of administration on the area under the plasma concentraton-time curve. *Journal of Pharmaceutical Sciences*, **58**, 71.

Houghton, G. W. & Richens, A. (1974) Rate of elimination of tracer doses of phenytoin at different steady-state serumphenytoin concentration in epileptic patients. *British Journal of Pharmacology*, **1**, 155–161.

Keiding, S., Johansen, K., Tonnesen, K. & Tygstrup, N. (1976) Michaelis–Menten kinetics of galactose elimination by the isolated perfused pig liver. *American Journal of Physiology*, **230**, 1302–1313.

Kornhauser, D. M., Wood, A. J. J., Vestal, R. E., Wilkinson, G. R., Branch, R. A. & Shand, D. G. (1978) Biological determinants of propranolol disposition in man. *Clinical Pharmacology and Therapeutics*, **23**, 165–174.

Levy, G. & Yacobi, A. (1974) Effect of protein binding on the elimination of warfarin. *Journal of Pharmaceutical Sciences*, **63**, 805–806.

Meikel, A. W., Jubiz, W., Matsukura, S., West, C. D. & Tyler, F. H. (1969) Effect of diphenylhydantoin on the metabolism of metyrapone and release of ACTH in man. *Journal of Clinical Endocrinology*, **29**, 1553–1558.

Nies, A. S., Shand, D. G. & Wilkinson, G. R. (1976) Altered hepatic blood flow in drug disposition. *Clinical Pharmacokinetics*, **1**, 135–155.

Pang, K. S. & Rowland, M. (1977a) Hepatic clearance of drugs. I. Theoretical considerations of a 'well-stirred' and a 'parallel tube' model. *Journal of Pharmacokinetics Biopharmaceutics*, **5**, 625–653.

Pang, K. S. & Rowland, M. (1977b) Hepatic clearance of drugs. II. Experimental evidence for acceptance of the 'well-stirred' model over the 'parallel tube' model using lidocaine in the perfused rat liver in situ preparation. *Journal of Pharmacokinetics and Biopharmaceutics*, **5**, 655–680.

Rane, A., Wilkinson, G. R. & Shand, D. G. (1977) Prediction of hepatic extraction ratio from in vitro measurement of intrinsic clearance. *Journal of Pharmacology and Experimental Therapeutics*, **200**, 420–424.

Rowland, M. (1972) Influence of route of administration on drug availability. *Journal of Pharmaceutical Sciences*, **61**, 70–74.

Rowland, M., Benet, L. Z. & Graham, G. G. (1973) Clearance concepts in pharmacokinetics. *Journal of Pharmacokinetics and Biopharmaceutics*, **1**, 123–136.

Shand, D. G., Cotham, R. H. & Wilkinson, G. R. (1976) Perfusion-limited effects of plasma drug binding on hepatic drug extraction. *Life Sciences*, **19**, 125–130.

Shand, D. G., Kornhauser, D. M. & Wilkinson, G. R. (1975) Effects of route of administration and blood flow on hepatic drug elimination. *Journal of Pharmacology and Experimental Therapeutics*, **195**, 424–432.

Shand, D. G. & Rangno, R. E. (1972) The disposition of propranolol. I. Elimination during oral absorption in man. *Pharmacology*, **7**, 159–168.

Stenson, R. E., Constantino, R. T. & Harrison, D. G. (1971) Interrelationships of hepatic blood flow, cardiac output and blood levels of lidocaine in man. *Circulation*, **43**, 205–211.

Wardell, W. M. (1974) Redistributional drug interactions: a critical examination of putative clinical examples. In *Drug Interactions*, ed. Moriselli, Cohen & Garratini, pp. 123–134. New York: Raven Press.

Wilkinson, G. R. (1975) Pharmacokinetics of drug disposition: hemodynamic considerations. *Annual Review of Pharmacology*, **15**, 11–27.

Wilkinson, G. R. (1976) Pharmacokinetics in disease states modifying body perfusion. In *The Effect of Disease States on Drug Pharmacokinetics*, ed. Benet, L. Z., pp. 13–32. Washington, DC: American Pharmaceutical Association.

Wilkinson, G. R. & Shand, D. G. (1975) A physiological approach to hepatic drug clearance. *Clinical Pharmacology and Therapeutics*, **18**, 377–390.

Winkler, K., Keiding, S. & Tygstrup, N. (1973) Clearance as a quantitative measure of liver function. In *The Liver: Quantitative Aspects of Structure and Function*, ed. Paumgartner, G. & Preisig, R., pp. 144–155. New York.

SOME ASPECTS OF THE RELATIONSHIP BETWEEN PLASMA DRUG LEVELS AND THEIR PHARMACOLOGICAL EFFECTS

Paul Turner

An important responsibility of a clinical pharmacologist involved in patient care is the organisation of a service for plasma drug level estimations, and the interpretation of such estimations in the contect of a particular patient's clinical state (Editorial, 1978). This depends upon the underlying principle that, for many drugs, there is a close relationship between their biological effects and their plasma concentrations, a subject which has been the subject of several recent comprehensive and authoritative reviews (for example, Davies and Prichard, 1973; Smith and Rawlins, 1973; Koch-Weser, 1975; Jellett, 1976).

Some factors determining this relationship

The relationship between the plasma level and biological effect of a drug depends upon the nature of its mechanism of action, its pharmacokinetics, the state of activity of the receptor, and other variables within the human subject which differ according to the drug and to the body systems involved. Some of these have been discussed in more detail elsewhere by Sjöqvist and Bertilsson (1973) and Turner (1977).

1. The drug should have a reversible action, its concentration at the receptor being in equilibrium with that in the extracellular water, and so with that in the plasma water. This, therefore, excludes those drugs which act non-reversibly, for example, by enzyme inhibition or by covalent bonding which persists after the drug has been eliminated from the rest of the body.

2. The development of tolerance at receptor sites should not be an important problem. Unfortunately, relatively little is known of the nature of tolerance to many different groups of drugs in man, and this represents an important limitation to a better understanding of concentration/response relationships over time.

3. The concentration of unbound drug in the plasma should reflect that of unbound drug at receptor sites. This indicates the importance of the 'free' or unbound component of the drug in plasma, which is biologically active.

4. The relationship between plasma level and response may change over time, particularly after a single dose. Several factors may account for this, including the production of major active or inactive metabolites, binding to tissues, and complex physiological homeostatic mechanisms. Studies designed to explore concentration/response relationships should allow time for drug distribution to occur, and preferably should use 'steady-state' conditions in which important metabolites have been allowed to equilibrate with the parent drug throughout the tissues.

5. Accurate, reproducible and specific methods for estimating drugs and their metabolites in body fluids must be available. Despite the sophistication of many assay techniques, large differences between laboratories in the results of simultaneous assays of some drugs such as phenytoin (Richens, 1975) raise serious doubts on the validity of much published literature on this subject.

6. There must be accurate, reproducible, safe and acceptable methods for recording drug effects in man. Development of methodology for estimating plasma levels has generally outstripped that for measurement of biological response, and concern has been expressed on the danger of an inappropriate emphasis on pharmacokinetic at the expense of pharmacodynamic aspects of drug action (Dollery, 1973; Turner, 1974).

7. The method of expression of pharmacological response and plasma level should be appropriate. For example, McDevitt and Shand (1975) showed that the beta-adrenoceptor blocking activity of propranolol was closely related to plasma concentration when the dose ratio -1 for antagonism of isoprenaline-induced tachycardia was used as the pharmacological test. When percentage reduction in exercise heart rate was used, however, it correlated closely with the log plasma concentration. The theoretical basis for these relationships has been reviewed by Levy (1966) and McDevitt and Shand (1975).

8. The rate of change of plasma level may markedly influence the biological effect. Morselli et al (1976) found significant and close relationships between the effects of amphetamine on blood pressure and its side-effects, on one hand, and its initial rate of entry into the circulation on the other, but no relationship with peak levels or area under the concentration curves. Garnham et al (1975) found that the central nervous adverse effects of indomethacin were markedly increased when its rate of absorption was accelerated by pretreatment with buffered aspirin, even though its plasma levels were lower than on other occasions when central effects were less.

9. Concentration–response relationships may not be constant over time. For example, Chan et al (1975) showed that pethidine binding to erythrocytes decreases with

increasing age, while plasma pethidine levels are higher for a given dose, and suggested that the increased incidence of adverse effects of pethidine in elderly patients depends on this change. Castleden et al (1977) found that the central effects of nitrazepam were more marked at a given plasma level in patients over 69 years, compared with young subjects under 40 years. They suggested that this was probably explained by an increased sensitivity of the ageing brain to the action of nitrazepam.

Indications for measuring drug levels in body fluids
When planning the establishment of a laboratory service for estimating a drug's level in body fluids, it is essential first to define the indications for which the estimations are requested in order that the most appropriate analytical technique may be chosen (Flouvat, 1976; Koch-Weser, 1977).

1. To monitor treatment with drugs which have a low therapeutic/toxicity ratio. This includes the aminoglycoside antibiotics, anticonvulsant drugs, digoxin, lithium and cardiac antidysrhythmic drugs, concentrations of which may be markedly influenced by changes in renal function.

2. In treatment with drugs which appear to have a therapeutic range or 'window' of plasma concentration. This has best been demonstrated with the antidepressive drug nortriptyline, where Äsberg and her colleagues (1971) found a narrow therapeutic range between about 50 and 150 ng/ml, above and below which response to treatment was less satisfactory. Although there have been some negative studies (Burrows, Davies and Scoggins, 1972; Burrows et al, 1974) most have confirmed these original findings with nortriptyline (Kragh-Sørensen, Äsberg and Eggert-Hansen, 1973; Kragh-Sørensen et al, 1976; Ziegler et al, 1976). A similar relationship may be found with protriptyline (Whyte et al, 1976; Biggs and Ziegler, 1977). The concentration effect relationship with other monoamine-reuptake inhibiting antidepressives is less clear (p. 168; Lader, 1974; Coppen et al, 1978).

3. For recognition of inherited characteristics of metabolic rates. This is especially important for those drugs which are acetylated (Drayer and Reidenberg, 1977), such as procainamide, hydrallazine, phenelzine, isoniazid, dapsone and some sulphonamides including sulphamethazine and salicylazosulfapyridine. Genetic slow acetylators are more likely than rapid acetylators to experience (a) earlier development of procainamide-induced antinuclear antibody; (b) earlier and more frequent development of procainamide-induced systemic lupus erythematosus (SLE); (c) hydrallazine-induced SLE; (d) spontaneous SLE; (e) drowsiness and nausea from phenelzine; (f) cyanosis, haemolysis and transient reticulocytosis from salicylazosulfapyridine; (g) polyneuropathy after isoniazid therapy. They are, of course, also more likely to experience greater therapeutic responses from similar doses.

Other inherited differences in drug metabolism are being recognised, for example, of hydroxylation of debrisoquine (Mahgoub et al, 1977) and their importance is being assessed.

4. In treatment with drugs which demonstrate 'saturable kinetics', where the dose/plasma level relationship is not linear, for example with phenytoin, (see p. 150).

5. As a guide to patient compliance, which is now recognised as being of major importance in the success of drug treatment. One of several methods of assessing compliance is measurement of urine, plasma or salivary drug levels to determine if the expected concentration is present. If the appropriate analytical technique is used, it

may also be possible to detect the presence of other drugs, the taking of which is not known by the prescribing doctor or admitted by the patient (Witts et al, 1977).

6. To assess bioavailability of drug preparations in which formulation may have a profound influence upon a drug's absorption and the quality of its therapeutic action (Turner, 1976).

7. To determine the influence of a patient's disease or other factors on drug absorption, disposition and excretion (Davies and Prichard, 1973).

8. As a guide to which of several pharmacological actions of a drug is responsible for a therapeutic or toxic effect. For example, propranolol has several pharmacological actions including beta-adrenoceptor blockade, local anaesthetic and antiserotoninergic activities. The concentrations required for these actions are different, and measurement of steady-state levels in patients receiving propranolol for hypertension, angina, dysrhythmias, hyperthyroidism, anxiety and psychoses may suggest the pharmacological mechanisms responsible for its therapeutic action in a particular indication (Turner, 1977).

9. To guide treatment in some drug overdosages. However, contrary to expectations, a high correlation between drug toxicity and plasma concentrations has been found with only few drugs. The mechanisms involved, and clinical implications have been reviewed by Prescott, Roscoe and Forrest (1973).

Use of saliva in drug monitoring
Mixed saliva, or spit, consists of parotid, submandibular, sublingual and minor gland secretions together with gingival fluid. Important features including pH, rate of flow, protein, carbohydrate, urea, electrolyte and enzyme content of mixed saliva and its components have been discussed in detail by Mason and Chisholm (1975), and methods for collecting the secretions of individual glands have been described by Stephen and Speirs (1976).

Generally speaking the concentration of a drug in saliva is proportional to the concentration of unbound, rather than to the total of bound and unbound drug in plasma. It is, however, clear that the dissociation constant and partition coefficient of the drug may also be important determinants in the case of weak acids and bases (Matin, Wan and Karan, 1974), the plasma/saliva ratio being markedly influenced by salivary pH. The latter is also dependent, at least in part, on rate of salivary flow, so that this may also be an important factor in determining salivary concentrations. Other factors that must be considered are (a) some substances such as lithium are actively secreted into saliva rather than by passive diffusion (Groth, Prellivitz and Jahnchen, 1974; Horning et al, 1977); (b) drug binding to salivary proteins may produce discrepancies in plasma/salivary ratios, as has been suggested for phenytoin (Reynolds et al, 1976); (c) drugs may bind to oral cell debris, either directly from the oral formulation in which they are administered, or after salivary excretion (Paxton, Whiting and Stephen, 1977). Such an effect is most likely to be seen with a highly lipid soluble drug such as propranolol, and Kaye et al (1977) found that contamination from this source interfered with salivary estimations for up to 2 h after oral administration of propranolol in tablet form; (d) salivary flow may be reduced in some patients, for example in endogenous depression, or by drugs with anticholinergic properties such as the monoamine-reuptake inhibiting antidepressive ('tricyclic') drugs, making it difficult to collect sufficient saliva for accurate drug estimations. If saliva flow is stimulated, it must be established that the materials used do not interfere with the drug estimation. For example, lemon flavoured sweets used to stimulate secretion were found to interfere with amitriptyline estimations (Jeffrey and Turner, 1978); and Taylor, Kaspi and Turner (unpublished observations) have found that highly lipid soluble drugs such as propranolol partition into hydrocarbon waxy strips, a material commonly chewed to stimulate salivary secretion. Nevertheless, and recognising these important potential complications, the advantages of salivary estimations of many drugs in terms of non-invasiveness in kinetic studies, for example, in children and in population studies such as West African villages have already been demonstrated (Fraser et al, 1976; Speirs, 1977; Horning et al, 1977).

REFERENCES

Äsberg, M., Crönholm, B., Sjöqvist, F. & Tuck, D. (1971) Relationship between plasma level and therapeutic effect of nortriptyline. *British Medical Journal*, iii, 331–334.

Biggs, J. T. & Ziegler, V. E. (1977) Protriptyline plasma levels and antidepressant response. *Clinical Pharmacology and Therapeutics*, 22, 269–273.

Burrows, G. D., Davies, B. & Scoggins, B. A. (1972) Plasma concentration of nortriptyline and clinical response in depressive illness. *Lancet*, ii, 619–623.

Burrows, G. D., Scoggins, B. A., Turecek, L. R. & Davies, B. (1974) Plasma nortriptyline and clinical response. *Clinical Pharmacology and Therapeutics*, 16, 639–644.

Castleden, C. M., George, C. F., Marcer, D. & Hallett, C. (1977) Increased sensitivity to nitrazepam in old age. *British Medical Journal*, i, 10–12.

Chan, K., Kendall, M. J., Mitchard, M., Wells, W. D. E. & Vickers, M. D. (1975) The effect of ageing on plasma pethidine concentration. *British Journal of Clinical Pharmacology*, 2, 197–302.

Coppen, A. et al (1978) Amitriptyline plasma-concentration and clinical effect. *Lancet*, i, 63–66.

Davies, D. S. & Prichard, B. N. C. (1973) *Biological Effects of Drugs in Relation to Their Plasma Concentrations*. Macmillan: London.

Dollery, C. T. (1973) Pharmacokinetics — master or servant? *European Journal of Clinical Pharmacology*, 6, 1–2.

Drayer, D. E. & Reidenberg, M. M. (1977) Clinical consequences of polymorphic acetylation of basic drugs. *Clinical Pharmacology and Therapeutics*, 22, 251–158.

Editorial (1978) The role of the clinical pharmacologist in district general hospitals. *British Journal of Clinical Pharmacology*, 5, 3–5.

Flouvat, B. (1976) Intérêt thérapeutique de la détermination des concentrations sanguines des médicaments. *Sciences et Techniques Pharmaceutiques*, 5, 67–76.

Fraser, H. S., Bulpitt, C. J., Kahn, C., Mould, G., Mucklow, J. C. & Dollery, C. T. (1976) Factors affecting antipyrine metabolism in West African villages. *Clinical Pharmacology and Therapeutics*, 20, 369–376.

Garnham, J. C., Raymond, K., Shotton, E. & Turner, P. (1975) The effect of buffered aspirin on plasma indomethacin. *European Journal of Clinical Pharmacology*, 8, 107–113.

Groth, V., Prellivitz, W. & Jahnchen, E. (1974) Estimation of pharmacokinetic parameters of lithium from saliva and urine. *Clinical Pharmacology and Therapeutics*, 16, 480–498.

Horning, M. G., Brown, L., Nawlin, J., Lertratanangkoon, K., Kellaway, P. & Zion, T. E. (1977). *Clinical Chemistry*, 23, 157–164.

Jeffrey, A. & Turner, P. (1978) Relationship between plasma and salivary concentrations of amitriptyline. *British Journal of Clinical Pharmacology*, 5, 268–269.

Jellett, L. B. (1976) Plasma concentrations in the control of drug therapy. *Drugs*, 11, 412–422.

Kaye, C. M., Orton, D., Taylor, E. A. & Brunel, C. (1977) Plasma–salivary ratios of acebutolol and propranolol. *British Journal of Clinical Pharmacology*, 4, 724P.

Koch-Weser, J. (1975) The serum level approach to individualisation of of drug dosage. *European Journal of Clinical Pharmacology*, 9, 1–8.

Koch-Weser, J. (1977) The value of serum concentration determinations in drug therapy. In *Advanced Medicine–Topics in Therapeutics*, 3, ed. Shanks, R. G., pp. 61–75. Tunbridge Wells: Pitman Medical.

Kragh-Sørensen, P., Äsberg, M. & Eggert-Hansen, C. (1973) Plasma nortriptyline levels in endogenous depression. *Lancet*, i, 113–115.

Kragh-Sørensen, P., Eggert-Hansen, C., Baastrup, P. C. & Hvidberg, E. F. (1976) Self-inhibiting action of notriptyline's antidepressive effect at high plasma levels. *Psychopharmacologia*, 45, 305–312.

Lader, M. (1974) Plasma concentrations of tricyclic antidepressive drugs. *British Journal of Clinical Pharmacology*, **1**, 281–283.

Levy, G. (1966) Kinetics of pharmacologic effects. *Clinical Pharmacology and Therapeutics*, **7**, 362–372.

Mahgoub, A., Idle, J. R., Dring, L. G., Lancaster, R. & Smith, R. L. (1977) Polymorphic hydroxylation of debrisoquine in man. *Lancet*, **ii**, 584–586.

Mason, D. K. & Chisholm, D. M. (1975) *Salivary Glands in Health and Disease*, pp. 42–50. London: W. B. Saunders.

Matin, S. B., Wan, S. H. & Karim, J. H. (1974) Pharmacokinetics of tolbutamide: prediction by concentration in saliva. *Clinical Pharmacology and Therapeutics*, **16**, 1952–1058.

McDevitt, D. G. & Shand, D. G. (1975) Plasma concentrations and time course of beta blockade due to propranolol. *Clinical Pharmacology and Therapeutics*, **18**, 708–713.

Morselli, P. L., Placidi, G. F., Maggini, C., Gomeri, R., Guazelli, M., de Lisio, G., Standen, S. & Tognoni, G. (1976) An integrated approach for the evaluation of psychotropic drug in man I. Studies on amphetamine. *Psychopharmacologia*, **46**, 211–217.

Paxton, J. W., Whiting, B. & Stephen, K. W. (1977) Phenytoin concentrations in mixed, parotid and submandibular saliva and serum, measured by radioimmunoassay. *British Journal of Clinical Pharmacology*, **4**, 185–189.

Prescott, L. F., Roscoe, P. & Forrest, J. A. H. (1973) Plasma concentrations and drug toxicity in man. In *Biological Effects of Drugs in Relation to Their Plasma Concentrations*, ed. Davies, D. S. & Prichard, B. N. C., pp. 51–82. Macmillan: London.

Reynolds, F., Ziroyanis, P. N., Jones, N. F. & Smith, S. E. (1976) Salivary phenytoin concentration in epilepsy and in chronic renal failure. *Lancet*, **ii**, 384–386.

Richens, A. (1975) Results of a phenytoin quality control scheme. In *Clinical Pharmacology and Anti-epileptic Drugs*, ed. Schneider, H., Janz, D., Gardner-Thorpe, C., Meinardi, H. & Sherwin, A. L., pp. 293–303. Berlin: Springer-Verlag.

Sjöqvist, F. & Bertilsson, L. (1973) Plasma concentrations of drugs and pharmacological response in man. In *Biological Effects of Drugs in Relation to Their Plasma Concentrations*, ed. Davies, D. S. & Prichard, B. N. C., pp. 25–40. London: Macmillan.

Smith, S. E. & Rawlins, M. D. (1973) *Variability in Human Drug Response*. Butterworth: London.

Speirs, C. F. (1977) Oral absorption and secretion of drugs. *British Journal of Clinical Pharmacology*, **4**, 97–100.

Stephen, K. W. & Speirs, C. F. (1976) Methods for collecting individual components of mixed saliva; the relevance to clinical pharmacology. *British Journal of Clinical Pharmacology*, **3**, 315–319.

Turner, P. (1974) Blood level or pharmacological response? *British Journal of Clinical Pharmacology*, **1**, 11.

Turner, P. (1976) Influence of formulation on a drug's activity. In *Advanced Medicine — Topics in Therapeutics 2*, ed. Turner, P., pp. 83–86. Tunbridge Wells: Pitman Medical.

Turner, P. (1977) Correlation between plasma levels and pharmacological effects. In *Advanced Medicine — Topics in Therapeutics 3*, ed. Shanks, R. G., pp. 50–52. Tunbridge Wells: Pitman Medical.

Whyte, S. F., MacDonald, A. J., Naylor, G. F. & Moody, J. P. (1976) Plasma concentrations of protriptyline and clinical effects in depressed women. *British Journal of Psychiatry*, **128**, 384–390.

Witts, D. J., Mulgirigama, D., Turner, P. & Pare, C. M. B. (1977) Some observations on patient compliance in an antidepressive trial. *Postgraduate Medical Journal*, **53**, Suppl. 1, 136–138.

Ziegler, V. E., Clayton, P. J., Taylor, J. R., Co, B. T. & Biggs, J. T. (1976) Nortriptyline plasma levels and therapeutic response. *Clinical Pharmacology and Therapeutics*, **20**, 458–463.

2. Prostaglandins

Alan Bennett

Research into prostaglandins (PGs) has moved at such a dramatic rate and in so many directions that *Recent Advances* are numerous, exciting and often potentially of great clinical significance. The field is now so extensive that only some areas can be covered in this chapter, even when the aspects chosen are restricted mainly to man.

Prostaglandin chemistry

Many reviews cover the basic chemistry of PGs, and this is not discussed here except where it relates to new information. Arachidonic acid metabolism produces many biologically potent substances, and the simplified basic scheme shown in Figure 2.1 is now known to occur.

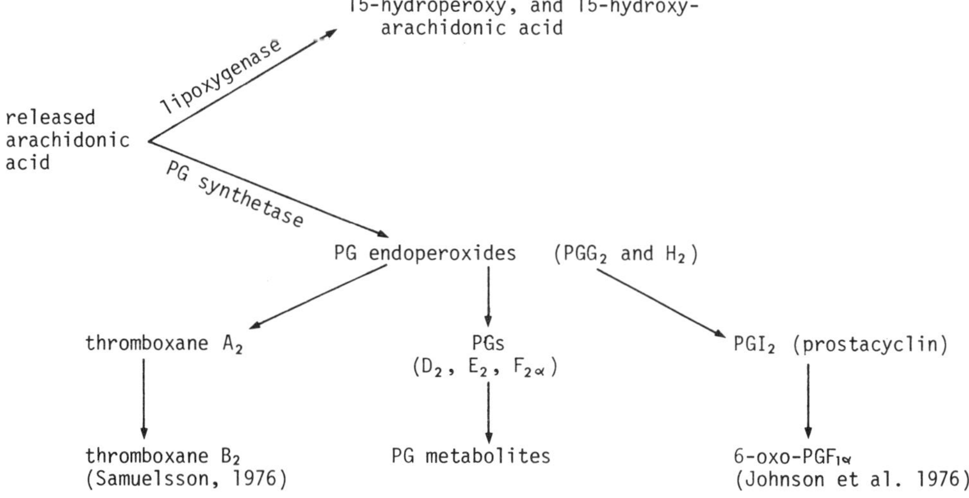

Fig. 2.1 Simplified scheme of arachidonic acid metabolism

Some tissues are thought to form predominantly PGs (e.g. ram seminal vesicles), some thromboxanes (e.g. platelets; Samuelsson, 1976), and some PGI₂ (blood vessel intima; Moncada et al, 1976). However, formation may depend on cofactor concentration: in vitro, ram seminal vesicle synthetase produces PGI₂ with low GSH concentrations whereas PGE₂ is formed with high GSH concentrations (Flower, personal communication). It is important to know which substances are formed in vivo, but no method can be guaranteed to give an accurate answer: perhaps a reasonable approximation can be obtained by homogenising tissues in an aqueous solution so that they provide their own substrate and cofactor material. Because PG endoperoxides, thromboxane A₂ (TXA₂) and PGI₂ are often considerably more potent than the 'primary'

PGD, E or F compounds, they may be more important biologically. However, since TXA$_2$ and PGI$_2$ are more quickly inactivated than PGs they may have to be generated continuously to exert a prolonged effect, and they must be able to reach appropriate sites of action before inactivation occurs. In some tissues TXA$_2$ or PGI$_2$ may be unimportant because they are not formed locally and do not reach the tissues through the circulation; in others they seem of great importance, as shown in the first topic discussed below.

PLATELET AGGREGATION

PGs seem likely to play a physiological role in platelet function. The platelet cyclo-oxygenase (which converts arachidonic acid into endoperoxides) was deficient in a subject with defective haemostasis due to an abnormal platelet release mechanism. Addition of PGG$_2$ restored the response (Malmsten et al, 1975).

It has been known for many years that PGE$_1$ inhibits aggregation of human blood platelets whereas PGE$_2$ tends to have the opposite effect. Willis et al (1974) and others obtained evidence that platelet aggregation occurs due to formation of the unstable but potent PG endoperoxide PGH$_2$. Subsequently, Hamberg, Svensson and Samuelsson (1975) showed that during thrombin-induced aggregation of human blood platelets substantial amounts of TXA$_2$ (Fig. 2.2) are produced. This substance potently causes both platelet aggregation and vasoconstriction, but is quickly broken down (half-life of about 30 s in aqueous solution) to TXB$_2$ (Fig. 2.2) which has low biological activity in many systems.

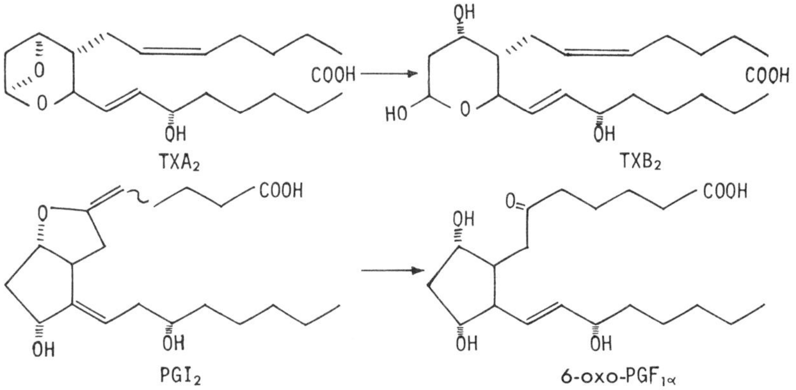

Fig. 2.2   The structures of thromboxane A$_2$ and B$_2$, PGI$_2$ and 6-oxo-PGF$_{1\alpha}$

Another exciting finding is the discovery of PGI$_2$, recorded in an excellent account by Moncada and Vane (1977). PGI$_2$ (Fig. 2.2) is a potent but unstable substance (half-life about 2 min. in neutral aqueous solution at room temperature; converted to 6-oxo-PGF$_{1\alpha}$). It is formed in the vascular endothelium, by an enzyme found in the microsomal fraction. In contrast, to TXA$_2$, minute amounts of PGI$_2$ inhibit platelet aggregation and cause vasodilatation. Moncada and Vane (1977) suggest that when platelets are damaged they form and release PG endoperoxides which aggregate platelets both directly and after conversion into TXA$_2$. However, the endothelium generates PGI$_2$ from the released endoperoxides so that the net pro- and antiaggregatory and vascular effects cancel each other. It seems that only the endoperoxide released within the platelets is converted to TXA_2: little TXB_2 is formed when PGG_2 is incubated with platelets (Malmsten et al, 1975). It is suggested that when the intima is destroyed or detached, the platelets start adhering to the subendothelial layers. These do not produce PGI_2, but contain collagen and other pro-aggregatory substances which, together with endoperoxides and TXA_2, cause platelet aggregation. Similarly, damage of the endothelium by plaque formation might reduce PGI_2 synthesis and increase the tendency for blood to clot. It may also be important that 15-hydroperoxy-arachidonic acid, formed from arachidonic acid by lipoxygenase (Fig. 2.1), selectively inhibits formation of PGI_2; excessive lipid peroxidation occurs in various conditions, possibly including hyperlipidaemia accompanying atherosclerosis (Slater, 1972). Moncada and Vane (1977) postulate that these aspects are important in various other conditions such as inflammation where PGI_2 is anti-inflammatory and lipid peroxides redirect metabolism to pro-inflammatory PGs.

The insubstantial effects of aspirin on most aspects of thrombosis in man, despite the potent effects of aspirin on platelets in vitro, may be explained by these results. Aspirin blocks formation of endoperoxides, and thus the formation of both TXA_2 and PGI_2, and when the effects of these substances are balanced, aspirin would be expected to have little net effect on thrombosis. A means of changing the balance between production of TXA_2 and PGI_2 might therefore be desirable, and one way is to block selectively the formation of TXA_2, e.g. with imidazole (Moncada et al, 1977). However, if the balance has previously been upset in favour of TXA_2, then a beneficial effect of aspirin would be expected. This may explain the tendency of aspirin to prevent myocardial infarction (Boston Collaborative Drug Surveillance Group, 1974; Jick and Miettinen, 1976), though the data are by no means conclusive.

PGI_2 may have other roles in the vascular system, such as vasodilatation. The ability of indomethacin to cause vasoconstriction is consistent with this. Impaired formation of PGI_2 (or other vasodilator PGs) might be involved in some types of hypertension (Moncada and Vane, 1977).

PERIPHERAL VASCULAR DISEASE

Carlson and Eriksson (1973) described preliminary results showing that intra-arterial injections of minute quantities of PGE_1 into the legs of patients with severe peripheral vascular disease greatly improved patient well-being and usually obviated the need for surgery. Other investigators have confirmed that PGE_1 usually gives immediate pain relief, often increases blood flow and sometimes heals ischaemic ulcers (see review by Carlson and Olsson, 1977). Unfortunately, PGE_1 is not commercially available for treating patients, and PGE_2, which is available for obstetric use, tends to aggregate platelets whereas PGE_1 has the reverse effect. The extent to which improvement depends on vasodilatation rather than an effect on platelets is not clear.

PGs IN BREAST TUMOURS AND THEIR RELATION TO BONE METASTASES

Human breast tumours, in common with other tumours, synthesise PG-like material during homogenisation in aqueous solution; the amounts are much higher than obtained from benign tumours or normal breast tissue (Bennett et al, 1975, 1977).

Breast cancers often metastasise to bone, and several pieces of evidence indicate that this may be causally related to PGs. Some PGs are potent bone-resorbing agents (first shown by Klein and Raisz (1970) and subsequently confirmed by various groups), which act by stimulating osteoclasts. Growth of dental cysts in the human jaw probably involves PGs (Harris et al, 1973). Recent data show that most PG metabolites have little bone-resorbing activity, but 13, 14-dihydro-PGE$_2$ has about one-third the activity of PGE$_2$ (Tashjian, Tice and Sides, 1977; Raisz, Dietrich and Simmons, 1977; Rowe, Bennett and Harris, unpublished). PGG$_2$ and PGH$_2$ are also active (Raisz et al, 1977), but PGI$_2$ and 6-oxo-PGF$_{1\alpha}$ seem relatively weak bone-resorbing agents (Rowe, Bennett and Harris, unpublished).

Primary breast tumours producing the most PG-like material during homogenisation are associated with the highest incidence of bone metastases as indicated by skeletal scintigraphy (Bennett et al, 1975, 1977). A similar association also occurs with tumours which destroy bone during in vitro culture. In addition to PG-like substances, these tumours also release a non-dialyable bone-resorbing material (Dowsett et al, 1976a). Lung, kidney, and prostate tumours, which also commonly spread to bone, produce substantial amounts of prostaglandin-like material (Bennett et al, unpublished).

Certain tumours injected in rats and rabbits destroy bone, but continuous treatment of the animals with aspirin or indomethacin which inhibit PG synthesis, reduces the tumour PG content (Voelkel et al, 1975; Galasko and Bennett, 1976) and prevents or reduces the bone destruction (Powles et al, 1973; Galasko and Bennett, 1976). This provides a rationale for treating skeletal metastases in patients with aspirin-like drugs (see later).

The precise association between PGs and bone metastases is not fully understood, but there are certain possibilities:

a. Tumour cells entering the bone might release PGs which initiate bone resorption and enable metastases to form; PGs released into the circulation from the primary breast tumour would probably not have much effect on bone since they are substantially inactivated during passage through certain vascular beds, particularly the lungs. To be most effective on the arterial side of the circulation, the PGs would presumably have to be released after a site of inactivation, as might occur from some lung metastases (Barrowman et al, 1975). However, metabolism by the lungs does not seem as great in man as in some animals: Golub et al (1975) found that almost 70 per cent of injected PGE$_1$ is cleared in a single passage through human lung, compared with 90 to 95 per cent in rabbit and dog (Ferreira and Vane, 1967), but they did not study PGE$_2$ or PGF compounds.

b. Tumour PGs might in some undefined way increase the dispersion of malignant cells from the primary tumour or affect the other aspects of their spread throughout the body, thus increasing the number of bone metastases.

c. PGs may interact with other bone-resorbing material released by tumour cells (e.g. the non-dialysable bone-resorbing agent described by Dowsett et al (1976a) which might be osteoclast activating factor). In conditions such as pain and inflammation PGs increase the response to other released substances.

d. The above aspects involve a role for PGs formed by tumour cells. By contrast, tumour cells might induce bone to form PGs. Various substances seem capable of doing this, since aspirin inhibits collagenase activity (Dowsett et al, 1976b), and resorbing substances such as parathyroid extract and osteoclast activating factor, increase the PG content of mouse calvaria (Rowe, Bennett and Harris, 1978). Osteoclasts are involved in early, but not late, bone destruction (Galasko, 1976). If PGs released by human tumour cells stimulate osteoclasts, early bone destruction would probably be inhibited by aspirin-like drugs. The later phase might not involve PGs, but this has not been tested.

Before advocating treatment of cancer patients with aspirin-like drugs we must consider other effects seen in laboratory animals. PGE compounds reduce tumour growth in vitro (Jaffe, 1974) and in vivo (Santoro, Philpott and Jaffe, 1976) and increase cell differentiation (Prasad, 1972). However, they either decrease (Plescia, Smith and Grinwich, 1975) or increase (Loose and di Luzio, 1973) the immune response which many believe to be important in defence by the host. The effect of PG synthetase inhibitors on tumour growth or spread to soft tissues in animals also varies. In mice, aspirin inhibits soft tissue metastases from various injected tumours (Gasic et al, 1973), and indomethacin inhibits primary tumour growth (Plescia et al, 1975; Strausser and Humes, 1975). Although these drugs reduce bone destruction in rats or rabbits, they neither reduce the numbers of pulmonary metastases nor increase survival time (Powles et al, 1973; Galasko and Bennett, 1976). However, in another mouse model flurbiprofen reduced tumour growth, particularly when combined with radiotherapy and chemotherapy, and tended to prolong survival (Bennett et al, 1978).

The extent to which these animal studies can be extrapolated to man is unclear, particularly since great species and tumour differences exist. It is not known whether some differences reflect variations in tumour antigenicity, or whether results with injected tumour cells can be compared with the growth and spread of spontaneous tumours. Nevertheless, since aspirin-like drugs either inhibit or do not significantly affect tumour growth or spread in animals, it seems ethical to use these drugs in cancer patients. Furthermore, many cancer patients with rheumatic disorders presumably receive continuous therapy with PG synthetase inhibitors, some occasionally take such drugs for minor ailments, and others receive aspirin to relieve radiation-induced diarrhoea (Mennie et al, 1975; see later). These facts justify the studies to investigate the influence of aspirin-like drugs on bone metastases in breast cancer patients currently being conducted by Powles (personal communication) and ourselves. Another way of assessing drug safety in cancer patients might be to determine the incidence and spread of the disease in people with rheumatic disorders who have received long-term therapy with PG synthetase inhibitors.

Hypercalcaemia
The ability of PGs to resorb bone has already been discussed. In addition, they seem to be involved in some types of hypercalcaemia such as that associated with lung and other tumours. PGE and F compounds are substantially broken down in a single passage through the pulmonary circulation, so that in animals large amounts would not normally reach the arterial circulation unless they are released distal to the lungs. Nevertheless, prolonged intravenous infusion of PGE_2 in rats causes hypercalcaemia (Tashjian et al, 1975). As discussed earlier, less PG seems to be inactivated in human lungs; it remains to be seen whether enough can survive to exert an effect on the arterial side of the circulation, or whether biologically active metabolites are formed. The bone-resorbing activity of 13,14-dihydro-PGE_2 has already been mentioned. PGs seem likely to be involved in bone resorption in patients with hypercalcaemia associated with some

solid (non-haematological) tumours, since urinary levels of PGE metabolites are high and their hypercalcaemia is reduced by aspirin or similar drugs (Seyberth et al, 1975). Indeed, raised excretion of metabolite can precede the onset of hypercalcaemia. The PG may come from the tumour, but another possibility is that the tumour produces material which stimulates bone to release PG. As discussed earlier, parathyroid extract and osteoclast activating factor increase PG synthesis in bone (Rowe et al, 1978).

PATENCY OF THE DUCTUS ARTERIOSUS

Infants with certain congenital cardiac defects require surgery to improve pulmonary blood flow, but the period prior to surgery is critical. Various animal experiments have shown that PGE_1 or PGE_2 dilate the ductus arteriosus. Elliott, Starling and Neutze (1975) therefore infused PGE_1 into two infants with cyanotic congenital heart disease and obtained an increase in arterial blood oxygen saturation. Others have used the technique and it seems possible to avoid unwanted effects (Heymann and Rudolph, 1977).

By contrast, in prematurely born infants with respiratory distress syndrome, a patent ductus often complicates the clinical course. Indomethacin given orally or rectally often causes permanent closure of the ductus and disappearance of the symptoms within one day of starting treatment. However, the authors warn against uncontrolled clinical application because possible effects on the kidney and elsewhere have not been fully evaluated (Friedman et al, 1976; Heymann, Rudolph and Silverman, 1976).

THE DISTRIBUTION OF PGs IN THE GUT IN RELATION TO FUNCTION AND DISEASE

The question of PG distribution is not straightforward. PGs are generally thought to be formed as required and are not stored in cells, although large amounts occur in human seminal plasma. There are presumably 'basal' amounts of PGs in tissues released for example during normal function, damage or cell death. Since PGs are readily formed when cells are damaged, such as during extraction procedures, it is not possible to obtain exact measurement of basal amounts. Homogenisation of tissues in solutions which prevent PG synthesis and breakdown give some indication of this, but it may be impossible to eradicate abnormal PG formation before enzyme activity is inhibited. In any case, it is probably more important to measure the ability of tissues to synthesise PGs, for example by homogenising tissues in aqueous solution (Bennett, Stamford and Unger, 1973). Using homogenisation of sections cut through the gut wall, substantial amounts of PGE_2-like material have been demonstrated in extracts of human gastric mucosa, but less biological activity was found in gastric muscle (Bennett et al, 1973). Recent studies show a different distribution of PGs in human ileum and colon. The amounts of biological assay (PGE_2 equivalents/g; rat stomach strip bioassay) are: gastric antral mucosa $>$ colon muscle $>$ gastric body mucosa $\approx$ ileal mucosa $>$ colon mucosa $\approx$ gastric muscle $\approx$ ileal muscle. Unlike the stomach there was evidence for 'PGF-like' material in intestinal muscle and mucosa (Bennett, Stamford and Stockley, 1977). The characterisation of human gastrointestinal PGs has depended on chromatography, but the problem is that various metabolites run with the 'primary' PGE and F compounds. Recent mass spectrometric data on two extracts of human gastric mucosa show mostly

6-oxo-PGF$_{1\alpha}$ with small amounts of PGD$_2$, E$_2$, F$_{2\alpha}$ and TXB$_2$ (Bennett, Boot, Dawson, Mallen, Osborne and Stamford, unpublished). 6-oxo-PGF$_{1\alpha}$ co-chromatograms with PGE$_2$ in many systems, and probably accounts for most of the PGE$_2$-like material reported by Bennett et al (1973). Others with radioimmuno assay have also reported PGE$_2$ but the cross-reactivity of the antibody with 6-oxo-PGF$_{1\alpha}$ was not determined.

The roles of PGs in human normal secretory or absorptive processes are not known. They may be involved in mucus secretion, and their stimulation of intestinal secretion may be important in some diarrhoeal diseases (see later). PG-like material is also formed in the muscle layers and nerve plexuses, and there is evidence that PGs affect muscle tone, muscle responsiveness to other substances, and nerve-mediated effects (Bennett and Stockley, 1977). The reason for differences in PG content of muscle from different parts of the human gut is not clear. It is not yet known whether the muscle produces TXA$_2$ or PGI$_2$, or whether the same substances formed during homogenisation are produced in vivo.

In the following discussion, advances in PGs with regard to the gastrointestinal tract are described starting with the proximal regions and working distally.

Gastro-oesophageal reflux
It has been known for several years that in vitro PGE compounds usually relax the circular muscle of the alimentary tract whereas PGF compounds cause contraction. In the longitudinal muscle both classes of PG cause contraction. Dilawari et al (1975) studied normal subjects and patients with upper abdominal complaints, and obtained results similar to those in vitro: PGF$_{2\alpha}$ contracted the lower oesophageal sphincter, whereas PGE$_2$ was inhibitory on the pentagastrin-contracted sphincter. Furthermore, indomethacin increased the sphincter tone and the authors suggested that PGE helps reduce sphincter pressure. If the lower oesophagus becomes inflamed this might release PGE$_2$ which aids reflux by relaxing the sphincter. This may help explain the relief of 'upset stomach' by Alka Seltzer, a highly buffered form of sodium acetylsalicylate. An effect on the lower oesophageal sphincter should be considered in the use of PG analogues for peptic ulcer since sphincter relaxation might increase oesophageal reflux.

GASTRIC BLEEDING DUE TO ASPIRIN-LIKE DRUGS

Aspirin-like drugs cause small losses of blood from the gastric mucosa in many people, and massive bleeding occurs on rare occasions. The importance attached by many to the mucosal damage seems out of proportion to the vast amount of aspirin consumed, and the drug is relatively safe. The cause of the bleeding is not known. In man, acid output does not increase with aspirin-like drugs as it can in rats (Main and Whittle, 1973) and dogs (Bennett and Curwain, 1977), but back-diffusion of hydrogen ions occurs through the gastric mucosa and this might mask increased secretion. Some groups have postulated that aspirin may act by reducing vascular perfusion through an effect on PG synthesis (Bennett et al, 1973; Main and Whittle, 1973; Whittle, 1977). Reduction of blood flow occurs with aspirin in rats (Main and Whittle, 1973), but a similar finding in dogs (O'Brien and Silen, 1973) was not substantiated by others (see Bennett and Curwain, 1977). The answer may lie at least partly in another direction. Minute amounts of various PGs inhibit damage to the gastric and intestinal mucosa and the effect is not necessarily dependent on inhibition of acid secretion (Robert, 1977). As discussed by Bennett et al (1977) the protection might involve mucus secretion. Output of mucus is stimulated by PG-15(R)-15-methyl-E₂ methyl ester (Fung, Lee and Karim, 1974c) and in inflammatory disease where PGs are presumably released. Furthermore, aspirin and corticosteroids can damage the gastric mucosa, both drugs inhibit mucus secretion, and both inhibit PG formation (see later).

Inhibition of gastric secretion
In man PGE_1 or PGE_2 analogues i.v. or orally inhibit gastric acid secretion induced by all types of stimuli, and this property is therefore of potential value in treating peptic ulcers. Intrinsic PGs may normally inhibit acid secretion in rats and dogs, but some data tend to argue against such a role in man and suggest that PG analogues act by a pharmacological antisecretory mechanism (Bennett et al, 1973).

Trials with PG-15(R)-15-methyl-E₂ methyl ester in human subjects with gastric or duodenal ulcers indicate that pain is reduced and healing speeded (Fung, Karim and Tye, 1974a, b). This analogue is in fact a pro-drug which is converted by acid in the stomach to the active S configuration; the 15-methyl group inhibits degradation by PG-15-dehydrogenase so producing a potent compound. Similar studies have been done with 16,16-dimethyl-PGE_2 and other analogues in animals (see Bennett, 1976a, for references). The problem with these analogues is that the effective dose is close to that producing diarrhoea as a side effect. Many drug companies are seeking more selective analogues and a recently reported compound, $(\pm)$-15-deoxy-16α,Tβ-hydroxy-PGE_1 methyl ester, has relatively little unwanted gastrointestinal activity in dogs (Dajani et al, 1975).

The PG analogues will obviously have to compete with other antisecretory drugs such as the histamine H_2 receptor antagonist cimetidine. PG analogues might be successful because of their abilities to inhibit both acid secretion and mucosal damage, and because they depress gastrin release. However, H_2 blockers reduce pepsin secretion while PGE_1 does not (Engel, Scruggs and Wilson, 1973). Perhaps a combination of various drugs such as PG analogues, anticholinergics, H_2 receptor antagonists or liquorice derivatives might produce the best results.

DIARRHOEA

PGs stimulate intestinal fluid secretion and intestinal muscle, and cause diarrhoea when administered orally or parenterally to man. These findings have led to the suggestion that PG release might be involved in certain types of diarrhoea. The hypothesis that PGs might be involved in cholera (Bennett, 1971) was supported by some papers but claimed as nonsense by others. Critical analysis of these latter papers showed many to contain illogical reasoning and glaring errors of calculation or interpretation (Bennett and Charlier 1977). Recently, Wald et al (1977) confirmed the work of other groups that indomethacin substantially reduces fluid secretion induced by cholera toxin in rabbits. Their paper also describes stimulation of fluid secretion before a rise in cAMP levels, so that this nucleotide may not be the only mediator for fluid secretion. However, cGMP was not measured and it is not possible to comment on the importance of cAMP : cGMP ratio. The authors suggest that indomethacin might reduce the effect of cholera toxin by inhibiting synthesis of PG which activates a non-cAMP mechanism.

The action of bacterial endotoxin also seems likely to involve a PG pathway. There is substantial evidence ranging from the pyretic action of PGs to their release in canine endotoxin shock. Harper and Skarnes (1972) found that indomethacin prevented the diarrhoeagenic effect of *Salmonella enteritidis* endotoxin in mice. In addition, Herman and Vane (1975) showed that *E. coli* endotoxin injected i.v. in rabbits increases synthesis of PG-like material from the subsequently excised intestine. Infantile endotoxin diarrhoea can be fatal, and it is therefore important to determine the role of PGs. If they are involved, aspirin-like drugs may be of substantial benefit. Alternatively, nutmeg may be useful (see later).

Radiation diarrhoea

Patients receiving radiotherapy for cancer of the cervix sometimes develop diarrhoea which is resistant to the usual forms of treatment such as morphine and diphenoxylate. Mennie et al (1975) used a double-blind technique to confirm the beneficial effect of aspirin, and obtained a highly significant improvement in the diarrhoea. It seems likely that incidental radiation damage to the intestine causes PG release which in turn produces diarrhoea. Ionising radiation increases the prostaglandin-like activity extracted from various tissues of the mouse (Eisen and Walker, 1976).

Diarrhoea associated with endocrine tumours

This has been discussed by Bennett (1976a, b) and Jaffe and Condon (1976). Williams, Karim and Sandler (1968) suggested that PGs are involved in the diarrhoea of medullary carcinoma of the thyroid, although evidence for this was found only in a few patients and others have obtained variable results. The only patient in whom we have found clearly raised PG levels in peripheral venous blood (bioassay on the rat stomach strip) had medullary carcinoma of the thyroid with lung metastases (Barrowman et al, 1975). We extrapolated to man the ability of animal lungs to inactivate PGE and F compounds, and reasoned that the PG-like material was being released from metastases distal to the site of inactivation (Barrowman et al, 1975). The lower inactivation of PGE$_1$ in human lung discussed earlier may mean that this conclusion should be modified; it may account for increased amounts of PGE-like activity in peripheral venous blood detected by radioimmunoassay, but cross-reactivity with PG metabolites cannot be excluded. The high normal values in some studies (e.g. Jaffe and Condon, 1976) suggest either that some cross-reactivity did occur or that PGs were formed during sampling or extraction. Perhaps the blood of these patients has increased ability to form PGs during sampling and extraction. The source of the blood PGs is presumed to be the thyroid tumour, but perhaps some is liberated by the intestine during increased activity; PG-like material was released into the perfusate of vagally stimulated rat intestine (Radmanovic, 1972). Blood PGs might play a part in the diarrhoea associated with other tumours such as carcinoid and in the WDHA syndrome (watery diarrhoea, hypokalaemia and achlorhydria) but not in the non-endocrine diarrhoeas examined by Jaffe and Condon (1976).

Nutmeg, prostaglandins and diarrhoea

Fawell and Thompson (1973) reported that nutmeg effectively treated otherwise-resistant diarrhoea in a man with medullary carcinoma of the thyroid, and speculated that this involved an effect on PGs. Bennett, Gradidge and Stamford (1974) demonstrated that small amounts of nutmeg inhibited formation of PG-like material during homogenisation of human colonic mucosa, but unlike PG synthetase inhibitors nutmeg did not lower the tone of rat isolated gastric fundus. Although Shafran, Maurer and Thomas (1977) reported that nutmeg reduced serum PG in a patient with Crohn's disease it is not certain that this explains how nutmeg acts, and whether the active material is present in nutmeg or obtained after metabolic transformation. Nutmeg is used widely for diarrhoea in some parts of the world, such as India, and many reports have now appeared in Western medical journals testifying to its efficacy; the drug seems useful in treating diarrhoea resistant to other forms of medication. Excellent results have also been obtained in treating or preventing calf scour and bowel oedema in piglets (Stamford, Bennett and Greenhalf, unpublished). Nutmeg exerts central effects in man, and it might be that identification of the active principle would be therapeutically worthwhile.

INFLAMMATION

It has been recognised for several years that PGs are one group of substances that contribute to inflammation, and the topic has been reviewed extensively. However, complications arise because PGs have both pro-inflammatory and anti-inflammatory actions. The pro-inflammatory effects include vasodilatation, increased vascular permeability, increased pain response to other mediators, and possibly leucotaxis. The anti-inflammatory effects are thought to include inhibition of release of lysosomal enzymes and histamine. The pro-inflammatory effects presumably outweigh the anti-inflammatory effects, because PG synthetase inhibitors reduce the inflammatory response. However, other actions of the drugs may contribute to the overall effect. In pain, PGE_2 acts as a modulator and not as a mediator; it produces little pain itself but causes hyperalgesia and potentiates the response to histamine and bradykinin (Ferreira, 1972). The roles of other products of arachidonic acid metabolism have received little study. Modulation also seems important in the inflammatory response although here PGs also act partly as mediators. Some PGs may be released by other mediators such as bradykinin (Ferreira, Moncada and Vane, 1973). Many believe that the anti-inflammatory action of aspirin-like drugs is due to inhibition of prostaglandin synthesis. Kuehl et al (1977) studied an anti-inflammatory drug which, unlike aspirin and indomethacin, increased synthesis of PGE_2 and $PGF_{2\alpha}$. However, all the drugs reduced the formation of PGG_2 which is a hydroperoxy PG endoperoxide. They suggest that tissue damage is due to the free radical formed when PGG_2 is converted to PGH_2, rather than to the actions of the PGs. This is an interesting hypothesis, but PGE_2 is known to interact with other released substances and such effects should not be ignored. Slater (1972) has for several years suggested that free radicals play a part in tissue injury.

Actions of other anti-inflammatory drugs on the prostaglandin system
The actions of the anti-inflammatory steroids include an effect on PGs. Lewis and Piper (1975) and Chang, Lewis and Piper (1977) suggested that steroids inhibit the release but not the synthesis of PGs in the rabbit fat pad. Gryglewski et al (1975) concluded that corticosteroids reduce the formation of PGs; this may occur by inhibition of phospholipase A which releases arachidonic acid from phospholipids (Blackwell et al, 1977). Anti-inflammatory steroids appear to inhibit prostaglandin production by human synovium (Kantrowitz et al, 1975).

Gold salts which are used in rheumatoid arthritis, inhibited the formation of $PGF_{2\alpha}$ and increased the formation of PGE_2 from arachidonic acid by a sheep seminal vesicle preparation (Stone, Mather and Gibson, 1975). The authors suggested that the ratio of PGE to PGF may be important for normal function.

Sulphasalazine is used to maintain ulcerative colitis in remission. Butt et al (1974) showed that sulphasalazine inhibits PG formation by a ram seminal vesicle preparation. The drug is broken down by colonic bacteria into sulphapyridine and 5-aminosalicylic acid. Preliminary experiments indicate that both 5-aminosalicylic acid and sulphapyridine reduce the formation of PG-like material during homogenisation of human colonic mucosa, whereas sulphasalazine appears to have no effect (Bennett, 1976b). The anti-inflammatory effect of sulphasalazine may therefore be due to inhibition of PG synthesis but it is not clear to what extent this is due to the parent drug or its metabolites. It may be advantageous to use other PG synthetase inhibitors which are better tolerated, either alone or in combination with sulphasalazine. Perhaps a drug can be formulated which, like sulphasalazine, reaches the colonic mucosa, exerts a local action and then has a further effect after absorption.

BARTTER'S SYNDROME

The pathology of Bartter's syndrome includes hypokalaemic alkalosis, high plasma renin and aldosterone, juxtaglomerular cell hyperplasia, and renal potassium wasting, with a normal blood pressure which is poorly sensitive to angiotensin. Since the report by Fichman et al (1976) several authors have found raised blood PG levels in the disease, and have obtained a beneficial effect with aspirin-like drugs (Leading article, 1976).

The potential implications for prostaglandins in medicine are more exciting than ever, and their manipulation may possibly have many unconventional uses ranging from kidney disease to cancer. Drugs which selectively inhibit the conversion of PG endoperoxides to thromboxanes or the various prostaglandins may become important new treatments. Prostaglandin analogues are already being studied in various conditions, and those based on the endoperoxides are now available for experimental use in animals. Compounds related to TXA_2 and PGI_2 will no doubt be made. Prostaglandin receptor antagonists might be useful clinically, but the drugs reported so far have rather poor activity and selectivity, and none except polyphloretin phosphate has been given to man. No studies have yet been reported on drugs to inhibit receptors for PG endoperoxides, TXA_2 or PGI_2.

REFERENCES

Barrowman, J. A., Bennett, A., Hillenbrand, P., Rolles, K., Pollock, D. J. & Wright, J. T. (1975) Diarrhoea in medullary carcinoma of the thyroid: evidence for the role of prostaglandins and the therapeutic effect of nutmeg. *British Medical Journal*, iii, 11–12.

Bennett, A. (1971) Cholera and prostaglandins. *Nature*, **231**, 536.

Bennett, A. (1976a) Prostaglandins and the alimentary tract. In *Prostaglandins: Physiological, Pharmacological and Pathological Aspects.* pp 247–276. Lancaster: MTP Press Ltd.

Bennett, A. (1976b) Prostaglandins as factors in diseases of the alimentary tract. *Advances in Prostaglandin and Thromboxane Research*, ed. Samuelsson, B. & Paoletti, R., Vol. 2, pp. 547–555. New York: Raven Press.

Bennett, A. & Charlier, E. M. (1977) Evidence against the release of prostaglandin-like material from isolated intestinal tissue by pure cholera toxin. *Prostaglandins*, **13**, 431–436.

Bennet, A. & Curwain, B. P. (1977) Effects of aspirin-like drugs on canine gastric mucosal blood flow and acid secretion. *British Journal of Pharmacology*, **60**, 499–504.

Bennett, A., Gradidge, C. F. & Stamford, I. F. (1974) Prostaglandins, nutmeg and diarrhea. *New England Journal of Medicine*, **290**, 110–111.

Bennett, A., Stamford, I. F. & Stockley, H. L. (1977) Estimation and characterisation of prostaglandins in the human gastrointestinal tract. *British Journal of Pharmacology*, **61**, 579–586.

Bennett, A., Stamford, I. F. & Unger, W. G. (1973) Prostaglandin E_2 and gastric acid secretion in man. *Journal of Physiology*, **229**, 349–360.

Bennett, A., Houghton, J., Leaper, D. J. & Stamford, I. F. (1978). Tumour growth and response to treatment: beneficial effect of the prostaglandin synthesis inhibitor flurbiprofen. *Br. J. Pharmac.*, (in press).

Bennett, A., McDonald, A. M., Simpson, J. S. & Stamford, I. F. (1975) Breast cancer, prostaglandins and bone metastases. *Lancet*, **i**, 1218–1220.

Bennett, A., Charlier, E. M., McDonald, A. M., Simpson, J. S., Stamford, I. F. & Zebro, T. (1977) Prostaglandins and breast cancer. *Lancet*, **2**, 624–626.

Bennett, A. & Stockley, H. L. (1977) The contribution of prostaglandins in the muscle of human isolated small intestine to neurogenic responses. *British Journal of Pharmacology*, **61**, 579–586.

Blackwell, G. J., Flower, R. J., Nijkamp, F. P. & Vane, J. R. (1977) Phospholipase A_2 activity of guinea-pig perfused lungs: stimulation and inhibition by anti-inflammatory steroids. *British Journal of Pharmacology*, **59**, 441P.

Boston Collaborative Drug Surveillance Group (1974) Regular aspirin intake and acute myocardial infarction. *British Medical Journal*, **i**, 440–443.

Butt, A. A., Collier, H. O. J., Gardener, P. J. & Saeed, S. A. (1974) Effects of prostaglandin biosynthesis of drugs affecting gastrointestinal function. *Gut*, **15**, 344.

Carlson, L. A. & Eriksson, I. (1973) Femoral-artery infusion of prostaglandin E_1 in severe peripheral vascular disease. *Lancet*, **i**, 155–156.

Carlson, L. A. & Olsson, A. G. (1977) PGE_1 in peripheral artery disease. *Prostaglandins and Therapeutics*, Vol. 2, pp. 1–2. Upjohn Company.

Chang, J., Lewis, G. P. & Piper, P. J. (1977) Inhibition by glucocorticoids of prostaglandin release from adipose tissue in vitro. *British Journal of Pharmacology*, **59**, 425–432.

Dajani, E. Z., Driskill, D. R., Bianchi, R. G., Collins, P. W. & Pappo, R. (1975) Influence of the position of the side chain hydroxy group on the gastric antisecretory and anti-ulcer actions of E_1 prostaglandin analogs. *Prostaglandins*, **10**, 733–745.

Dilawari, J. D., Newman, A., Poleo, J. & Misiewicz, J. J. (1975) Response of the human cardiac sphincter to circulating prostaglandins $F_{2\alpha}$ and E_2 and to anti-inflammatory drugs. *Gut*, **16**, 137–143.

Dowsett, M., Easty, G. C., Powles, T. J., Easty, D. M. & Neville, A. M. (1976a) Human breast tumour-induced osteolysis and prostaglandins. *Prostaglandins*, **11**, 447–460.

Dowsett, M., Eastman, A. R., Easty, D. M., Easty, G. C., Powles, T. J. & Neville, A. M. (1976b) Prostaglandin mediation of collagenase-induced bone resorption. *Nature*, **263**, 72–74.

Eisen, V. & Walker, D. I. (1976) Effect of ionising radiation on prostaglandin-like activity in tissues. *British Journal of Pharmacology*, **57**, 527–532.

Elliott, R. B., Starling, M. D. & Neutze, J. M. (1975) Medical manipulation of the ductus arteriosus. *Lancet*, **i**, 140–142.

Engel, J. J., Scruggs, W. & Wilson, D. E. (1973) Failure of SC-19220 to affect prostaglandin E_1 (PGE_1) gastric antisecretory actions. *Prostaglandins*, **4**, 65–70.

Fawell, W. N. & Thompson, G. (1973) Nutmeg for diarrhea of medullary carcinoma of the thyroid. *New England Journal of Medicine*, **289**, 108–109.

Ferreira, S. H. (1972) Prostaglandins, aspirin-like drugs and analgesia. *Nature (New Biology)*, **240**, 200–203.

Ferreira, S. H. & Vane, J. R. (1967) Prostaglandins: their disappearance from and release into the circulation. *Nature* (Lond), **216**, 868–873.

Ferreira, S. H., Moncada, S. & Vane, J. R. (1973) Some effects of inhibiting endogenous prostaglandin formation on the responses of the cat spleen. *British Journal of Pharmacology*, **47**, 48–58.

Fichman, M. P., Telfer, N., Zia, P., Speckart, P., Golub, M. & Rude, R. (1976) Role of prostaglandins in the pathogenesis of Bartter's syndrome. *American Journal of Medicine*, **60**, 785–797.

Friedman, W. F., Hirschklaw, M. J., Printz, M. T., Pitlick, P. T. & Kirkpatrick, S. E. (1976) Pharmacologic closure of patent ductus arteriosus in the premature infant. *New England Journal of Medicine*, **295**, 526–529.

Fung, W. P., Karim, S. M. M. & Tye, C. Y. (1974a) Effect of 15(R)15 methyl prostaglandin E_2 methyl ester on healing of gastric ulcers. Controlled endoscopic study. *Lancet*, **ii**, 10–12.

Fung, W. P., Karim, S. M. M. & Tye, C. T. (1974b) Double-blind trial of 15(R)15 methyl prostaglandin E_2 methyl ester in the relief of peptic ulcer pain. *Annals of the Academy of Medicine (Singapore)*, **3**, 375–378.

Fung, W. P., Lee, S. K. & Karim, S. M. M. (1974c) Effect of prostaglandin 15(R)15 methyl-E_2-methyl ester on the gastric mucosa in patients with peptic ulceration—an endoscopic and histological study. *Prostaglandins*, 5, 465–472.

Galasko, C. S. B. (1976) Mechanisms of bone destruction in the development of skeletal metastases. *Nature*, 263, 507–508.

Galasko, C. S. B. & Bennett, A. (1976) Relationship of bone destruction in skeletal metastases to osteoclast activation and prostaglandins. *Nature*, 263, 508–510.

Gasic, G. J., Gasic, T. B., Galanti, N., Johnson, T. & Murphy, S. (1973) Platelet-tumor-cell interactions in mice. The role of platelets in the spread of malignant disease. *International Journal of Cancer*, 11, 704–718.

Golub, M., Zia, P., Matsuno, M. & Horton, R. (1975) Metabolism of prostaglandins A_1 and E_1 in man. *Journal of Clinical Investigations*, 56, 1404–1410.

Gryglewski, R. J., Panczenko, B., Korbut, R., Grodzinska, L. & Ocetkiewicz, A. (1975) Corticosteroids inhibit prostaglandin release from perfused mesenteric blood vessels of rabbit and from perfused lungs of sensitised guinea-pig. *Prostaglandins*, 10, 343–355.

Hamberg, M., Svensson, J. & Samuelsson, B. (1975) Thromboxanes: a new group of biologically active compounds derived from prostaglandin endoperoxides. *Proceedings of the National Academy of Sciences*, 72, 2994–2998.

Harris, M., Jenkins, M. V., Bennett, A. & Wills, M. R. (1973) Prostaglandin production and bone resorption by dental cysts. *Nature*, 245, 213–215.

Harper, M. J. K. & Skarnes, R. C. (1972) Inhibition of abortion and fetal death produced by endotoxin or prostaglandin $F_{2\alpha}$. *Prostaglandins*, 2, 295–309.

Herman, A. G. & Vane, J. R. (1975) Endotoxin and production of prostaglandins by the isolated rabbit jejunum. Influence of indomethacin. *Archives of International Pharmacodynamics*, 213, 328–329.

Heymann, M. A. & Rudolph, A. M. (1977) Ductus arteriosus patency maintained by PGE_1 infusion. *Prostaglandins and Therapeutics*, Vol. 2, p. 2. Upjohn Company.

Heymann, M. A., Rudolph, A. M. & Silverman, N. H. (1976) Closure of the ductus arteriosus in premature infants by inhibition of prostaglandin synthesis. *New England Journal of Medicine*, 295, 530–533.

Jaffe, B. M. (1974) Prostaglandins and cancer: an update. *Prostaglandins*, 6, 453–461.

Jaffe, B. M. & Condon, S. (1976) Prostaglandins E and F in endocrine diarrheagenic syndromes. *Annals of Surgery*, 184, 516–523.

Jick, H. & Miettienen, O. S. (1976) Regular aspirin use and myocardial infarction. *British Medical Journal*, i, 1057.

Johnson, R. A., Morton, D. R., Kinner, J. H., Gorman, R. R., McGuire, J. C. & Sun, F. F. (1976) The chemical structure of prostaglandin X (prostacyclin). *Prostaglandins*, 12, 915–928.

Kantrowitz, F., Robinson, D. R., McGuire, M. B. & Levine, L. (1975) Corticosteroids inhibit prostaglandin production by rheumatoid synovia. *Nature (London)*, 258, 737–739.

Klein, D. C. & Raisz, L. G. (1970) Prostaglandins: stimulation of bone resorption in tissue culture. *Endocrinology*, 86, 1436–1440.

Kuehl, F. A., Humes, J. L., Egan, R. W., Ham, E. A., Beveridge, G. C. & Van Arman, C. G. (1977) Role of prostaglandin endoperoxide PGG_2 in inflammatory processes. *Nature*, 265, 170–173.

Leading article (1976) Bartter's syndrome. *Lancet*, ii, 721–722.

Lewis, G. P. & Piper, P. J. (1975) Inhibition of release of prostaglandins as an explanation of some of the actions of anti-inflammatory corticosteroids. *Nature*, 254, 308–311.

Loose, L. D. & Di Luzio, N. R. (1973) Effect of prostaglandin E_1 on cellular and humoral immune responses. *Journal of Reticuloendothelial Society*, 13, 70–77.

Main, I. H. M. & Whittle, B. J. R. (1973) Effects of indomethacin on rat gastric acid secretion and mucosal blood flow. *British Journal of Pharmacology*, 47, 666.

Malmsten, C., Hamberg, M., Svensson, J. & Samuelsson, B. (1975) Physiological role of an endoperoxide in human platelets: hemostatic defect due to platelet cyclo-oxygenase deficiency. *Proceedings of the National Academy of Sciences*, 72, 1446–1450.

Mennie, A. T., Dalley, V. M., Dinneen, L. C. & Collier, H. O. J. (1975) Treatment of radiation-induced gastrointestinal distress with acetylsalicylate. *Lancet* 2, 942–943.

Moncada, S., Gryglewski, R., Bunting, S. & Vane, J. R. (1976) An enzyme isolated from arteries transforms prostaglandin endoperoxides to an unstable substance that inhibits platelet aggregation. *Nature*, 263, 663–664.

Moncada, S. & Vane, J. R. (1977) The discovery of prostacyclin (PGX): a fresh insight into arachidonic acid metabolism. *Biochemical Aspects of Prostaglandins and Thromboxanes*, Ed. Kharasch, N. & Fried, J. pp. 155–177. New York: Academic Press.

Moncada, S., Bunting, S., Mullane, K., Thorogood, P., Vane, J. R., Raz, A. & Needleman, P. (1977) Imidazole: a selective inhibitor of thromboxane synthetase. *Prostaglandins*, 13, 611–618.

O'Brien, P. & Silen, W. (1973) Effect of bile salts and aspirin on the gastric mucosal blood flow. *Gastroenterology*, 64, 246–253.

Plescia, O. J., Smith, A. H. & Grinwich, K. (1975) Subversion of immune system by tumor cells and role of prostaglandins. *Proceedings of the National Academy of Sciences*, 72, 1848–1851.

Powles, T. J., Clark, S. A., Easty, D. M., Easty, G. C. & Neville, A. M. (1973) The inhibition by aspirin and indomethacin of osteolytic tumour deposits and hypercalcaemia in rats with Walker tumour, and its possible application to human breast cancer. *British Journal of Cancer*, **28**, 316–321.

Prasad, K. N. (1972) Morphological differentiation induced by prostaglandin in mouse neuroblastoma cells in culture. *Nature (New Biology)*, **236**, 49–52.

Radmanovic, B. Z. (1972) Effect of prostaglandin E_1 on the peristaltic activity of the guinea-pig isolated ileum. *Archives of International Pharmacodynamics and Therapeutics*, **200**, 396–404.

Raisz, L. G., Dietrich, J. W. & Simmons, H. A. (1977) Effect of prostaglandin endoperoxides and metabolites on bone resorption in vitro. *Nature*, **267**, 532–534.

Robert, A. (1977) Effect of prostaglandins on gastrointestinal functions. In *Prostaglandins and Thromboxanes*, ed. Berti, F., Samuelsson, B. & Velo, G. P., pp. 287–313. New York: Plenum Press.

Rowe, D. J. F., Bennett, A. & Harris, M. (1978) Endogenous prostaglandin (PG) synthesis and osteolysis. *Journal of Dental Research* (in press).

Samuelsson, B. (1976) New trends in prostaglandin research. In *Advances in Prostaglandin and Thromboxane Research*. ed. Samuelsson, B. & Paoletti, R., Vol. 1, pp. 1–6. New York: Raven Press.

Santoro, M. G., Pilpott, G. W. & Jaffe, B. M. (1976) Inhibition of tumour growth in vivo and in vitro by prostaglandin E. *Nature*, **263**, 777–779.

Seyberth, H. W., Segre, G. V., Morgan, J. L., Sweetman, B. J., Potts, J. T. & Oates, J. A. (1975) Prostaglandins as mediators of hypercalcemia associated with certain types of cancer. *New England Journal of Medicine*, **293**, 1278–1283.

Shafran, I., Maurer, W. & Thomas, F. D. (1977) Prostaglandins and Crohn's disease. *New England Journal of Medicine*, **296**, 694.

Slater, T. F. (1972) *Free Radical Mechanisms in Tissue Injury*. London: Pion Ltd.

Stone, K. G., Mather, S. J. & Gibson, P. B. (1975) Selective inhibition of prostaglandin biosynthesis by gold salts and phenylbutazone. *Prostaglandins*, **10**, 241–251.

Strausser, H. R. & Humes, J. L. (1975) Prostaglandin synthesis inhibition: effect on bone changes and sarcoma tumor induction in BALB/c mice. *International Journal of Cancer*, **15**, 724–730.

Tashjian, A. H., Voelkel, E. F., Levine, L. & Goldhaber, P. (1972) Evidence that the bone resorption-stimulating factor produced by mouse fibrosarcoma cells is prostaglandin E_2. A new model for the hypercalcemia of cancer. *Journal of Experimental Medicine*, **136**, 1329–1343.

Tashjian, A. H., Voelkel, E. F., Wolfe, H. J. Gagel, R., DeLellis, R. A., Franklin, R. & Jackson, C. E. (1975) Cited by Voelkel et al, 1975.

Tashjian, A. H., Tice, J. E. & Sides, K. (1977) Biological activities of prostaglandin analogues and metabolites on bone in organ culture. *Nature*, **266**, 645–647.

Voelkel, E. F., Tashjian, A. H., Franklin, R., Wasserman, E. & Levine, L. (1975) Hypercalcemia and tumor-prostaglandins: the VX_2 carcinoma model in the rabbit. *Metabolism*, **24**, 973–986.

Wald, A., Gotterer, G. S., Rajendra, N. A., Turjman, N. A. & Hendrix, T. R. (1977) Effect of indomethacin on cholera-induced fluid movement, unidirectional sodium fluxes, and intestinal cAMP. *Gastroenterology*, **72**, 106–110.

Williams, E. D., Karim, S. M. M. & Sandler, M. (1968) Prostaglandin secretion by medullary carcinoma of the thyroid. *Lancet*, **i**, 22–23.

Willis, A. L., Vane, F. M., Kuhn, D. C., Scott, C. G. & Petrin, M. (1974) An endoperoxide aggregator (LASS), formed in platelets in response to thrombotic stimuli: purification, identification and unique biological significance. *Prostaglandins*, **8**, 453–507.

Whittle, B. J. R. (1977) Antisecretory prostaglandins and gastric mucosal erosions in the rat. In *Prostaglandins and Thromboxanes*, ed. Berti, F., Samuelsson, B. & Velo, G. P., pp. 315–322. New York: Plenum Press.

3. Selectivity of beta-adrenoceptor agonists and antagonists

Cyrus R. Kumana   Graham E. Marlin

INTRODUCTION

The unending goal of all therapeutics is to intervene in biological systems so as to produce benefit without giving rise to adverse effects. Generally, the more powerful an intervention, the more likely that several delicately balanced and interdependent biological mechanisms might also be affected — giving rise both to desirable and undesirable consequences. The use of drugs to influence the extent of adrenergic stimulation is no exception. The recent explosive increase in the use of these agents and the plethora of alternative drugs available means that the assessment of possible selective activity as applied in this context has important clinical and economic ramifications, quite apart from leading to a better understanding of drug action and disease.

Numerous drugs directly influencing beta-adrenoceptor stimulation (as opposed to indirectly acting drugs acting on adrenergic neurons) have been administered to man. Their actions have been deemed potentially desirable, potentially harmful or indifferent. In truth, however, such description must depend upon the prevailing circumstances. Whatever their therapeutic pros and cons, their differing pharmacological properties have been ascribed to the extent to which these agents possess (a) *agonist and/or antagonist activity*, (b) *receptor specificity and* (c) *tissue selectivity*. The specificity of beta-adrenoceceptor agonist and antagonist drugs refers to their ability to influence the beta-adrenoceptor and only that receptor and not any final common pathway mediating the effect. The naturally occurring catecholamines are agonists lacking specificity in this sense, since as described in Ahlquist's original work (1948), they influence both alpha- and beta-adrenoceptors, though to differing extents. The term selectivity, when used with respect to these drugs, refers to their relative predilection to influence beta-receptor mediated effects in different organs and tissues. The distinction between 'receptor specificity' and 'tissue selectivity' has currently become blurred, as according to one school of thought 'tissue selectivity' may, in fact, be explained in terms of different degrees of specificity towards subtypes of beta-receptors.

The ability to stimulate receptors in the lung is generally viewed as a favourable property — as by giving rise to bronchodilatation, ventilation would be facilitated; conversely, pulmonary beta-receptor blocking activity is considered an adverse property impeding air flow and capable of precipitating asthma in persons dependent on sympathetic stimulation to maintain airway patency. With regard to the heart — antagonism of its beta-receptors is made use of extensively in the treatment of ischaemic heart disease, hypertension and tachyarrhythmias. In contrast (except in very special situations), stimulation of cardiac beta-receptors is generally avoided if at all possible, since serious side effects including angina, cardiac infarction and tachycardias may ensue. It follows that amongst beta-receptor stimulant drugs, those primarily influencing the pulmonary airways rather than the heart are considered desirable and termed selective agonists. Amongst beta-adrenoceptor blocking agents, those which affect cardiac receptors and spare receptors in the lungs have similarly been considered to have pharmacological advantages, and have been termed selective antagonists.

From the foregoing discussion, it should not be concluded that an ideal selective antagonist (i.e. one that produced cardiac beta-adrenoceptor blockade exclusively) could never be harmful. During near maximal exercise or in the presence of myocardial disease, sympathetic cardiac stimulation may be critical (viz. both rate and force of contraction of the heart) — in which case cardiac beta-adrenoceptor blockade could reduce cardiac output and produce heart failure. Similarly, an ideal selective agonist (producing pulmonary beta-adrenoceptor stimulation exclusively) might conceivably have deleterious effects in certain circumstances. Uniform pulmonary bronchodilatation, though increasing total ventilation, could nevertheless give rise to regional imbalances in ventilation and perfusion. Selective agonism thus far available also produces pulmonary vasodilation which may have a more important role in such an effect (see p. 38); and even if the extent of arterial Po_2 reduction may be trivial (Palmer and Diament, 1969), its failure to rise in the face of increased ventilation is itself noteworthy.

Mechanism of selectivity

With respect to drugs directly influencing beta-adrenoceptors, there are two main explanations for the phenomenon of 'tissue selectivity'. It may arise from different degrees of 'specificity' towards stereospecific subtypes of beta-receptors. Alternatively, it may be ascribed to the physicochemical properties of different organs and tissues which may affect the ability of any given agent to reach the receptors. In the sense that the physicochemical properties of the environment surrounding beta-receptors in different tissues may differ, it might still be arguable to refer to these as different types of beta-receptors.

Tissue selectivity and beta-receptor subtypes

A hypothesis by Lands et al (1967) that there were two beta-receptor populations; $beta_1$ subserving lipolysis and cardiac stimulation and $beta_2$ subserving bronchodilatation and vasodilatation seemed to offer a ready explanation for tissue selectivity. These workers based their conclusions on the observation that 15 sympathomimetic amines used to evoke accepted beta-receptor mediated responses in a series of isolated tissues and intact animals, gave two orders of potency. The applicability of the $beta_1$- and $beta_2$-receptor hypothesis to man was supported by Collier and Dornhorst (1969), who showed that the activity ratio of two beta-receptor agonists (isoprenaline and isoetharine), when tested for the changes they produced in human volunteers, also fell into two distinct groups. Thus, the activity ratios for increases in pulse rate, increases in respiratory minute volume and decreases in diastolic blood pressure were all highly comparable and about three-fold greater than the ratio for increase in forearm blood flow. The latter ratio was of the same order as that obtained in other human work with respect to bronchodilatation (Herschfus et al, 1951). Further support for the $beta_1$ and $beta_2$ hypothesis seemed to be provided by the development of many new beta-adrenoceptor agonist and antagonist drugs, which have their predominant action on tissues purported to have one or other type of beta-receptor. Nevertheless, several objections to the $beta_1$ and $beta_2$ hypothesis exist:

1. An obvious criticism of the original work by Lands and co-workers (1967) was the use of different species to study different responses — so that the differences in potency ratios could have been due to species differences rather than differences in receptors. The same criticism could not be levelled at Ahlquist's work (1948), as his studies involved several different tissues from each of several species and included a comparison of responses on given organs from different species.
2. The potency rank orders encountered did not fall exactly into two, but involved a statistical analysis from which it was inferred that two distinct potency orders were involved. It must be admitted, however, that unlike the device of ranking used by Ahlquist (1948), a parametric correlation coefficient was used so that substantial potency differences were unlikely to be obscured.
3. Other studies (Furchgott, 1967; Levy and Wilkenfeld, 1969) have indicated the non-homogeneity of beta-receptor types, and the existence of at least three subtypes has been proposed.
4. The fact that to date not a single antagonist or agonist appears to possess absolute tissue selectivity (i.e. 'selectivity' is invariably relative), favours the existence of only one type of receptor, whose extent of activation in different tissues may depend on many variables. This could, however, be ascribed to mixtures of $beta_1$- and $beta_2$-receptors existing in different tissues in different proportions provided that in any given tissue both types of receptors mediated the same response.

Tissue selectivity and physicochemical factors
Propranolol, which is the prototype of non-selective beta-adrenoceptor antagonists, has a high degree of lipid solubility. In contrast, practolol, which is the most widely acknowledged 'selective' antagonist, is very water soluble and lacking in appreciable lipid solubility. This difference may account for observations in animals that after intravenous or oral administration of propranolol, it accumulates preferentially (in the form of parent compound and metabolites) in the lungs (Hayes and Cooper, 1971) and to a much lesser extent in the heart (about five-fold less); whereas practolol accumulates in the lungs and heart to approximately the same extent (Scales and Cosgrove, 1970). These studies also revealed that compared with other organs, the brain (which is largely lipid tissue) acquired a relatively high concentration of propranolol, second only to that in the lung. Compared with propranolol, the relative inability of practolol to give rise to pulmonary effects and its reported lesser tendency to produce side effects such as vivid dreams may thus be reflecting the different extents to which these drugs can penetrate tissues with different physicochemical characteristics and not any differences between tissue receptors. Similar work on animals with oxprenolol, another non-selective antagonist like propranolol and with similar lipid solubility (Hellenbrecht et al, 1973) also reveals preferential distribution to the lungs, about five-fold that to the heart (Riess et al, 1970). However, with this drug, distribution into brain was minimal, so that physicochemical tissue penetrating characteristics taken in isolation cannot account for all aspects of drug distribution.

Substances in solution do not cross biological membranes readily by passive diffusion unless (a) they have appreciable lipid solubility and (b) they are un-ionised. Even highly lipophilic non-polar molecules lose their lipid solubility on ionisation. Precisely these two physicochemical properties of a series of beta-adrenoceptor antagonists and partial agonists have been correlated against non-specific activity as well as beta-receptor blocking activity in a number of in vitro systems (Pratesi, Grana and Villa, 1968; Hellenbrecht et al, 1973). Indeed, whatever the activity being tested, the best correlation was found when a function incorporating both lipid solubility and pKα values together was used. To account for selectivity in these terms, (a) it should be realised that lungs behave as a much more lipid tissue than heart and (b) that what matters for any given drug is the ratio of its pulmonary presence/cardiac presence (P/C). Antagonists such as propranolol having high penetrating characteristics (lipid solubility) would have high P/C ratios and turn out to be non-selective, whilst those with poor penetrability characteristics would have a low ratio and thus be 'cardioselective', even though cardiac penetrating ability would also be reduced — so that greater plasma concentrations would be required to produce any given cardiac effect. In keeping with such a prediction, it has been observed that for any given degree of cardiac beta-adrenoceptor blocking activity in man, the plasma concentrations of practolol are in the order of 23 to 28 times those of propranolol (Bodem et al, 1973; Kumana et al, 1974, 1975). Moreover, unbound drug ratios must have been much higher as propranolol is highly protein bound. With respect to agonists, it would be predicted that those with high tissue penetrating ability (lipid solubility, etc.) would have high P/C ratios and be 'selective' agonists, and conversely, those with poor penetrating characteristics would be associated with low P/C ratios and non-selectivity.

It does not necessarily follow that to produce a given effect either with agonists or antagonists, those with high penetrating ability would only require to be present at low plasma concentrations and vice versa. Clearly, if an agent's innate beta-receptor influencing activity was low, then even if it had very good penetrating properties, the drug would still need to be present in very high concentrations around the receptors, and hence may require relatively higher concentrations in plasma, and possibly may have to be given in larger doses than intrinsically more active substances with lesser penetrating properties. This may explain why a simple correlation between any single pharmacological activity of beta-adrenoceptor antagonists and physicochemical properties has not been found (Levy, 1968).

The so-called differences in beta-receptor subtype revealed by manipulating the chemical structure of agonists and antagonists (and there is an enormous literature on this subject) also involve alterations in the physicochemical properties of these drugs. Nevertheless, in considering a physicochemical hypothesis to explain tissue selectivity, a number of related outstanding issues need to be resolved:

1. For beta-adrenoceptor agonists, any correlation between physicochemical characteristics (functions incorporating lipid solubility, pKₐ values, etc.) and the degree of selectivity is not yet available. Similarly it remains to be seen to what extent the physicochemical characteristics of the newer beta-adrenoceptor antagonists correlate with the extent of tissue selectivity.
2. Particularly in man, minor differences in selectivity are difficult to measure (unlike physicochemical characteristics) and the most appropriate function of lipid solubility and pKₐ values determined from animal work may not be appropriate in humans.
3. Whenever substantial amounts of active metabolites are formed in vivo, any attempt to correlate in vivo selectivity with the physicochemical characteristics of the parent drug would be misleading.
4. The fact that a drug is concentrated in a particular organ, does not imply that it

necessarily has a substantial access to relevant receptors. Tissue binding could well be non-specific, and rather than net accumulation in any organ it is the presence of free drug in the immediate environment of the receptors that matters. It follows that crude measurements of total fat in any given tissue would not necessarily be helpful in predicting responsiveness to drugs even if lipid solubility, etc., did determine tissue selectivity.

5. Stereospecificity does not influence drug distribution. As opposed to any non-specific actions, beta-receptor mediated responses unquestionably involve stereospecificity (Biel and Lum, 1966; Howe and Shanks, 1966; Levy and Richards, 1966; Patil, 1968), and it is this characteristic which may help to discriminate between the alternative hypotheses. Thus, if distribution characteristics rather than beta-receptor differences are to account for tissue selectivity, then non-specific pharmacological properties might also manifest predictable selectivity, so long as drug molecules executing non-specific actions are also in equilibrium with the environment of the beta-receptors. It remains to be determined therefore, whether a selective antagonist will also turn out to have relatively weak 'membrane stabilising activity' on bronchial and vascular smooth muscle, and conversely, whether the non-specific actions of selective agonists will also be relatively more marked in these tissues.

Conceivably both physicochemical differences between beta-receptor environments in different tissues as well as steric differences in the 'receptors' themselves may together account for selectivity (Pratesi, Villa and Grana, 1975) and the two may even be interdependent. Regardless of whether or not tissue distribution is a crucial factor determining selectivity, it may nevertheless be of prime importance to the development of long-term complications. For example, in animals at least, secretory glands tend to accumulate very much higher concentrations of practolol than other tissues (Scales and Cosgrove, 1970), a fact which may be of particular relevance to some of its known long-term complications in humans such as keratoconjunctivitis sicca.

Other mechanisms to explain tissue selectivity. Coexisting ability to influence alpha-receptors could also affect the degree of selectivity manifest by beta-adrenoceptor angonists and antagonists. In the airways the existence of alpha-receptors (stimulation of which produces bronchoconstriction) has been suspected for some time (Fleisch, Maling and Brodie, 1970). Assuming that the heart is relatively devoid of alpha-receptors compared to the bronchi, an antagonist with a combined action on beta- and alpha-receptors might produce relatively less bronchoconstriction than a pure beta-adrenoceptor blocker whilst having the same cardiac effect. Labetalol, a combined beta- and alpha-adrenoceptor antagonist, can be considered to manifest a type of selectivity by this means without true beta-receptor selectivity (Richards, 1976). Conversely, beta-receptor agonists which can also stimulate alpha-receptors may have to be administered in relatively greater amounts to produce a given degree of bronchodilatation and may hence produce greater degrees of cardiac stimulation than beta-receptor agonists devoid of action on alpha-receptors. The latter drugs might thus exhibit selective agonism.

Connolly and Batten (1970) suggested that *partial agonist activity (PAA)* might be a factor influencing the 'cardioselectivity' of beta-adrenoceptor antagonists. Thus, whenever sympathetic stimulation of the airways was of a low order such as at rest then antagonists with PAA (e.g. practolol) may produce very little net reduction in bronchial beta-receptor stimulation. However, such a mechanism is unlikely to be important in accounting for selectivity as oxprenolol (which has PAA) is non-selective whilst atenolol (which virtually lacks PAA) is generally regarded as selective (see p. 49).

INDIVIDUAL TISSUES AND SELECTIVITY

Regrettably, in clinical practice, the term 'selectivity' as generally applied to drugs which influence beta-adrenoceptor function is misleading in many ways as follows:

1. When applied to agonist drugs, it refers to their ability to stimulate pulmonary beta-adrenoceptors and spare those in the heart; whilst in the context of antagonists, 'selectivity' implies a lack of effect on the lungs, but presence of effect on the heart.
2. Beta-receptors may mediate several different types of responses in any given tissue. For example, in the lungs, their stimulation gives rise to bronchodilatation, increased mucociliary clearance and reduced bronchoconstrictor mediator release following allergic reactions in the lung (see p. 37). Therefore, it may not be correct to assume that any given drug has a preferential effect or lack of effect on the lungs as a whole, when selectivity may only have been shown for one aspect of beta-receptor function. To date, almost all the work on 'selectivity' and the lungs, whether in animals or in humans, has been on that aspect which concerns bronchodilatation. Similarly, for most agents presence or absence of activity on the heart, has usually been inferred from the influence on chronotropic rather than inotropic cardiac responses.
3. Selectivity is not an absolute (i.e. all or nothing) characteristic, but as already mentioned, it refers to the ability of these agents to influence certain tissues more than others. Thus, increasing the dose of such drugs (which are essentially competitively acting) will generally produce discernible effects even on the tissues they are considered to spare (Lertora et al, 1975; Kumana et al, 1977; Oh, 1977).
4. There has been a tendency to apply to humans conclusions based on animal investigation. Patterns of tissue selectivity differ between species, whilst in some species tissue selectivity is not readily manifest at all.
5. It may yet be premature to accede that all selective agents invariably have the same pattern of selectivity for different tissues.

A more appropriate and accurate way of describing these drugs would be to express their activity or lack of activity on a number of peripheral organs or metabolic processes by precisely specifying the responses concerned. Such activity or lack of activity requires to be related to the corresponding properties of a standard agent, whilst ensuring that both the standard and test drugs are given in such a way as to have equivalent potentially therapeutic effects. For example, relative to propranolol, given to produce a certain degree of cardiac beta-blockade, an antagonist giving rise to the same cardiac effect could be described as bronchosparing, equibronchoactive or more bronchoactive. Conversely, relative to isoprenaline administered so as to produce a certain pulmonary effect, agonists producing equivalent effect could be described as cardiosparing, equicardioactive or more cardioactive.

To many workers, including the present authors, the subdivision of beta-receptors into two stereospecific subtypes to account for selectivity is an attractive concept. However, the use of terms such as beta$_1$ or beta$_2$ in this sense may yet be premature and it is important that such nomenclature should not become dignified by the passage of time unless the hypothesis on which it is based can be verified and the various objections outlined above reasonably satisfied.

Table 3.1   Beta-adrenoceptors and tissue selectivity in man

Response Preferentially influenced by selective antagonist Preferentially spared by selective agonist (Beta$_1$-receptor mediated)	Response Preferentially influenced by selective agonist Preferentially spared by selective antagonist (Beta$_2$-receptor mediated)
↑ Heart rate and contractility [a] ↑ BP [b] Often but not necessarily related ↑ Renin release [c] ↑ Ventilation [d]	Bronchodilation [a] Vasodilation [a] — including coronary arteries [e] ↑ Muscle tremor [f] ↑ Lipolysis [g] [h] ⋆? ↑ Pancreatic insulin release and hypokalaemia [g] ↑ Rise of blood glucose after hypoglycaemia [i] ? Relaxation of gravid uterus [j] ?

⋆ Contrary to the view of Lands (1969)
?Evidence not clear
[a] Fitzgerald (1972)
[b] Davidson et al (1976)
[c] Hamer (1976)
[d] Collier and Dornhorst (1969)
[e] Frick and Virtanen (1976)
[f] Marlin and Turner (1975b)
[g] Goldberg et al (1975)
[h] Harms and Vandermeer (1975)
[i] Deacon, Karunanayake and Barrett (1977)
[j] Anderson, Ingemarsson and Persson (1973)

Notwithstanding all these considerations, in an attempt to be clinically relevant, a tentative scheme relating beta-adrenoceptors and tissue selectivity is given in Table 3.1. Possible within tissue selectivity, if any, as for example between beta-receptor mediated cardiac inotropy and chronotropy, is not considered. From a practical point of view, it emerges that in contrast to responses mediated through beta-receptors in the heart, those mediated through bronchial and vascular beta-receptors generally reveal a similar sensitivity both to stimulation by agonists and inhibition by antagonists. Thus, beta-receptors in the latter tissues at least, appear to share some common characteristic distinguishing them from those in the heart.

SELECTIVE AGONISM

The chief clinical application of beta-adrenoceptor agonists is in the treatment of reversible airways obstruction in asthma. This is achieved by (1) stimulation of beta-adrenoceptors in bronchial smooth muscle giving rise to bronchodilation, and possibly also by (2) inhibiting the release of bronchoconstrictor substances (Assem, 1971; Orange et al, 1971) following type I (reaginic) antigen–antibody interactions (Turner-Warwick, 1971; Pepys, 1973), and (3) accelerating the clearance of mucus from the tracheobronchial tree (Foster et al, 1976). Because of their actions on beta-adrenoceptors elsewhere, these agents are also used in the treatment of acute anaphylaxis and occasionally they are given to suppress premature labour. Their relative potency has usually been described with reference to their action on bronchial smooth muscle. Not surprisingly, the term selectivity used in this context refers to an ability to evoke bronchial beta-adrenoceptor stimulation with little or no stimulation of beta-adrenoceptors in other tissues.

In the treatment of asthma, it is desirable that the actions of beta-adrenoceptor agonists be confined to pulmonary beta-adrenoceptors, so as to avoid unwanted side effects from unnecessary stimulation of beta-adrenoceptors in other organs. Currently feasible pharmacologically selective agonism, whilst producing bronchodilatation, may nevertheless give rise to muscle tremor, hypokalaemia and unwanted cardiac effects. Indeed such agonism appears not to discriminate between bronchial beta-adrenoceptors and those in skeletal muscle, pancreas and peripheral vasculature (see Table 3.1). In this context, it is not entirely clear to what extent the suspected cardiotoxicity of beta-adrenoceptor agonists is due to stimulation of cardiac beta-adrenoceptors or to other complex events. The problem has been well reviewed by D'Arcy and Griffin (1972), and the relevant arguments may be summarised as follows:

1. During the late 1960s, an epidemic of sudden deaths was encountered in asthmatic patients using excessive doses of sympathomimetic bronchodilators. Failure to use steroid treatment at an earlier stage may also have been relevant to their deaths, since autopsies on these individuals frequently revealed airways almost totally plugged up with mucus.
2. When ECG evidence has been available, isoprenaline associated sudden deaths in asthmatics were noted to be due to ventricular asystole, not fibrillation.
3. Studies in dogs predictably revealed that administration of isoprenaline increased cardiac rate and contractility, and large doses ultimately produced ventricular fibrillation. However, when dogs were made hypoxic, isoprenaline administration produced bradycardia, diminished cardiac contractility and an accentuated hypotensive effect; moreover, deaths were due to asystole and occurred after very small doses.
4. Numerous studies attest that in asthmatics, administration of beta-adrenoceptor agonists sometimes give rise to paradoxical reductions in arterial P_{O_2}, the reductions being marked in some individuals. Such effects may be ascribed to vasodilatation in underventilated regions of the lung and/or excessive ventilation of underperfused lung tissue. In other words, beta-adrenoceptor agonists may exaggerate inequalities in the distribution of ventilation and perfusion by steal phenomena both in the pulmonary circulation and in the pulmonary airways.
5. Such reductions in arterial P_{O_2} have been encountered after both non-selective and selective agonists.
6. Inhalation of isoprenaline (to produce bronchodilatation) together with phenylephrine (to stimulate alpha-receptor mediated pulmonary vasoconstriction so as to oppose beta-receptor mediated vasodilatation) does not appear to worsen ventilation/perfusion ratios.

These observations are compatible with the notion that the potential cardiotoxicity of beta-adrenoceptor agonists is of two kinds. First, there is toxicity associated with cardiac beta-adrenoceptor stimulation — which is presumably responsible, at least in part, for the tachycardias encountered in asthmatic patients, and which may be theoretically attenuated by using selective (cardiosparing) agonists. Secondly, there may be indirect toxicity associated with hypoxaemia — and because of the sigmoid oxyhaemoglobin dissociation curve, any given tendency to reduce arterial P_{O_2} would produce greater reductions in arterial O_2 content in patients who were already hypoxaemic. Predictably, this form of cardiotoxicity would occur both with non-selective and selective agents, since only vascular and/or bronchial beta-receptors are likely to be involved.

Determination of selectivity

In assessing the therapeutic value of beta-adrenoceptor agonists, it is essential to determine their selectivity as this will reflect to some degree their margin of safety. On the other hand, their potency may not be related to their therapeutic safety, since a more powerful bronchodilator effect might be accompanied by an equally more powerful, undesirable cardiac effect. The selectivity of any given beta-adrenoceptor agonist is best determined in man by administering equipotent bronchodilating doses of the test drug and a standard agent (usually the non-selective beta-adrenoceptor agonist isoprenaline), and establishing dose–response curves for each drug while comparing their effects on other tissues, especially the heart. Such studies should use bronchodilating doses which intersect the straight part of their respective sigmoid log dose–response curves, thus avoiding comparison of doses producing either subminimal or supramaximal responses.

Bronchomotor tone is minimal in healthy man and is controlled by the parasympathetic nervous system (Nadel, 1975). High doses of bronchodilator and bronchoconstrictor drugs are required to produce measurable changes in bronchial calibre. To demonstrate these, direct measurement of airways resistance by whole body plethysmography is necessary because of its increased sensitivity over tests of forced expiration. The degree of bronchodilatation possible in the normal subject will also be limited by the mechanical properties of the lung. However, when bronchomotor tone is increased, the effects of bronchodilators are more easily demonstrable. Thus, beta-adrenoceptor agonists are usually tested with respect to their influence on bronchoconstricted airways, and this is also the only clinical situation in which the drugs are used therapeutically. Beta-adrenoceptor agonists may be evaluated as follows:

1. *Bronchial provocation in healthy subjects*. Histamine, cholinergic drugs and other agents will produce bronchoconstriction in susceptible healthy subjects (Kamburoff, Griffin and Bianco, 1972; Benson, 1975). Histamine constricts bronchial smooth muscle locally, but like cholinergic drugs it is also capable of inducing vagally mediated bronchoconstriction through reflex mechanisms (Nadel, 1975). Beta-adrenoceptor agonists will reverse this bronchoconstriction which bears sufficient resemblance to human asthma to be of value in the assessment of new drugs in healthy sensitive subjects before their administration to asthmatics.

2. *Bronchial provocation in asthmatic patients*. Most asthmatic patients in remission demonstrate bronchial hyperreactivity to histamine, cholinergic drugs and exercise (Benson, 1975). Thus, the degree to which post-exercise bronchoconstriction is inhibited by beta-adrenoceptor agonists has proved to be a reproducible and physiological means of studying agonists (Anderson et al, 1975).

3. *Asthmatic patients with moderate reversible airways obstruction*. The evaluation of bronchodilators in asthma is complicated by the natural variability of the disease and of a patient's response from day to day. The efficacy of a bronchodilator depends not only upon the degree of airways obstruction, but also upon the phase of the disease, i.e.

'non-responsive' acute phase and 'responsive' recovery phase (Hume and Gandevia, 1957; Pain and Read, 1963). The asthmatics selected for drug studies should be in a steady state of moderate airways obstruction. It should also be possible to safely withdraw maintenance bronchodilator treatment prior to administration of the test drugs so as to avoid interference.

Mechanisms of selectivity

Pharmaceutical. When beta-adrenoceptor agonists are deposited into the tracheobronchial tree by inhalation, selectivity of action results (Walker et al, 1972; Davies, 1975). If delivered by metered pressurised aerosol more than 90 per cent of the dose is swallowed. Although only less than 10 per cent is absorbed from the lung, this small dose is sufficient to produce peak bronchodilatation of rapid onset despite no detectable plasma drug level. Drug which is swallowed may be conjugated and inactivated in the gut wall (e.g. isoprenaline by sulphatase enzymes), or absorbed and distributed throughout the body producing very low drug levels elsewhere compared to the airways. Drugs such as isoprenaline and rimiterol, which are substrates for the enzyme catechol-O-methyl transferase (COMT) will also be partly metabolised and inactivated during absorption from the bronchi before reaching the systemic circulation. Thus when administered by pressurised aerosols in recommended doses, even pharmacologically non-selective agonists usually produce negligible cardiovascular side effects, unless excessive doses are being used. Following delivery by intermittent positive pressure ventilation (IPPV) proportionately higher plasma drug levels are achieved initially than by pressurised aerosol suggesting that a greater percentage of the dose is deposited in the lung (Shenfield et al, 1973). It follows that systemic effects upon other tissues are likely to be greater by IPPV than by pressurised aerosol. Administration of the drug by IPPV produces similar bronchodilatation to when delivered by other methods of nebulisation without positive pressure (Webber, Shenfield and Paterson, 1974). However, Choo-Kang and Grant (1975) have claimed that in asthmatic patients with severe airways obstruction (pre-treatment $FEV_1 < 0.751$), a beta-adrenoceptor agonist delivered by IPPV may provide some additional benefit.

Pharmacological. This may be referred to as true selectivity and can best be demonstrated when the drug is administered i.v., whereby it is equally available to all beta-adrenoceptor sites in the body via the circulation. Such selectivity is demonstrable by comparing the test drug with a standard agent and measuring tissue responses when time has been allowed for the respective drugs to equilibrate and distribute into the tissues (Paterson, Courtenay Evans and Prime, 1971; Svedmyr, Malmberg and Thiringer, 1972; Marlin and Turner, 1975a, b).

Following the principles outlined, Marlin and Turner (1975a, b) have determined the relative potencies of three beta-adrenoceptor agonists for their effects on the bronchus, heart, peripheral vasculature and skeletal muscle (Table 3.2). When peak bronchodilator and heart rate responses of equimolar doses of the three drugs were compared, isoprenaline for an equal bronchodilator action increased the heart rate 2 and 2.5 times more than rimiterol and salbutamol respectively, demonstrating the relative selectivity of the latter two drugs. However, the heart rate increase produced by beta-adrenoceptor agonists by the parenteral route, as well as being due to direct cardiac

Table 3.2   The relative potencies of intravenous rimiterol, salbutamol and isoprenaline for forced expiratory volume in 1 s (FEV_1), heart rate, pulse pressure and skeletal muscle tremor in healthy subjects with histamine-induced bronchoconstriction [a] and asthmatic patients [b]

	Potency ratios compared with isoprenaline			
	FEV_1	Heart rate	Pulse pressure	Tremor
Healthy subjects with histamine-induced bronchoconstriction				
Rimiterol	6.7	13.6	11.1	9.4
Salbutamol	4.8	10.1	6.9	7.5
Asthmatic patients				
Rimiterol	8.0	16.0	13.6	7.8
Salbutamol	4.6	12.0	8.7	3.7

In all instances isoprenaline is more potent than each drug comparing equimolar doses
[a] Marlin and Turner (1975a)
[b] Marlin and Turner (1975b)

beta-adrenoceptor stimulation, might also be related to reflex tachycardia initiated by a fall in mean blood pressure due to stimulation of beta-adrenoceptors in vascular smooth muscle (Dunlop and Shanks, 1968). Moreover, the tachycardia produced by i.v. isoprenaline even after pre-treatment with atropine was incompletely blocked by practolol (Brick et al, 1968), whereas after inhaled isoprenaline the same dose of practolol produced complete blockade (Palmer et al, 1969). This supports the concept that the heart rate response following parenteral administration of beta-adrenoceptor agonists involves both cardiac and peripheral vascular beta-adrenoceptors. According to receptor theory, differences in potency ratios indicate that the drugs are acting upon different populations of beta-adrenoceptors (Jenkinson, 1973; Schild, 1973). However, if the physiological parameters measured are determined by the responses of more than one type of tissue receptor (e.g. adrenergic and cholinergic), then differences in potency ratios may not necessarily support the existence of different subtypes of beta-receptors. Table 3.2 which summarises the studies of Marlin and Turner (1975a, b) shows that all three drugs produced similar peripheral vascular effects and suggests that the differences in their chronotropic cardiac effects were predominantly due to their differing activities on the cardiac beta-adrenoceptors. The relative potencies for bronchodilatation and skeletal muscle tremor were of similar magnitude, suggesting a similar affinity for these receptors. With respect to pulse pressure increase, the relative potencies for these drugs were intermediate to those for bronchial and cardiac effects. Assuming that the bronchus and peripheral vasculature are populated by similar beta-adrenoceptors, these results support the concept that pulse pressure is under the dual control of cardiac ($beta_1$) and peripheral-vascular ($beta_2$) adrenoceptors. Although the potency ratios were similar in healthy subjects and asthmatic patients (Table 3.2), it cannot be assumed that during asthmatic attacks, the airways of the patients will react in the same way. The bronchus possesses numerous receptors, e.g. alpha- and beta-adrenoceptors, cholinergic, histaminic and other receptors, all of which interact to maintain overall bronchial tone. It is possible, however, that these receptors may be abnormal in nature and distribution in asthma, thus altering bronchial responsiveness.

INDIVIDUAL DRUGS AND SELECTIVE AGONISM IN MAN

By structural modifications to the basic catecholamine molecule and by determination of the structure–activity relationships of the compounds formed, numerous so-called beta$_2$-adrenoceptor stimulating drugs have been developed. The properties of these drugs are shown in Table 3.3. Drugs which suffer a 'first pass' metabolism effect in the gut wall, e.g. sulphate conjugation, will be inactive by the oral route, e.g. isoprenaline, rimiterol. The potency of an oral drug may be increased by the formation of an active metabolite, e.g. salmefamol (Evans, Shenfield and Paterson, 1974). The path of metabolism also determines the duration of action of the drug, so that drugs which are substrates for COMT have a short duration of effect, e.g. isoetharine, isoprenaline and rimiterol.

Table 3.3 The properties of beta-adrenoceptor agonists

Drug	Duration of action by inhalation (h)	Routes of administration	Reference reviewing selectivity in man
Non-selective agonist			
Isoprenaline	1½–2	i, p	Paterson et al (1971)
Selective agonists (beta$_2$>beta$_1$)			
Orciprenaline	3–4	i, o, p	McEvoy, Vall-Spinosa and Paterson (1973)
Salbutamol	4–6	i, o, p	Paterson et al (1971)
Isoetharine	1½–2	i, o, p	Thiringer, Bergh and Svedmyr (1971)
Terbutaline	4–6	i, o, p	Arner et al (1970)
Rimiterol	1½–2	i, p	Marlin and Turner (1975a, b)
Salmefamol	4–6	i, o	Shenfield and Paterson (1973)
Fenoterol	4–6	i, o, p	Shenfield and Paterson (1973)

i, inhalational; o, oral; p, parenteral (usually intravenous)

SELECTIVE ANTAGONISM

Beta-adrenoceptor blocking drugs are all competitive antagonists that can be further characterised according to whether or not they also have: quinidine-like or so-called membrane stabilising activity (MSA); partial agonist activity (PAA); tissue selectivity; and alpha-adrenoceptor blocking activity. One of these, namely 'tissue selectivity', may be clinically relevant, and the following pages attempt to review its importance, if any, with special reference to antagonism which is cardiac rather than bronchial. A discussion of vasosparing properties is also included.

The wide variety of both common and rare clinical disorders in which beta adrenoceptor blocking drugs are used (Table 3.4) and the numerous alternative antagonists available make a powerful case for assessing the importance of using selective or non-selective agents in any given situation. A corollary of this concerns their long-term use in patients with ischaemic heart disease, which has recently been reviewed by Fitzgerald (1976). Thus, numerous trials attest to their anti-anginal effects, whilst some studies also indicate that when used prophylactically in patients surviving myocardial infarction, they also reduce mortality and morbidity. Therefore, it is especially regrettable that in many studies throughout the world comparing medical and surgical treatment of angina, medical therapy has been uncontrolled and involved the use of inadequate and often token doses of beta-blocking drugs. All else being equal,

Table 3.4   Therapy with beta-adrenoceptor antagonists [a,b,c]

Established indications	Uses not well defined
Angina	Psychiatric uses
Cardiac arrhythmias	Anxiety
Hypertension	Alcohol withdrawal
Phaeochromocytoma	Schizophrenia
Hyperthyroidism	Glaucoma
Obstructive cardiomyopathy	Management of labour
Tetralogy of Fallot	
Migraine	
Tremor	

[a] *Postgraduate Medical Journal* (1976)
[b] *Lancet* (1974)
[c] Phillips (1976)

discovery of safe, selective antagonists (i.e. with lesser potential adverse pharmacological properties), might encourage the judicious use of adequate doses, and if these were justified, they might in turn reduce mortality and morbidity as well as the costs and inconvenience of undertaking surgery. Furthermore, the most promising post-infarction prophylactic trial (Green et al, 1977), which was also the best designed and included the largest number of patients (3053 in all) involved the selective antagonist, practolol (see p. 47). Therefore, it remains to be determined whether all beta-blocking drugs, or only selective antagonists, or perhaps practolol alone can confer the beneficial effects.

With respect to using these drugs in man, *assessment of selectivity* and its *clinical significance* have been discussed in a number of reviews (Dollery, Paterson and Conolly, 1969; Fitzgerald, 1972, 1975; Beumer, 1974; George, 1975; McDevitt, Shanks and Pritchard, 1976), and highlights from these and other communications are summarised in the following sections.

Problems of assessing the selectivity of beta-adrenoceptor antagonists in man

1. The tissue sparing properties of what are referred to as selective antagonists are not absolute but relative. That this becomes more evident with increasing doses has been confirmed in studies on man (Formgren, 1976; Kumana et al, 1977; Oh, 1977). Therefore any given antagonist must be assessed by comparison with a dose or doses of a non-selective agent (such as propranolol) given to produce the same desirable effect (usually a given degree of cardiac beta-blockade). Ideally, comparison with a known selective agent should also be included. In this way, dosing with the test drug no longer becomes arbitrary, and it can be shown whether the system used to make the assessment can indeed discriminate between a known selective and a known non-selective agent (Kumana et al, 1974, 1975). Furthermore the doses of drugs selected for comparison should not produce near maximal responses, as in that case inadvertent use of supramaximal doses could mask any possible selectivity (Lertora et al, 1975).

2. Doses of different drugs reported to be therapeutically equivalent in any one small group of individuals may not be equivalent in another group, particularly when the agents involved are substantially metabolised and taken orally. Depending on the

drug, systemic bioavailability and binding to plasma and other proteins may vary considerably due to dose dependent and dose independent factors (Shand, 1976; Johnson and Regardh, 1976). Though in logarithmic terms such differences may not be great, ideally any anticipated therapeutic equivalence should be confirmed.

3. The timing of measurements relative to dosing may be critical. For example, even after allowing for plasma concentrations, the full cardiac beta-adrenoceptor blocking activity of practolol takes hours to develop, so that effect appears to increase with decreasing plasma level of drug (Kumana and Kaye, 1974). Similarly, pulmonary beta-blocking activity may also evolve slowly (Kumana et al, 1974, 1975). Presumably this is due to time taken for drugs to reach receptors; and allowance for such 'distribution time' should be made before undertaking comparisons.

4. Single oral dose studies may not be applicable to the situation after chronic oral dosing, and conclusions from studies carried out after single intravenous doses may not be applicable to the situation after single oral doses. These and other problems related to pharmacokinetics have been reviewed by Shand (1976) with special reference to propranolol. Conclusions from studies carried out in healthy volunteers may be inapplicable in diseased states. To assess the clinical relevance of selectivity, ideal studies should be carried out after chronic oral dosing of patients, as this is the way beta-blocking drugs are generally used. However, with rare exceptions (Formgren, 1976), for logistic reasons such studies are seldom performed.

5. Both in normal volunteers and in asthmatics, there is very considerable interindividual variation in sensitivity to the measurable pulmonary effects of beta-blocking drugs (McNeill, 1971). Therefore, within subject investigations are required unless a large number of individuals can be studied.

6. Many tests purported to reflect airway function lack reproducibility (McCarthy, Craig and Cherniak, 1975), and the ensuing variation mitigates against obtaining significant results.

7. Asthmatics are generally more sensitive to the bronchopulmonary effects of these drugs than normal persons. Arguably, therefore, studies of selectivity on them might be more sensitive as well as more clinically relevant. However, the extent to which their airway calibre depends on sympathetic stimulation may vary from time to time, and hence the effects of drugs may also be variable. Some workers also feel that all these agents are contraindicated in asthmatics, and that even whilst they are being closely supervised, it is ethically unjustifiable to submit them to the risk of a distressing asthmatic attack. Others are prepared to assess new agents in asthmatics, but are not prepared to give a non-selective agent for comparison. Presumably such workers are biased in expecting the test agent to be selective, and if it was indeed shown to have little or no adverse pulmonary influence, the sensitivity of the particular test system used would still be open to suspicion.

8. It is likely that the airways of healthy individuals (as opposed to asthmatics) are not being constantly subjected to a significant degree of sympathetic stimulation. Therefore, just as cardiac beta-blocking activity is more sensitively tested in the presence of sympathetic agonism, so too beta-adrenoceptor antagonism elsewhere should be similarly assessed. To this end, endogenous stimulation or a pharmacological agonist may be used, and the respective pros and cons of these two alternative approaches are reviewed by George (1975) and by McDevitt (1977), and two specific examples (namely vigorous exercise and i.v. isoprenaline) are contrasted in Table 3.5.

Table 3.5

Endogenous sympathetic stimulation using vigorous exercise [a,b,c,d,e]	Pharmacological sympathetic stimulation using i.v. isoprenaline [b,c,f,g]
1. Physiological	1. Not a naturally occurring catecholamine
2. Cardiorespiratory physiological stimulation is accompanied by parasympathetic withdrawal. Therefore, further compensatory reduction in parasympathetic activity less likely to be important during assessment of beta-blockade	2. Direct and reflex cardiac acceleration may occur, so that heart rate response may be unsuitable for equating cardiac beta-blockade of differingly selective drugs
3. Near maximal tolerable agonism obtainable; in which case heart rate may differ up to 60 or more beats/min, depending on the extent of beta-blockade	3. No theoretical upper limit to agonism, as it may always be countered by more antagonist. However heart rate increases usually have to be confined to <25 beats/min because of alarming palpitations
4. Exercise induced increases in plasma catecholamines and their absolute concentrations themselves are greater in beta-blocked than non-medicated individuals. [h] The assumption that the extent of agonism in the two groups is equivalent may be inaccurate, but assuming that the amines measured were largely of adrenal origin — the important neurological component of agonism may yet remain substantially the same	4. Apparently equivalent responses arising through nerve stimulation and pharmacological agonism may not be influenced to the same degree by pharmacological antagonists [g,i]
5. Near exhausting exercise requires utmost subject cooperation. Even after training some subjects find difficulty in simultaneously performing lung function tests. Besides this, tests performed during vigorous exercise as opposed to rest may need different interpretation [j]	5. Requires minimal cooperation from subject

[a] Chamberlain, Turner and Sneddon (1967)
[b] Coltart and Shand (1970)
[c] Bodem et al (1973)
[d] Kumana et al (1974)
[e] Carruthers, Shanks and McDevitt (1976)
[f] Paterson et al (1970)
[g] Taylor et al (1976)
[h] Irving et al (1974)
[i] Ablad, Carlsson and Ek (1973)
[j] Kumana and Ruffin (1978)

9. Indirect means of inferring selectivity involve basic assumptions, and hence may be misleading. For example, the bronchosparing property of antagonists is often assumed when they appear to be vasosparing — and the label 'selective' applied. Apart from the use of direct methods such as plethysmography (Briant et al, 1973), vascular effects have also been indirectly inferred from differences in effect on the heart rate response to exercise and to isoprenaline respectively. Thus the heart rate increase after isoprenaline involves cardiac beta-receptor stimulation and reflex effects from beta-receptor mediated vascular dilation. Compared with non-selective antagonists, selective (vascular sparing) ones may be much less effective in attenuating such heart rate responses with doses producing fairly similar attenuation of beta-receptor mediated heart rate responses to exercise. Such findings are reported by Taylor et al (1976), but these authors doubt the above reasoning, as the results with isoprenaline occurred independently of the diastolic BP.

Significance of bronchopulmonary selectivity

Asthma

It is by no means clear that the bronchoconstrictive property of beta-adrenoceptor antagonists are unacceptable. In North America, where propranolol is the only generally available antagonist, asthmatic reactions attributed to this non-selective drug have not been a problem. However, this may be misleading, as (a) the doses of propranolol generally used (in the author's opinion) are smaller than those used in Europe, as are the dosage recommendations (*US Pharmacopoeia*, 1975; *British Pharmacopoeia* 1973), (b) already well-known effects may get under-reported, and (c) recourse to coronary artery surgery probably occurs more readily. The following broad generalisations help to define the issues:

1. All of these drugs affect tests of airway function adversely, even in non-asthmatics, though selective agents may only be seen to do so when large doses producing relatively greater degrees of cardiac beta-blockade are given (Kumana et al, 1977).
2. Asthmatics given non-selective or selective antagonists are more prone to develop acute attacks than normal individuals and their propensity to do so increases with increasing doses of drug.
3. Very rarely, administration of these drugs to persons denying any past history of asthma may nevertheless precipitate an attack.
4. Asthmatics (and non-asthmatics) are less liable to develop wheezing when given selective rather than non-selective drugs.
5. If a beta-adrenoceptor antagonist has to be given despite an asthmatic problem, it is reasonable to choose a selective agent and if necessary also prescribe a selective beta-adrenoceptor agonist to be taken by inhalation.

Chronic obstructive lung disease

To date, there is no clear information on the use of these agents (whether selective or non-selective) in persons having other forms of obstructive airways disease. It is well known that patients with bronchitis and/or emphysema may be prone to intermittent wheezing and that occasionally their airway function seems to depend on pharmacological and presumably also on endogenous sympathetic support. Even so, available evidence, admittedly from short-term studies (Stone, Keltz and Samortin, 1971; Nordstrom, MacDonald and Gobel, 1975), suggests that tests of airway function are no more liable to be adversely influenced than in normals and that symptomatic deterioration does not occur. It should be appreciated, however, that the ventilatory reserve of such patients is likely to be reduced. Moreover, as beta-adrenoceptor agonists enhance bronchial mucociliary clearance (Foster et al, 1976), the corresponding effects of antagonists are likely to be adverse. The clinical significance of such actions is unknown and may remain unappreciated if the ensuing consequences develop insidiously. Whether so-called 'selective antagonists' may also be selective in this respect remains to be seen. A further consideration in chronic obstructive lung disease derives from the finding that propranolol reduces the ventilatory response to CO_2 in normal volunteers (Mustchin et al, 1976). It is possible that propranolol which enters the CNS exerts its influence on the central respiratory centres. In that event, antagonists lacking lipid solubility (which may yet turn out to be the most crucial property conferring selectivity) may well be safer than other drugs in the presence of CO_2 retention.

Though there may not be a great need for selective antagonism, all else being equal, selective antagonists seem preferable to non-selective antagonists, particularly if they must be used in asthmatics. Clinically deleterious effects in patients with other forms of obstructive lung disease are not documented, though there are theoretical grounds for expecting them and critical evaluation is awaited. Till then, it might also be prudent to exercise special caution when prescribing any beta-adrenoceptor antagonists to these patients.

Significance of vascular selectivity

There is no hard evidence that selective as opposed to non-selective beta-adrenoceptor antagonists have clinically important differences with respect to their actions on blood vessels. However, depending on the circumstances, theoretical grounds for preferring selective (i.e. non-vasoconstrictive) antagonism may exist as follows:

1. Independent of their PAA and MSA, selective blockers possibly produce less reduction in cardiac output for a given negative chronotropic response than non-selective blockers, presumably because the latter, being more inhibitory to beta-receptor mediated vasodilation, also raise peripheral resistance to a greater extent (Gibson, 1974).
2. Selective antagonists might in theory produce less side effects such as cold extremities, Raynaud's syndrome, and symptoms due to peripheral vascular disease; and some workers make it a policy to prescribe selective beta-blockers under such circumstances (Zacharias, 1976a), though the latter should not be regarded as entirely safe in this respect (Roger et al, 1976).
3. They may give rise to lesser degrees of coronary artery vasoconstriction (Frick and Virtanen, 1976).
4. In patients with phaeochromocytomas, it is advised that treatment of cardiac tachyarrhythmias with beta-blockers should not be given unless adequate alpha-receptor blockade has already been achieved. This is based on the fact that blockade of vascular beta-receptors before alpha-receptor blockade may increase BP (Prichard and Ross, 1966). By extension of this line of reasoning, selective (i.e. non-vasoconstrictive) rather than non-selective antagonists might be preferable in this disorder. On the other hand, when used in treating patients with migraine, it may be reasonable to expect that a non-selective (i.e. vasconstrictive) antagonist might be preferable. This is because migrainous headache is commonly ascribed to pulsatile dilatation of extracranial arteries. Critical studies to evaluate this are lacking.

INDIVIDUAL DRUGS AND SELECTIVE ANTAGONISM IN MAN

Practolol

It is regrettable that the long-term use of this agent, which was the most widely used and acknowledged selective beta-adrenoceptor antagonist (Shanks, 1976), has been associated with ocular, peritoneal, dermatological and other complications (*British Medical Journal*, 1975). Though uncommon, some of these side effects have proved serious, so that long-term therapy with practolol has ceased. These reactions are not due to beta-adrenoceptor blockade itself. Indeed, though documented, they appear to be much rarer after other antagonists and cross-reactions with practolol do not necessarily occur (Cubey and Taylor, 1975; Holt and Waddington, 1975; Furhoff, Nordlander and

Peterson, 1976; Zacharias, 1976b; *British Medical Journal*, 1977). Therefore, in seeking out safer alternative drugs, grounds for optimism exist, but it must be remembered that selective antagonists other than practolol have not been in extensive use until recently and it remains to be seen whether they will turn out to be safer.

Atenolol *(Tenormin)*

The selectivity of this agent is attested by within subject indirect (Taylor et al, 1976; Conway et al, 1976) and direct (Marlin et al, 1975; Vilsvik and Schaanning, 1976) studies. The last and most rigorous of these was performed on asthmatics and found atenolol to be at least as free of effects on airway function as practolol in doses producing slightly more cardiac beta-blockade, though a non-selective agent was not given for comparison.

Metoprolol *(Betaloc, Lopressor)*

Indirect evidence of vasosparing properties was provided by Taylor et al (1976). Studies on asthmatics by Skinner et al (1976), Singh et al (1976) and Formgren (1976), seem to confirm that it also has relatively little effect on tests of airway function. The first of these, which compared i.v. doses of metoprolol and propranolol, used resting heart rate changes to infer equivalence of cardiac beta-blocking activity which could be misleading. The second report, which involved comparing the effects of metoprolol, propranolol and other active drugs, assumed that the doses of active drugs used had equivalent cardiac effects from observations in healthy volunteers (not in the patients themselves), and regrettably the extent of within patient comparison was not entirely clear. The final study utilised chronic oral dosing in hypertensive patients who were also asthmatic. Metoprolol had no more adverse effect on airway function than practolol in doses which appeared to be equally effective in lowering blood pressure. A major flaw in the latter study was that before undertaking the measurements, bronchodilator therapy was not restricted or controlled. Other work in asthmatics has incorporated i.v. pharmacological agonism to compare i.v. (Johnsson, Svedmyr and Thiringer, 1975) and oral (Thiringer and Svedmyr, 1976) doses of metoprolol and other antagonists. Though single blind, the oral study by comparing effects after relatively larger doses of metoprolol (in terms of cardiac activity) provides convincing evidence for its selectivity. A study of patients with chronic obstructive lung disease (Tivenius, 1976) also found that when given orally metoprolol had less pulmonary effect than propranolol, the doses used having been reported to be equicardioactive in other work though not confirmed to be so in the patients in that investigation. The overall conclusion from a within-subject study comparing the cardiac and pulmonary effects of propranolol and metoprolol in healthy volunteers at rest and during exercise, is also in keeping with metoprolol being selective (Kumana and Ruffin, 1978).

Tolamolol

There is indirect evidence of its vasosparing properties (Taylor et al, 1976). Its effects on the airways of healthy volunteers and asthmatics suggest that it is relatively bronchosparing compared to propranolol (Dierckx, Gillard and Gossart, 1976; Steen et al, 1976), but the cardiac equivalence of the doses used was not adequately confirmed. Clinical studies with this agent have been suspended.

Acebutolol *(Sectral)*

Contrary to results from in vitro work (Harms 1976), a within subject i.v. study comparing its cardiac and pulmonary beta-blocking effects with those of propranolol and practolol, found that only practolol was convincingly selective (Kumana et al, 1975). Previous studies involving its bronchopulmonary effects (reviewed in the latter communication) inferred that acebutolol was selective, but this was on the basis of inappropriate comparisons. Moreover, in man acebutolol does not appear to selectively spare vascular beta receptors (Briant et al, 1973). It should be appreciated, however, that after oral dosing the extent of metabolite formation is much greater than after i.v. doses (Winkle et al, 1977) and since animal work suggests that the metabolite is active, selectivity after i.v. and oral dosing may not be equatable.

Pindolol *(Prindolol)*

A number of studies based on healthy volunteers and on patients with obstructive airways disease given oral and intravenous doses of various beta-blocking drugs (Kal-

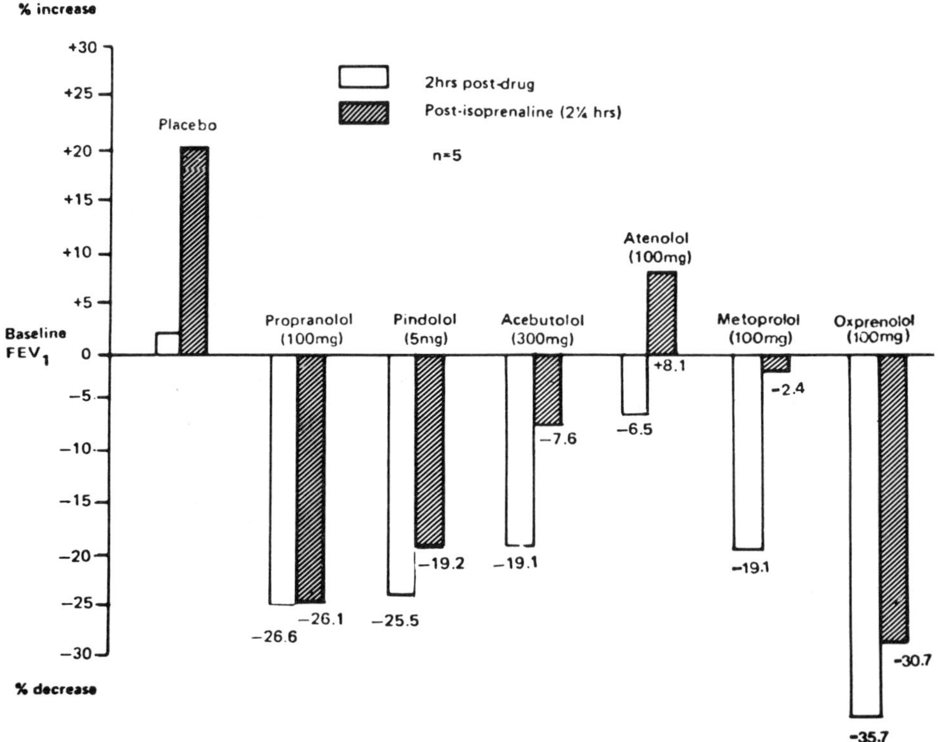

Fig. 3.1   In a within-patient single blind investigation different beta-blockers were given orally in doses considered to produce equivalent cardiac blockade. The patients had reversible airways disease and were all termed 'responders' to beta-blocking medication. The active drugs alone (white blocks) all had an adverse though variable effect on forced expiratory volume in 1 s (FEV₁). This variation was presumably due to differing baseline FEV₁ values, differing degrees of endogenous sympathetic stimulation of the airways as well as differences in the selectivity of the drugs. In the presence of more substantial sympathetic stimulation such as produced by isoprenaline inhalation (hatched blocks), metoprolol and atenolol appear to be the most selective. However, as the agonist was given by inhalation, the dose being delivered and hence the response could also have varied according to the extent of pre-existing airway obstruction. (Modified from Figures 2 and 3, Benson et al, 1977).

tenbach et al, 1970; Beumer and Hardonk, 1971; Ulmer and Palmer, 1976), have suggested that pindolol may have a relatively trivial effect on airway function. These investigations suffered from one or more of the following drawbacks: failure to substantiate that the various antagonists were producing equivalent cardiac beta-blockade, failure to conduct within-subject comparison whilst dealing with small numbers, failure to take account of time that might be necessary to develop pulmonary effects, use of non-blind and/or non-randomised protocols. Under the circumstances their conclusions, though promising, must still be regarded as sub-judice until the results from more rigorous trials become available.

It is difficult to appreciate the relative selectivity of these various agents to each other. For example, in one investigation (Decalmer et al, 1977) it could be inferred that metoprolol was relatively selective or relatively non-selective depending on the particular airway function test used as a yardstick. Another source of confusion is that the results from very similar studies often appear to conflict (Decalmer et al, 1977; Benson et al, 1977). A further problem is the logistic difficulty of conducting within-subject comparative studies with so many drugs. The work of Benson et al (1977) attempts such a comparison, and though suffering from being a single blind, unbalanced assessment of only five patients and involving inhalation of isoprenaline (rather than i.v. injection), it nevertheless gives some overall perspective (Fig. 3.1). However, these authors do not state whether baseline FEV_1 values before each beta-blocking agent were essentially the same, as otherwise it may not be valid to compare reductions in FEV_1. Moreover, the differing pulmonary responses to inhaled isoprenaline could arguably be due to differences in the dose delivered (depending on the pre-existing extent of airway obstruction), rather than to differing degrees of pulmonary beta-blockade. With these reservations their findings taken as a whole as well as those from studies involving fewer drugs (refer individual drugs) suggest that atenolol and metoprolol are the most selective.

REFERENCES

Ablad, B., Carlsson, E. & Ek, L. (1973) Pharmacological studies of two new cardioselective adrenergic beta-receptor antagonists. *Life Sciences*, **12**, 107–119.

Ahlquist, R. P. (1948) A study of the adrenotropic receptors. *American Journal of Physiology*, **153**, 586–600.

Anderson, K. E., Ingemarsson, I. & Persson, C. G. A. (1973) Relaxing effects of beta-receptor stimulators in isolated gravid human myocardium. *Life Sciences*, **13**, 335–344.

Anderson, S. D., Silverman, M., Konig, P. & Godfrey, S. (1975) Exercise-induced asthma. *British Journal of Diseases of the Chest*, **69**, 1–39.

Arner, B., Bertler, A., Karlefors, T. & Westling, H. (1970) Circulatory effects of orciprenaline, adrenaline and a new sympathomimetic T-receptor-stimulating agent, terbutaline, in normal human subjects. *Acta medica scandinavica*, Suppl., **512**, 25–32.

Assem, E. S. K. (1971) Inhibition of allergic reactions by beta-adrenergic stimulants. *Postgraduate Medical Journal*, **47**, Suppl. on Saltutand, 31–33.

Benson, M. K. (1975) Bronchial hyperreactivity. *British Journal of Diseases of the Chest*, **69**, 227–239.

Benson, K. M., Berrill, W. T., Cruickshank, J. M. & Sterling, G. M. (1977) Cardioselective and non-cardioselective beta blockers in reversible obstructive airways disease. *Postgraduate Medical Journal*, **53**, Suppl. 3, 143–147.

Beumer, H. M. (1974) Adverse effects of beta-adrenergic receptor blocking drugs on respiratory function. *Drugs*, **7**, 130–138.

Beumer, H. M. & Hardonk, H. J. (1971) Zur Wirkung beta-adrenerg blockierender Substanzen bei Asthma bronchiale. *Medizinische Klinik*, **66**, 1804–1807.

Biel, J. H. & Lum, B. K. B. (1966) The beta adrenergic blocking agents. Pharmacology and structure activity relationships. *Progress in Drug Research*, **10**, 46–89.

Bodem, G., Brammell, H. L., Weil, J. V. & Chidsey, C. A. (1973) Pharmacodynamic studies of beta adrenergic antagonism induced in man by propranolol and practolol. *Journal of Clinical Investigation*, **52**, 747–754.

Briant, R. H., Dollery, C. T., Fenyvesi, T. & George, C. F. (1973) Assessment of selective T-adrenoceptor blocked in man. *British Journal of Pharmacology*, **49**, 106–114.

Brick, I., Hutchison, K. J., McDevitt, D. G., Roddie, I. C. & Shanks, R. G. (1968) Comparison of the effects of I.C.I. 50,172 and propranolol on the cardiovascular responses to adrenaline, isoprenaline and exercise. *British Journal of Pharmacology*, **34**, 127–140.

British Medical Journal (1975) Editorial: Side effects of practolol. **ii**, 577–578.

British Medical Journal (1977) Editorial: Hazards of non-practolol beta-blockers. **i**, 529–530.

British Pharmacopoeia (1973) p. 398. London: Her Majesty's Stationery Office.

Carruthers, S. G., Shanks, R. G. & McDevitt, D. G. (1976) Intrinsic heart rate on exercise and the measurement of beta-adrenoceptor blockade. *British Journal of Clinical Pharmacology*, **3**, 991–999.

Chamberlain, D. A., Turner, P. & Sneddon, J. M. (1967) Effects of atropine on heart-rate in healthy man. *Lancet*, **ii**, 12–15.

Choo-Kang, Y. F. J. & Grant, I. W. B. (1975) Comparison of two methods of administering bronchodilator aerosol to asthmatic patients. *British Medical Journal*, **ii**, 119–120.

Collier, J. G. & Dornhorst, A. C. (1969) Evidence for two different types of beta receptors in man. *Nature*, **223**, 1283–1284.

Coltart, D. J. & Shand, D. G. (1970) Plasma propranolol levels in the quantitative assessment of beta adrenergic blockade in man. *British Medical Journal*, **iii**, 731–734.

Connolly, C. K. & Batten, J. C. (1970) Comparison of the effects of alprenolol and propranolol on specific airway conductance in asthmatic subjects. *British Medical Journal*, **ii**, 515–576.

Conway, F. J., Fitzgerald, J. D., McAinsh, J., Rowlands, D. J. & Simpson, W. T. (1976) Human pharmacokinetic and pharmacodynamic studies on atenolol (ICI 66,082), a new cardioselective beta-adrenoceptor blocking drug. *British Journal of Clinical Pharmacology*, **3**, 267–272.

Cubey, R. Bevis & Taylor S. H. (1975) Ocular reaction to propranolol and resolution on continued treatment with a different beta-blocking drug. *British Medical Journal* **4**, 327–328.

D'Arcy, P. F. & Griffin, J. P. (1972) Cardiotoxicity of isoprenaline and other sympathomimetic amines. In *Iatrogenic Diseases*, Ch. 5, pp. 52–53. London: Oxford University Press.

Davidson, C., Thadani, U., Singleton, W. & Taylor, S. H. (1976) Comparison of antihypertensive activity of beta-blocking drugs during chronic treatment. *British Medical Journal*, **ii**, 7–9.

Davies, D. S. (1975) Pharmacokinetics of inhaled substances. *Postgraduate Medical Journal*, **51**, Suppl. 7, 69–75.

Deacon, S. P., Karunanayake, A. & Barrett, D. (1977) Acebutolol, atenolol and propanolol and metabolic responses to acute hypoglycaemia in diabetics. *British Medical Journal*, **ii**, 1255–1257.

Decalmer, P. B., Chattergee, S. S., Croxson, R. S, & Cruickshank, J. M. (1977) Cardioselective and non-cardioselective beta blockers in reversible obstructive airways disease. *Postgraduate Medical Journal*, **53**, Suppl. 3, 147–148.

Dierckx, J. P., Gillard, C. & Gossart, R. (1974) Clinical trial of a new beta-blocking agent, tolamolol (UK-6558): Its effect on the respiratory function of healthy subjects and asthmatic patients. *Clinical Experiences with Tolamolol, a Cardioselective Beta-blocking Agent*. Proceedings of a symposium held at The Royal College of Physicians. London: Excerpta Medica.

Dollery, C. T., Paterson, J. W. & Conolly, M. E. (1969) Clinical pharmacology of beta-receptor-blocking drugs. *Clinical Pharmacology and Therapeutics*, **10**, 765–799.

Dunlop, D. & Shanks, R. G. (1968) Selective blockade of adrenoceptive beta receptors in the heart. *British Journal of Pharmacology*, **32**, 201–208.

Evans, M. E., Shenfield, G. M. & Paterson, J. W. (1974) The clinical pharmacology of salmefamol. *British Journal of Clinical Pharmacology*, **1**, 391–397.

Fitzgerald, J. D. (1972) Cardioselective beta-adrenergic blockade. *Proceedings of the Royal Society of Medicine*, **65**, 761–764.

Fitzgerald, J. D. (1975) The evaluation of beta adrenergic blocking drugs in man. In *Kardiale Sympathikolyse als Therapeutisches Prinzip*, ed. Lydtin, H. & Meesmann, W. Stuttgart: Georg Thieme Verlag.

Fitzgerald, J. D. (1976) The effect of beta-adrenoreceptive antagonists on the morbidity and mortality in cardiovascular disease. *Postgraduate Medical Journal*, **52**, 770–781.

Fleisch, H. J., Maling, H. M. & Brodie, B. B. (1970) Evidence for existence of alpha adrenergic receptors in the mammalian trachea. *American Journal of Physiology*, **218**, 596–599.

Formgren, H. (1976) The effect of metoprolol and practolol on lung function and blood pressure in hypertensive asthmatics. *British Journal of Clinical Pharmacology*, **3**, 1007–1014.

Foster, W. M., Bergofsky, E. H., Bohning, D. E., Lippmann, M. & Albert, R. E. (1976) Effect of adrenergic agents and their mode of action on mucociliary clearance in man. *Journal of Applied Physiology*, **41**, 146–152.

Frick, M. H. & Virtanen, K. S. (1976) Beta blockade and coronary circulation. *American Heart Journal*, **91**, 536–537.

Furchgott, R. F. (1967) The pharmacological differentiation of adrenergic receptors. *Annals of the New York Academy of Sciences*, **139**, 553–570.

Furhoff, A. K., Nordlander, P. & Peterson, C. (1976) Cross sensitivity between propranolol and other beta blockers. *British Medical Journal*, i, 831.

George, C. F. (1975) Problems in assessing beta-adrenoceptor antagonism in man. *British Journal of Clinical Pharmacology*, 2, 3–4.

Gibson, D. G. (1974) Pharmacodynamic properties of beta adrenergic receptor blocking drugs in man. *Drugs*, 7, 8–38.

Goldberg, R., van As, M., Joffe, B. I., Krut, L., Bersohn, I. & Seftel, H. C. (1975) Metabolic responses to selective beta-adrenergic stimulation in man. *Postgraduate Medical Journal*, 51, 53–58.

Green, K. G. et al (1977) Multicentre international study: supplementary report. Reduction in mortality after myocardial infarction with long-term beta-adrenoceptor blockade. *British Medical Journal*, ii, 419–421.

Hamer, J. (1976) Renin and beta-adrenoceptor blockade — the mechanism of the hypotensive effect? *British Journal of Clinical Pharmacology*, 3, 425–427.

Harms, H. H. (1976) Isoproterenol Antagonism of Cardioselective Beta Adrenergic Receptor Blocking Agents: A comparative study of human and guinea pig cardiac and bronchial beta adrenergic receptors. *J. of Pharmacol and Exp. Thera.* 199, No. 2, 329.

Harms, H. H. & Vandermeer, J. (1975) Isoprenaline antagonism of cardioselective beta adrenergic receptor blocking agents on human and rat adipocytes. *British Journal of Clinical Pharmacology*, 2, 311–315.

Hayes, A. & Cooper, R. G. (1971) Studies on the absorption, distribution and excretion of propranolol in rat, dog and monkey. *Journal of Pharmacology and Experimental Therapeutics*, 176, 302–311.

Hellenbrecht, D., Lemmer, B., Wiethold, G. & Grobecker, H. (1973) Measurement of hydrophobicity, surface activity, local anaesthesia, and myocardial conduction velocity as quantitative parameters of the non-specific membrane affinity of nine beta adrenergic blocking agents. *Naunyn-Schmiedeberg's Archives of Pharmacology*, 277, 211–226.

Herschfus, T. A., Bresnick, E., Levinson, L. & Segal, S. M. (1951) A new sympathomimetic amine (Neosuprel) in the treatment of bronchial asthma. *Annals of Allergy*, 9, 1769–1773.

Holt, P. J. A. & Waddington, E. (1975) Oculocutaneous reaction to oxprenolol. *British Medical Journal*, ii, 539–540.

Howe, R. & Shanks, R. G. (1966) Optical isomers of propranolol. *Nature*, 210, 1336–1338.

Hume, K. M. & Gandevia, B. (1957) Forced expiratory volume before and after isoprenaline. *Thorax*, 12, 276–278.

Irving, M. H., Britton, B. J., Wood, W. G., Padgham, C. & Carruthers, M. (1974) Effects of beta adrenergic blockade on plasma catecholamines in exercise. *Nature*, 248, 531–533.

Jenkinson, D. H. (1973) Classification and properties of peripheral adrenergic receptors. *British Medical Bulletin*, 29, 142–147.

Johnson, G. & Regardh, C. G. (1976) Bioavailability of beta-adrenoceptor blocking drugs. *British Journal of Clinical Pharmacology*, 3, 1064–1065.

Johnsson, G., Svedmyr, N., Thiringer, G. (1975) Effects of i.v. Propranolol and Metoprolol and their interactions with isoprenaline on pulmonary function, heart rate and blood pressure in asthmatics. *Europ. J. Clin. Pharmacol*, 8, 175–180.

Kaltenbach, M., Becker, H. J., Mitrou, P., Petersen P., Kober, G., Meier-Sydow, J., Krehan, L., Guldner, N., Dierkesmann, R. & Böhnlau, V. (1971) Comparable doses of different beta-blockers in man, their effects on haemodynamics, heart rate, peripheral blood flow, heart size, bronchial resistance and angina pectoris. In *Proceedings of a Symposium held in Frankfurt*, ed. Kaltenbach, M. & Lichtlen, P., pp. 198–205, 230. Stuttgart: Georg Thieme Verlag.

Kamburoff, P. L., Griffin, J. P. & Bianco, S. (1972) The use of histamine-induced bronchoconstriction as a method of investigating bronchodilator drugs in man. *British Journal of Diseases of the Chest*, 66, 21–26.

Kumana, C. R. & Kaye, C. M. (1974) An investigation of the relationship between beta-adrenoceptor blockade and plasma practolol concentration in man. *European Journal of Clinical Pharmacology*, 7, 243–248.

Kumana, C. R., Marlin, G. E., Kaye, C. M. & Smith, D. M. (1974) New approach to assessment of cardioselectivity of beta blocking drugs. *British Medical Journal*, iv, 444–447.

Kumana, C. R., Kaye, C. M., Leighton, Mo., Turner, P. & Hamer, J. (1975) Cardiac and pulmonary effects of acebutolol. *Lancet*, ii, 89–93.

Kumana, C. R., Kaye, C. M., Leighton, M. & Marlin, G. E. (1977) An investigation of 'absolute plasma level effect relationships' and absolute cardioselectivity with respect to beta adrenoceptor blockade. *European Journal of Clinical Pharmacology*, 12, 7–14.

Kumana, C. R. & Ruffin, R. (1978) Application of 'flour volume curves' to assess the selectivity of beta adrenoceptor antagonists drugs. *British Journal of Clinical Pharmacology* (in press).

Lancet (1974) Editorial: Delaying premature labour. ii, 875–876.

Lands, A. M., Arnold, A., McAuliff, J. P., Luduena, F. P. & Brown, T. G., Jr. (1967) Differentiation of receptor systems activated by sympathomimetic amines. *Nature*, 214, 597–598.

Lertora, J. J. L., Mark, A. L., Johannsen, U. J., Wilson, W. R. & Abboud, F. M. (1975) Selective beta receptor blockade with oral practolol in man. *Journal of Clinical Investigation*, 56, 719–724.

Levy, B. & Wilkenfeld, B. E. (1969) An analysis of selective beta receptor blockade. *European Journal of Pharmacology*, **5**, 227–234.

Levy, J. V. (1968) Myocardial and local anesthetic actions of beta-adrenergic receptor blocking drugs: relationship to physicochemical properties. *European Journal of Pharmacology*, **2**, 250–257.

Levy, J. V. & Richards, V. (1966) Inotropic and chronotropic effects of a series of beta adrenergic blocking drugs: some structure activity relationships. *Proceedings of the Society for Experimental Biological Medicine*, **122**, 373–379.

Marlin, G. E. & Turner, P. (1975a) Comparison of the T_2-adrenoceptor selectivity of rimiterol, salbutamol and isoprenaline by the intravenous route in man. *British Journal of Clinical Pharmacology*, **2**, 41–48.

Marlin, G. E. & Turner, P. (1975b) The relative potencies and T_2-selectivities of intravenous rimiterol, salbutamol and isoprenaline in asthmatic patients. *International Journal of Clinical Pharmacology and Biopharmacy*, **12**, 158–169.

Marlin, G. E., Kumana, C. R., Kaye, C. M., Smith, D. M. & Turner, P. (1975) An investigation into the cardiac and pulmonary beta-adrenoceptor blocking activity of ICI 66,082 in man. *British Journal of Clinical Pharmacology*, **2**, 151–157.

McCarthy, D. S., Craig, D. B. & Cherniack, R. M. (1975) Intraindividual variability in maximal expiratory flow volume and closing volume in asymptomatic subjects. *American Review of Respiratory Disease*, **112**, 407–411.

McDevitt, D. G. (1977) An assessment of beta adrenoceptor blocking drugs in man. *British Journal of Clinical Pharmacology*, **4**, 413–426.

McDevitt, D. G., Shanks, R. G. & Prichard, B. N. C. (1976) The clinical pharmacology of beta adrenergic blocking drugs. *Journal of the Royal College of Physicians*, **2**, 21–57.

McEvoy, J. D. S., Vall-Spinosa, A. & Paterson, J. W. (1973) Assessment of orciprenaline and isoproterenol infusions in asthmatic patients. *American Review of Respiratory Disease*, **108**, 490–500.

McNeill, R. S. (1971) The effect of beta-antagonists on the bronchi. *Postgraduate Medical Journal*, **47**, Suppl. on Advances in Adrenergic Beta-receptor Therapy, 14–16.

Mustchin, C. P., Gribbin, H. R., Tattersfield, A. E. & George, C. F. (1976) Reduced respiratory responses to carbon dioxide after propranolol: a central action? *British Medical Journal*, **ii**, 1229–1231.

Nadel, J. A. (1975) Parasympathetic regulation of lungs and airways. *Postgraduate Medical Journal*, **51**, Suppl. 7, 86–90.

Nordstrom, L. A., MacDonald, F. & Gobel, F. L. (1975) Effect of propranolol on respiratory function and exercise tolerance in patients with chronic obstructive lung disease. *Chest*, **67**, 287–292.

Oh, V. M. S. (1977) Relationship of cardioselectivity to plasma proctolol concentrations in man. *British Journal of Clinical Pharmacology*, **4**, 722.

Orange, R. P., Kaliner, M. A., Laraia, P. J. & Austen, K. F. (1971) Immunological release of histamine and slow reacting substance of anaphylaxis from human lung. II. Influence of cellular levels of cyclic AMP. *Federation Proceedings*, **30**, 1725–1729.

Pain, M. C. F. & Read, J. (1963) Patterns of response to bronchodilator in young patients with asthma. *Australasian Annals of Medicine*, **12**, 216–220.

Palmer, K. N. V. & Diament, M. L. (1969) Effect of salbutamol on spinometry and blood–gas tensions in bronchial asthma. *British Medical Journal*, **i**, 31–32.

Palmer, K. N. V., Legge, J. S., Hamilton, W. F. D. & Diament, M. L. (1969) Effect of selective T-adrenergic blocker in preventing falls in arterial oxygen tension following isoprenaline in asthmatic subjects. *Lancet*, **ii**, 1092–1093.

Paterson, J. W., Conolly, M. E., Dollery, C. T., Hayes, A. & Cooper, R. G. (1970) The pharmacodynamics and metabolism of propranolol in man. *Pharmacologia Clinica*, **2**, 127–133.

Paterson, J. W., Courtenay Evans, R. J. & Prime, F. J. (1971) Selectivity of bronchodilator action of salbutamol in asthmatic patients. *British Journal of Diseases of the Chest*, **65**, 21–38.

Patil, P. N. (1968) Steric aspects of adrenergic drugs. VIII. Optical isomers of beta adrenergic receptor antagonists. *Journal of Pharmacology and Experimental Therapeutics*, **160**, 308–314.

Pepys, J. (1973) Immunopathology of allergic lung disease. *Clinical Allergy*, **3**, 1–22.

Phillips, C. I. (1976) Beta-blockers in the treatment of chronic simple glaucoma. *British Medical Journal*, **i**, 584.

Postgraduate Medical Journal (1976), **52**, Suppl. 4, 35–180.

Pratesi, P., Grana, E. & Villa, L. (1968) Molecular properties and biological activity of catecholamines and certain related compounds. In *Physico-Chemical Aspects of Drug Action*, ed. Ariens, E. J., pp. 283–294, Oxford: Pergamon Press.

Pratesi, P., Villa, L. & Grana, E. (1975) Molecular geometry and binding capacity in the series of beta-adrenergic compounds. *Il Frarmaco-Ed.Sc.* **30**, 315.

Prichard, B. N. & Ross, E. J. (1966) Use of propranolol in conjunction with alpha receptor blocking drugs in phaeochromocytoma. *American Journal of Cardiology*, **18**, 394–398.

Richards, D. A. (1976) Pharmacological effects of Labetalol in man. *British Journal of Clinical Pharmacology*, **3**, Suppl. 3, 721–723.

Riess, W., Rajagopalan, J. G., Imhof, P., Schmid, K. & Kaberle, H. (1970) Metabolic studies with oxprenolol in animals and man by means of radio tracer techniques and GLC-analysis. *Postgraduate Medical Journal*, **46**, Suppl. on Oxprenolol, 32–39.

Roger, J. C., Sheldon, C. D., Lerski, R. A. & Livingstone, W. R. (1976) Intermittent claudication complicating beta-blockade. *British Medical Journal*, **i**, 1125.

Scales, B. & Cosgrove, M. B. (1970) The metabolism and distribution of the selective adrenergic beta blocking agent practolol. *Journal of Pharmacology and Experimental Therapeutics*, **175**, 338–347.

Schild, H. O. (1973) Receptor classification with special reference to T-adrenergic receptors. In *Drug Receptors*, ed. Rang, H. P., pp. 29–36. London: Macmillan.

Shand, D. G. (1976) Pharmacokinetics of propranolol — a review. *Postgraduate Medical Journal*, **52**, Suppl. 4, 22–25.

Shanks, R. G. (1976) The properties of beta adrenoceptor antagonists. *Postgraduate Medical Journal*, **52**, Suppl. 4, 14–20.

Shenfield, G. M. & Paterson, J. W. (1973) Clinical assessment of bronchodilator drugs delivered by aerosol. *Thorax*, **28**, 124–128.

Shenfield, G. M., Evans, M. E., Walker, S. R. & Paterson, J. W. (1973) The fate of nebulised salbutamol (albuterol) administered by intermittent positive pressure respiration to asthmatic patients. *American Review of Respiratory Disease*, **108**, 501–505.

Singh, B. N., Phil, D., Whitlock, M. L., Comber, R. H., Williams, R. H. & Harris, E. A. (1976) Effects of cardioselective beta adrenoceptor blockade on specific airways resistance in normal subjects and in patients with bronchial asthma. *Clinical Pharmacology and Therapeutics*, **19**, 493–501.

Skinner, C., Gaddie, J., Palmer, K. N. V. & Kerridge, D. F. (1976) Comparison of effects of metoprolol and propranolol on asthmatic airway obstruction. *British Medical Journal*, **i**, 504.

Steen, S. N., Clifton, J. F., Ziment, I. & Thomas, J. S. (1976) Double-blind study of tolamolol and propranolol in patients with bronchospastic disease. *Clinical Experiences with Tolamolol, a Cardioselective Beta-blocking Agent*. Proceedings of a symposium held at the Royal College of Physicians. London: Excerpta Medica.

Stone, D. J., Keltz, H. & Samortin, T. (1971) The effect of beta-adrenergic inhibition on respiratory gas exchange and lung function. *American Review of Respiratory Disease*, **103**, 503–515.

Svedmyr, N., Malmberg, R. & Thiringer, G. (1972) The effect of a new adrenergic T$_2$-receptor-stimulating agent (rimiterol, R798) in patients with chronic obstructive lung disease. *Scandinavian Journal of Respiratory Diseases*, **53**, 302–313.

Taylor, S. H., Thadani, U., Davidson, C., Singleton, W. & Myint, S. (1976) Comparative activity of beta-adrenoreceptor antagonists in man. *Clinical Experiences with Tolamolol, a Cardioselective Beta-blocking Agent*. Proceedings of a symposium held at the Royal College of Physicians. London: Excerpta Medica.

Thiringer, G., Bergh N. P. & Svedmyr (1971) A comparative study of the effects of isoetharine and some other adrenergic beta stimulators in chronic obstructive lung disease. *Scand. J. Resp. Dis.*, **52**, 183–91.

Thiringer, G. & Svedmyr N. (1976) Interaction of orally administered metoprolol, practolol and propranolol with isoprenaline in asthmatics. *Europ. J. Clin. Pharmacol*, **10**, 163–170.

Tivenius, L. (1976) Effects of multidoses of metoprolol and propranolol on ventilatory function in patients with chronic obstructive lung disease. *Scandinavian Journal of Respiratory Disease*, **57**, 190–196.

Turner-Warwick, M. (1971) Provoking factors in asthma. *British Journal of Diseases of the Chest*, **65**, 1–20.

Ulmer, W. T. & Palmer, K. (1976) Propranolol und Pindolol bei chronisch-obstruktiver Atemwegserkrankung. *Deutsche Medicinische Wochenschrift*, **101**, 1765–1768.

US Pharmacopoeia (1975) Vol. XIX, p. 422. Eastern Pa.: Mack Publishing Co.

Vilsvik, J. S. & Schaanning, J. (1976) Effect of atenolol on ventilatory and cardiac function in asthma. *British Medical Journal*, **ii**, 453–455.

Walker, S. R., Evans, M. E., Richards, A. J. & Paterson, J. W. (1972) The clinical pharmacology of oral and inhaled salbutamol. *Clinical Pharmacology and Therapeutics*, **13**, 861–867.

Webber, B. A., Shenfield, G. M. & Paterson, J. W. (1974) A comparison of three different techniques for giving nebulised albuterol to asthmatic patients. *American Review of Respiratory Disease*, **109**, 293–295.

Winkle, R. A., Meffin, P. J., Ricks, W. B. & Harrison, D. C. (1977) Acebutolol metabolite plasma concentration during chronic oral therapy. *British Journal of Clinical Pharmacology*, **4**, 519–522.

Zacharias, F. J. (1976a) Patient acceptability of propranolol and the occurrence of side effects. *Postgraduate Medical Journal*, **52**, Suppl. **4**, 87–89.

Zacharias, F. J. (1976b) Cross sensitivity between propranolol and other beta blockers. *British Medical Journal*, **i**, 1213.

4. Antihypertensive drugs*

David Robertson   Alan S. Nies

Although hypertension has been recognised as a disease for about a century (Mahomed, 1874), the major advances in treatment have occurred in the past two decades. The principal advance during the last 10 years has been in the individualisation of antihypertensive therapy. It is now clear that antihypertensive therapy lowers the incidence of hypertensive complications and improves survival although the development of atherosclerotic coronary artery disease and the incidence of sudden death remain unchanged (Wolff and Lindeman, 1966; Veterans' Administration, 1967, 1970, 1972). The value of therapy is most apparent in persons with diastolic blood pressures greater than 104 mmHg but persons with diastolic blood pressures in the range 90 to 104 probably also benefit, particularly if there is evidence of cardiovascular or renal disease. The value of therapy is least well established in white women with mild hypertension. It is possible that long-term studies correlating clinical course with such parameters as plasma renin activity or serum catecholamines will permit the identification of subgroups at greater or lesser risk of hypertensive complications at a given level of blood pressure. Until such conclusive data is in, it seems prudent to initiate therapy in patients whose diastolic blood pressures are consistently greater than 95 mmHg.

THE PHYSIOLOGY OF BLOOD PRESSURE REGULATION

The principal determinants of blood pressure are the autonomic nervous system and the renin–angiotensin–aldosterone system. In the face of a wide range of stresses, these systems can maintain blood pressure within the normal range (Guyton et al, 1972).

The autonomic nervous system

The sympathetic nervous system
The adrenergic neurotransmitter noradrenaline is synthesised in the neuron from tyrosine in three steps. The tyrosine is first hydroxylated to dopa by tyrosine hydroxylase (Nagatsu, Levitt and Udenfriend, 1964). Dopa is then decarboxylated to dopamine by aromatic-l-amino acid decarboxylase. Finally the dopamine is taken up into a specialised granule where it is hydroxylated and stored as noradrenaline (Von Euler and Hillarp, 1956). In the adrenal medulla and the para-aortic bodies, the cytoplasmic enzyme phenylethanolamine-N-methyltransferase methylates some of the norepinephrine to adrenaline (Axelrod, 1962).

The rate-limiting step in the above sequence is the initial one catalysed by tyrosine hydroxylase. For full activity, tyrosine hydroxylase requires molecular oxygen, iron, and a reduced pteridine cofactor. By competing with the pteridine cofactor for the

* Supported in part by USPHS Grants GM15431 and GM00113.

oxidised form of the enzyme, noradrenaline is able to exert end-product feedback inhibition of its own synthesis (Spector et al, 1967; Weiner et al, 1972). Other catecholamines may also inhibit this step in the same way.

The noradrenaline in the adrenergic neuron is located primarily in the storage granules. A nerve action potential causes release of intragranular noradrenaline into the synaptic cleft toward adrenergic receptor sites. If the innervated tissue is arteriolar or venous smooth muscle, the effect is to induce constriction in most circumstances. The major mechanism terminating the action of the released noradrenaline is re-uptake by active transport from the extracellular space back into the cytoplasmic pool and ultimately into another storage granule. However, before it reaches the granule some of the noradrenaline is degraded by mitochondrial monoamine oxidase and the inactive products are released from the neuron (Kopin, 1964; Dahlström, Fuxe and Hillarp, 1965; Carlsson, 1966; de Champlain, Mueller and Axelrod, 1969; Burn, 1976). Once the noradrenaline is released from the neuron into the synaptic cleft where its physiological effect occurs, it may also escape into the circulation and be metabolised by catechol-O-methyltransferase and appear in the urine as normetanephrine.

Since the activity of almost all the sympathetic nervous system depends upon this scheme of events at the neuronal level, pharmacological agents which interfere with any steps in the sequence may alter sympathetic activity and hence blood pressure. Since noradrenaline is the neurotransmitter in many parts of the central nervous system as well, it should be anticipated that most agents affecting noradrenaline synthesis will at high dosages have central side effects in addition to their effect on the sympathetic nervous system. Reserpine, for example, can interfere with the ATP-magnesium dependent transport mechanism for noradrenaline leading to depletion of its intragranular stores (Dahlstöm et al, 1965; Carlsson, 1966; de Champlain et al, 1969). On the other hand guanethidine because of its low lipid solubility is excluded from the central nervous system and acts only on the peripheral sympathetic neuron by binding to storage granules, depleting their noradrenaline and thus preventing adequate translation of nerve impulses into effective noradrenaline release (Cass and Spriggs, 1961; Chang, Costa and Brodie, 1965; Oates et al, 1971).

Stimulation of the sympathetic nervous system results in (a) acceleration of heart rate, (b) constriction of arteriolar resistance vessels and venous capacitance vessels, and (c) release of renin. Such stimulation occurs in a wide variety of ordinary circumstances in normal man: it can for example be brought on by startle, by pain, by anxiety, by mental arithmetic, by upright posture, and by physical exertion. The acceleration in heart rate serves to increase cardiac output. Constriction of arterioles causes increased resistance. Constriction of venous capacitance vessels causes increased return of blood to the right heart which in turn contributes to the increased cardiac output. The release of renin and its subsequent production of angiotensin also serves to increase arteriolar resistance. Since blood pressure is directly proportional to cardiac output and resistance, all these effects of sympathetic stimulation serve to elevate that parameter.

It is clear that not all the stimuli mentioned above affect the pulse and blood pressure in exactly the same way. This is because a number of cardiovascular reflexes may be brought into play by sympathetic activation. The resultant of all these factors may attenuate the manifestations of sympathetic stimulation.

The heart. At rest, the heart is under the control of both sympathetic and parasympathetic influences. Abolition of parasympathetic effects by atropine usually accelerates the heart rate more than abolition of sympathetic influences by propranolol will slow it (Linden, 1963). With physical exertion or any of the other sympathetic stimuli cited above, the sympathetic influence on the heart becomes more marked. This is manifested by both increased heart rate and increased force of contraction. With age many stimuli such as upright posture seem to have less effect on the heart, and the nearly 20 beat/min increment in heart rate observed in young people on standing contrasts with the 10 to 15 beat/min increment found in middle and old age (Hellström, 1961; Strandell, 1964).

Peripheral vascular resistance. The arteriolar constriction of sympathetic stimulation is primarily a manifestation of alpha-adrenergic activity. While most vascular beds respond to sympathetic stimulation with an increase in resistance, the blood vessels supplying the brain have a capacity for autoregulation that permits cerebral blood flow to remain essentially unchanged in the face of wide swings in blood pressure (Purves, 1972). This probably accounts for the fact that antihypertensive therapy reduces rather than increases strokes in hypertensive patients, and it may also explain why mental function often remains remarkably good in patients with very low blood pressures due to massive haemorrhage.

Venous capacitance. Blood return to the right heart depends on such factors as intrathoracic pressure, skeletal muscle contraction, and the capacity of veins in the periphery to pool blood. The increased venous tone attending sympathetic stimulation can be dramatic; when venous volume is temporarily stabilised by tourniquet and sympathetic activation brought about by mental arithmetic or a deep breath, pressure increases of 10 to 20 mmHg in the venous system are readily achieved in normal man. Blockade of this venous tone can be demonstrated in patients on guanethidine; when maximally treated with guanethidine, the venous pressure increase in the situation described above is less than 5 mmHg. When venous tone is blocked, postural hypotension is usually a significant problem until sufficient intravascular volume is accumulated to occupy the increased venous capacity (Walter et al, 1975).

The parasympathetic nervous system
The syncope of acute emotional trauma and the vasovagal reactions sometimes seen in healthy young men with venipuncture are usually accompanied by bradycardia and represent activation of the parasympathetic nervous system. Conversely, the administration of the parasympatholytic agent atropine will usually raise both heart rate and blood pressure at certain dosage levels. While such parasympathomimetic drugs as bethanechol and methacholine lower blood pressure in some individuals, they are not used in antihypertensive therapy because of side effects and the unreliability of the salutary effect on blood pressure observed in most patients.

The renin–angiotensin–aldosterone system
The second major system for blood pressure regulation is the renin–angiotensin–aldosterone system. Renin is a proteolytic enzyme produced in the renal cortex by specialised cells at the afferent arteriole of the glomerulus. Renin acts on a leucyl–leucyl bond in a plasma alpha-2-globulin to release angiotensin I, a decapeptide that is then

rapidly hydrolysed to the octapeptide angiotensin II by converting enzyme. In the adrenal cortex, angiotensin II may be converted to the heptapeptide angiotensin III, a potent stimulator of aldosterone release (Goodfriend and Peach, 1975; Meyer, 1976; Bravo, Khosla and Bumpus, 1976).

The baroreceptor theory of renin release postulates that a decrease in renal perfusion pressure decreases the stretch of the afferent arteriole, signaling the juxtaglomerular cells to secrete renin. This mechanism is supported by abundant experimental evidence (Blaine, David and Prewitt, 1971).

The distal tubule is near the glomerular vessels at the macula densa, a group of specialised tubular cells. The entire structure of the juxtaglomerular cells and the macula densa is the 'juxtaglomerular apparatus'. The macula densa is felt to be a chemoreceptor where information regarding tubular fluid's composition is transferred to the juxtaglomerular cells. The exact stimulus for renin release sensed by the chemoreceptor is unknown, but appears to be related to the sodium chloride concentration in the tubular fluid. Whether high or low sodium chloride concentration is the stimulus is still a matter of debate (Oparil and Haber, 1974).

The third mechanism responsible for renin release is the sympathetic nervous system. Stimulation of the renal nerves results in renin release; the release is blocked by beta-adrenergic blockers. Although it is difficult to be certain that beta-receptor stimulation in vivo directly acts to stimulate renin release as distinguished from indirect effects on the systemic and renal vasculature, experiments in isolated kidneys, kidney slices, and cell suspensions indicate that beta-adrenergic receptor stimulation will release renin, independent of vascular effects (Michelakis, Caudle and Liddle, 1969; Weinberger, Aoi and Henry, 1975).

Through these mechanisms, many stimuli can provoke the release of renin. Hypotension, upright posture, anaesthesia, and surgery are all associated with elevation of plasma renin activity (Robertson and Michelakis, 1972). The list of drugs causing elevation of plasma renin activity is growing rapidly. In addition to the diuretics and the arteriolar dilators, even such drugs as chlorpromazine (Robertson and Michelakis, 1975) and levodopa (Michelakis and Robertson, 1970) will increase renin activity in certain situations.

The release of renin is normally controlled by several negative feedback loops. The 'short' loop is a direct suppression of renin by angiotensin II. The 'medium' loop is a feedback resulting from the vasoconstriction produced by angiotensin II, which increases renal perfusion pressure. The 'long' loop acts in concert with the 'medium' loop through the release of aldosterone, with subsequent sodium and water retention resulting in increased effective blood volume and renal perfusion.

THE PATHOPHYSIOLOGY OF HYPERTENSION

When hypertensive subjects are studied, it is usually not possible to identify the cause of their disease. However, about 10 to 20 per cent will have an identifiable cause of their hypertension. Since some of these forms of hypertension are curable, it is important to identify patients with secondary hypertension.

Essential hypertension

The dichotomy based on renin status
When the many secondary causes of hypertension have been ruled out by appropriate

studies there remain the 80 per cent of patients for whom no aetiology is apparent. The word 'essential' in its now somewhat archaic sense of 'non-secondary' is still used to describe these patients. The essential hypertensive patients are themselves now known to be heterogeneous on the basis of several haemodynamic and humoral characteristics. Of these perhaps the most useful is categorisation on the basis of renin status (Table 4.1) This categorisation has been alleged to have aetiologic (Liddle, 1975; Esler et al, 1977), prognostic (Laragh, 1976), and therapeutic (Hollifield et al, 1976) significance.

Table 4.1   Categorisation of essential hypertension by renin status

Characteristic		LREA [a]	NREH/HREH [a]
1.	Plasma renin activity (definition)	Low	Higher
2.	Age	Older	Younger
3.	Frequency in Caucasian hypertensives	20%	55%
4.	Frequency in Afro-American hypertensives	40%	
5.	Blood pressure lowering with aminoglutethimide	+++	—
6.	Blood pressure lowering with spironolactone	+++	+
7.	Blood pressure response to saralasin	May be pressor	May be depressor
8.	Diuretic responsive	+++	+
9.	Propranolol responsive	+	+++
10.	Phenoxybenzamine responsive	+	+++

[a] NREH = normal renin essential hypertension
LREH = low renin essential hypertension
HREH = high renin essential hypertension

Using varying criteria, many centres around the world have identified in their hypertensive populations a group whose plasma renin level is subnormal and remains so in spite of provocation by upright posture and acute diuresis. This seems to constitute about one-fifth of Caucasian hypertensives but perhaps as many as 50 per cent of a randomly selected population of American Blacks (Hollifield, 1976).

The low renin essential hypertensive (LREH) patients differ from the normal and high renin hypertensive (NREH and HREH) patients in that they are somewhat older. This has led some to postulate that LREH is in fact an end-stage process, perhaps more related to duration of hypertension than chronological age. In a frequency distribution study of 81 patients with essential hypertension, a continuum of PRA levels was documented that did not seem to divide readily into distinct subpopulations of LREH and NREH (Padfield et al, 1975). There was a significant negative correlation between renin and age in this group, as there has been in all large series. The lack of bimodality in the continuum of PRA levels and the negative age correlation constitute the principal arguments in favour of the hypothesis that NREH is eventually modulated into LREH, presumably as a result of some long-term effect of hypertension on the kidney (Brown et al, 1974).

Since PRA is low in primary aldosteronism and in the presence of excessive mineralocorticoid activity, it has been suggested that LREH patients have an excess of an unidentified 'cryptic' mineralocorticoid. Aminoglutethimide, which inhibits the first step in the biosynthesis of all adrenal steroids, will lower the blood pressure in LREH but not in HREH or NREH (Woods et al, 1969). Furthermore, spironolactone, a specific antagonist of mineralocorticoid activity is a more effective antihypertensive in patients with LREH than in those with HREH or NREH (Carey et al, 1972). However, other diuretics are also effective, perhaps as effective as spironolactone in LREH, underscoring the volume-dependent nature of this disease (Sennett, 1974).

Unfortunately, efforts to identify the cryptic mineralocorticoid in LREH have thus far not succeeded (Liddle, 1975) although several groups are continuing a systematic search for it. Because it has proved so difficult to identify, other aetiologies of LREH have been considered. Recent great interest in the prostaglandins and the observation that indomethacin, an inhibitor of their synthesis, reduces PRA in certain clinical situations (Frölich et al, 1976) has raised the possibility that imbalance or other abnormality in prostaglandin synthesis or metabolism might somehow be related to the syndrome. Because of present methodological limitations, the role of the prostaglandins in hypertension has not yet been fully assessed. Finally, it is also possible that the low PRA in LREH patients could have a neurological basis. It is known that in untreated Parkinson's disease, renin levels are subnormal (Michelakis and Robertson, 1970). Parkinsonian patients, many of whom have low blood pressures, might be expected to have had a compensatory elevation in PRA. Their failure to do so and the limited response of their PRA levels to postural stimulation suggest a neurologic basis for their reduced PRA.

The discovery of inhibitors of the pressor effects of angiotensin such as saralasin led to the expectation that renin-dependent and non-renin-dependent varieties of hypertension could be separated. Although it was hoped that the significant depressor response to saralasin would identify renovascular hypertension, it is now clear that some patients with HREH or NREH also respond in this way, and with sufficient sodium depletion, LREH subjects may exhibit a qualitatively similar response (Gavras et al, 1976). Because the 'antagonist' saralasin also has some weak agonistic properties, some patients with LREH will actually have an increase in blood pressure during the infusion (Hollifield, 1976, Anderson, Streeten and Dalakos, 1977).

The converting enzyme inhibitor (SQ-20881), a nonapeptide which blocks the generation of angiotensin II from angiotensin I, does not show the pressor activity sometimes seen when LREH patients are administered saralasin (Erdös, 1976). While saralasin is dependent on sodium depletion for its effect, converting enzyme inhibitor appears often to work regardless of the sodium balance. The blood pressure response to angiotensin blockade with converting enzyme inhibitor has been suggested as an alternative to categorisation by the renin–sodium index (Case et al, 1976).

Now that the volume-dependent nature of LREH is widely appreciated, studies have confirmed that initial therapy of LREH patients is readily accomplished by diuretics (Sennett, 1974). Not uncommonly, with adequate chronic diuretic therapy the LREH patients will have an elevation of their PRA levels into the normal range.

The role of the sympathetic nervous system
The notion that hypertension develops in response to a nervous temperament has long been fixed in the popular imagination. With the rapid acceleration in our understanding of events at the neuronal level in the 1950s and 1960s, great strides in treating hypertension by agents acting on the nervous system were made. However, efforts to incriminate the autonomic nervous system as the cause of essential hypertension were generally not successful (Sjoerdsma, 1961; Crout, Pisano and Sjoerdsma, 1961; Brunjes, 1964).

In the 1970s technological improvements have permitted a re-evaluation of the role of the sympathetic nervous system in human hypertension. Of greatest importance has been the evolution of accurate and rapid methods for the determination of serum noradrenaline, adrenaline, and dopamine (Engelman, Portnoy and Sjoerdsma, 1970; Passon and Peuler, 1973).

When early studies of urinary catecholamines and their metabolites showed little evidence of hyperexcretion in unselected patients with essential hypertension (Crout et al, 1961; Brunjes, 1964), subgroups were sought in whom the sympathetic nervous system seemed especially likely to play a role. Phaeochromocytoma had long been recognised as a catecholamine-dependent cause of hypertension. A subgroup that would appear to have many characteristics of catecholamine excess is that of the borderline or labile hypertensive patients (Julius and Esler, 1975). Borderline hypertension is generally said to exist in a subject in whom blood pressure is intermittently above 150/90 but occasionally normal. Patients with minimal persistent blood pressure elevations are sometimes also included. Clinicians have long noted that some of these patients have characteristics suggestive of both alpha- and beta-receptor stimulation.

There are several haemodynamic and humoral characteristics of borderline hypertension that could be explained by excessive sympathetic nervous system activity. While cardiac output is normal in established hypertension (Freis, 1960) it is raised in a significant number of subjects with borderline hypertension, but not all (Julius et al, 1975). When the significantly raised resting heart rate in this group is released from autonomic influences by both atropine and propranolol, it tends to settle into the same 'intrinsic' rate as control subjects on these medications, thus suggesting a neurogenic cause of the elevated rate. An increased ratio of stroke volume to central blood volume in borderline hypertension (Tarazi et al, 1974) also suggests a neurogenic basis. In the same group some have found a reduced plasma volume (Dissman et al, 1967) or a central redistribution of total blood volume (Safar et al, 1973), both consistent with a neurogenic aetiology.

Plasma noradrenaline levels correlate in most circumstances with sympathetic nervous system activity in that they are raised by circumstances that are known to stimulate the sympathetic nervous system such as upright posture, sodium depletion, pain, isometric handgrip exercise and treadmill exercise. Plasma noradrenaline is raised in some patients with hypertension whether labile or sustained (Louis, Doyle and Anarckar, 1973; DeQuattro et al, 1976) but not in all; indeed some hypertensive patients have serum noradrenaline levels that are lower than the mean for the general population. Many of the apparent discrepancies in noradrenaline levels obtained in various laboratories may relate partially to differences in sodium balance, age, method of sampling (venipuncture versus indwelling catheter), and renal function. These factors do not, however, account for all the abnormalities noted in essential hypertensive patients. If *serum* noradrenaline levels are a correlate of sympathetic nervous activity, *urinary* noradrenaline, to the extent that it reflects the integration of fluctuating serum levels of noradrenaline across time, might be expected to provide a less variable parameter of sympathetic function. However, while some subjects with hypertension have elevated urinary noradrenaline (Cuche et al, 1974), others clearly do not (Engelman et al, 1970; Weidmann et al, 1977).

The metabolites of noradrenaline and adrenaline by the enzyme catechol-O-methyltransferase are normetanephrine and metanephrine. These metabolites are present in several-fold greater concentrations in the urine than noradrenaline and adrenaline. While early studies suggested there was little difference in the excretion of these metabolites by hypertensive patients and by normal subjects (Sjoerdsma et al, 1961; Crout et al, 1961), more recently increased excretion of normetanephrine has been seen (Wolf et al, 1965; Stott and Robinson, 1967; Nestel and Doyle, 1968). Vanillylmandelic acid has generally paralleled normetanephrine excretion with some studies documenting normal levels in hypertension (Sjoerdsma, 1961; Crout et al, 1961) with others finding subnormal levels (Brunjes, 1964) or increased levels (Wolf et al, 1965; Nestel and Doyle, 1968).

Most of the investigations to date have evaluated the biochemical indicators of the function of the adrenergic nervous system by measuring total catecholamines or norepinephrine. There has been less attention to adrenaline because normal and low levels of adrenaline or its urinary metabolite, metanephrine, have been difficult to measure with precision. Nevertheless, many patients with early hypertension have features suggesting a greater increase in beta-adrenergic activities (cardiac, renin release). This raises the possibility that the ratio of adrenaline to noradrenaline might be increased in these patients. The newly developed sensitive and specific methods for measuring both normetanephrine and metanephrine by a stable isotope dilution method are permitting accurate determination of the relative levels of these urinary metabolites of adrenaline and noradrenaline (Robertson et al, 1977).

While urinary catecholamines and their metabolites have been the focus of much work in efforts to implicate the sympathetic nervous system in hypertension, data generated must be interpreted with caution: such urinary parameters represent the 'final common pathway' of events occurring throughout the body — brain, adrenal medulla, spinal cord — and probably do not reflect sympathetic activity alone. However it has been proposed that most urinary noradrenaline is in fact derived from blood vessels (Spector, Tarvel and Berkowitz, 1971) and O-methylation is the primary route of metabolism for noradrenaline released by nerve stimulation.

Some of these problems are circumvented by the use of tritiated noradrenaline (which because of limited penetration into adrenal medulla and brain, equilibrates primarily with the noradrenaline in the cardiovascular system) (Gitlow et al, 1969). Patients with essential hypertension have more tritiated noradrenaline and noradrenaline metabolites in their urine during the 24 h following an intravenous dose of the drug than do normal subjects or patients with renovascular hypertension (Gitlow et al, 1969; Wolf, 1971). This was interpreted to mean that noradrenaline turnover was increased in patients with essential hypertension.

Another approach has been to look at serum and urinary levels of cyclic AMP. Although it is uncertain exactly how urinary cyclic AMP excretion reflects beta-adrenergic activity, they are correlated and, at least in borderline hypertensive patients, cyclic AMP excretion is normal in the supine posture but abnormally raised with assumption of upright posture (Hamet, Kuchel and Genest, 1973). The five-fold increase in plasma cyclic AMP induced in normal subjects by insulin-hypoglycaemia is diminished in low renin hypertensive patients and enhanced in high renin hypertensive patients (Lowder, Hamet and Liddle, 1976). An imbalance in vascular tissue levels of cyclic AMP and cyclic GMP has been proposed as a mechanism of hypertension (Amer, 1975).

The recognition that renin release is at least partially under neural control (Vander,

1965) and that its release in response to certain stimuli is attenuated by propranolol therapy (Michelakis and McAllister, 1972) suggested to some that the high renin essential hypertensive patients — excluding by definition those with renal parenchymal or renovascular disease — might have increased adrenergic tone as a cause for their disease. Patients with the highest plasma renin activities do appear to respond most readily to propranolol (Bühler et al, 1973; Hollifield et al, 1976), and patients with low renin activities tend to respond only to higher doses of propranolol. Another line of evidence that high renin essential hypertension may be a hyperadrenergic state is the relatively greater response of blood pressure to phenoxybenzamine and phentolamine in this subgroup than in the low renin hypertensives (Hollifield et al, 1977, unpublished observations; Esler et al, 1977).

In patients with high-renin borderline hypertension, alpha-blockade with intravenous phentolamine reduced peripheral vascular resistance and blood pressure more than in those with normal or low renin levels (Julius and Esler, 1975). Preliminary blockade with intravenous propranolol in these patients reduced plasma renin activity but not blood pressure until phentolamine was given (Esler et al, 1977). The blood pressure change was immediate with phentolamine and occurred without a significant further change in plasma renin activity. This suggests a dissociation, at least in the high renin essential hypertensive subgroup between plasma renin activity and blood pressure.

In spite of the rapidly accelerating evidence that at least some patients with essential hypertension have a neurogenic component to their disease, the role of the central nervous system in modulating that component remains poorly understood. Recent experimental evidence confirms that suprapontine mechanisms are important even in such simple reflexes as the baroreceptor–heart rate reflex (Korner, 1976). Neurogenic hypertension can now be induced in animals by lesions in the nucleus tractus solitarii (Nathan and Reis, 1977) as well as by section of afferents from the carotid sinus and aortic arch baroreceptors (Chalmers, Korner and White, 1967). The relation of these findings to human essential hypertension is still unknown.

Renovascular hypertension
Five per cent of patients with hypertension have renovascular hypertension. By producing decreased renal perfusion pressure on the stenotic side, the normal renin–angiotensin feedback loop is interrupted triggering increased renin from the involved side. This increased renin in turn suppresses renin release from the uninvolved side. It is still uncertain if renin release is sufficient to account for the increase in arterial pressure through the generation of angiotensin II and release of aldosterone.

The hypertension resulting from renal artery stenosis is a consequence of both increased cardiac output and peripheral vascular resistance as might be expected from excessive angiotensin II generation (Tarazi, Frölich and Dustan, 1973). However, plasma renin activity is not consistently elevated during chronic renovascular hypertension, and there are other diseases (e.g. cirrhosis) where high plasma renin activity, angiotensin II, and aldosterone concentrations in plasma are not associated with hypertension. Thus our understanding of the pathogenesis of the syndrome is incomplete (Brackett et al, 1968; Bianchi et al, 1970; Oparil and Haber, 1974; Peart, 1975). Recent experiments utilising the angiotensin II blocker, saralasin, indicate that early renovascular hypertension probably is largely due to circulating angiotensin II. However, chronic renovascular hypertension is additionally related to other factors, such as an expanded extracellular volume. In patients with renovascular hypertension the acute effects of blockade of angiotensin II do not result in lowering blood pressure if the subject is not salt depleted (Gavras et al, 1975; Streeten et al, 1975). Whether additional humoral mediators of hypertension are also released by the kidney in renovascular hypertension is undetermined (Mizukoshi and Michelakis, 1972; MacDonald, Boyd and Peart, 1975; Skeggs et al, 1977).

The diagnosis of renal artery stenosis depends upon renal function tests, renal arteriography and evaluation of plasma renin activity. The presence of an abdominal or flank bruit raises the likelihood of renal artery stenosis to 50 per cent but does not establish the diagnosis since essential hypertensive patients may also have bruits as atherosclerosis becomes severe. While the presence of a surgically correctable stenosis depends on arteriographic demonstration of the lesion, functional significance of the stenosis usually is assessed by split renal function tests and measurements of the differential in renal venous plasma renin activities (Howard and Connor, 1962; Stamey, 1963). In spite of the controversy regarding the aetiological role of renin in renovascular hypertension, assessment of renin production by each kidney is a useful diagnostic test. When the renal venous renin activity from the kidney with the arterial stenosis is >1.5 times that from the uninvolved side, surgical correction of the renal artery stenosis is likely to be accompanied by lowered blood pressure (Michelakis et al, 1967; Dean and Foster, 1973; Hunt et al, 1974). Stimulation of renin release by upright posture, salt depletion, or vasodilator drugs can maximally increase the difference in renin activity from the two kidneys (Mannick, Huros and Hollander, 1969; Michelakis and Simmons, 1969; Strong et al, 1971). If either renal venous renin determinations or differential renal function tests are positive, operative treatment will be successful in up to 90 per cent of patients (60–70 per cent cures; 20–30 per cent more easily managed with drugs). Of those patients cured by surgery, either the renal venous renins or the differential renal function tests will be falsely negative in about 20 per cent. The number of patients who have both tests falsely negative is unknown, since such patients receive operative treatment (Dean and Foster, 1973). When renal artery lesions are segmental or bilateral, split function tests are often not helpful. However, sampling blood from a renal vein draining the portion of the kidney supplied by a stenotic segmental artery can help to identify significant stenosis that may otherwise be missed (Schambelan et al, 1974).

The presence of high levels of circulating angiotensin in blood would be expected to blunt the response of infused (exogenous) angiotensin II, since receptor sites would presumably be occupied by the endogenous angiotensin. However in practice such a test has not been a reliable predictor of renovascular hypertension (Genest, 1968).

An alternative test is the administration of the angiotensin blocker saralasin. A decrease in arterial pressure produced by infusion of saralasin implies that the blood pressure elevation is dependent in part on angiotensin II. Response to the blocking analogue can be determined in the clinic, and if positive, hospital admission for the more definitive and invasive tests could follow. The results with saralasin appear promising and a positive test correlates well with other evidence for renovascular hypertension in many patients (Marks, Maxwell and Kaufman, 1975; Streeten et al, 1975). However, some patients with high renin essential hypertension also respond with a lowering of blood pressure.

If medical therapy were as effective as surgery and if medical compliance were never a problem, surgery would not be advocated. Unfortunately some patients with renal artery stenosis do not respond adequately to medical therapy and others have gradual loss of renal function or complications of drug therapy. At the present time, there are insufficient data to outline rigid criteria for surgery in renal artery stenosis.

THE PHARMACOLOGY OF ANTIHYPERTENSIVE DRUGS

Drugs that alter central sympathetic nervous system activity

Clonidine

Clonidine is a centrally acting antihypertensive agent that resembles alpha-methyldopa in its clinical effects. Its hypotensive effect can be achieved by microgram quantities of drug. No other antihypertensive drug in wide clinical use is effective in such minute dosages. While the acute peripheral effects of the drug are vasoconstrictor, it also inhibits sympathetic outflow from the central nervous system and increases the depressor effects of baroreceptor stimulation (Kobinger and Walland, 1972a, b). Alpha-adrenergic receptors are now postulated to exist in the cardiovascular control system of the medulla; when stimulated, they inhibit peripheral sympathetic activity, when blocked they cause increased sympathetic outflow (Van Zweiten, 1973; Haeusler, 1975). Clonidine stimulates these central alpha-receptors and the hypotensive effect of the drug can be reversed by the alpha-adrenergic blocker tolazoline (Merguet et al, 1968). The peripheral alpha-mediated vasoconstriction predominates transiently when the drug is given intravenously, and the blood pressure may actually rise (Mroczek, Davidov and Finnerty, 1973). In other circumstances the central effect predominates.

Reduction in sympathetic activity reduces blood pressure, lowers heart rate, and decreases the urinary excretion of catecholamines (Hökfelt, Hedeland and Dymling, 1970). Plasma renin activity is also reduced (Hökfelt et al, 1970); Reid et al, 1975; Pettinger et al, 1976). Cardiac output is lowered though a slight reduction in peripheral vascular resistance occurs (Onesti et al, 1971). The reduction in renal vascular resistance permits maintenance of renal blood flow at control levels (Brod et al, 1972). Exercise-induced changes in blood pressure, cardiac output, heart rate, stroke volume and peripheral resistance are qualitatively normal after clonidine though quantitatively reduced.

Little is known about the pharmacokinetics of clonidine. The half-life in five normal subjects averaged 12 h but ranged from 6 to 24 h and the duration of action in patients was from 4 to 24 h (Pettinger, 1975; Dollery et al, 1976). Peak plasma levels of radioactivity following oral administration of radiolabelled clonidine occur at 2 to 4 h. The tricyclic antidepressant desipramine interferes with the antihypertensive effect of clonidine (Briant, Reid and Dollery, 1973; Reid, Briant and Dollery, 1973; Raftos et al, 1973; Bucher et al, 1973; Hoefke and Warnke-Sachs, 1974).

Clonidine therapy can provide a sustained antihypertensive effect similar to alpha-methyldopa over long periods of time. Tolerance is rare if concomitant diuretic therapy is given. Sedation and dry or 'parched' mouth are the most common side effects. In general they are more severe with clonidine than with alpha-methyldopa but individual patients may tolerate clonidine better (Conolly et al, 1972). With continued therapy most side effects abate somewhat, but the decreased salivation usually continues. Constipation and impotence have also occasionally been reported but orthostatic hypotension is rare (Hoobler and Sagastume, 1971; Onesti et al, 1971).

The most serious side effect of the drug has been the report of a withdrawal syndrome following sudden cessation of chronic therapy (Conolly et al, 1972). It may occur between 8 and 36 h following the last dose of clonidine and is characterised by anxiety, headache, abdominal pain, tachycardia, sweating and nausea. The blood pressure may rapidly reach pretreatment levels and occasionally can even surpass these levels. Although the pathology of this syndrome is uncertain, many of the side effects suggest sympathetic overactivity. Elevated serum and urinary levels of catecholamines have been documented in clonidine withdrawal and the blood pressure elevation responds to alpha-adrenergic blockers (Hökfelt et al, 1970; Conolly et al, 1972; Hansson et al, 1973).

The incidence of clinically significant clonidine withdrawal is not yet established. Although it clearly occurs in only a minority of patients, it is incumbent on the prescribing physician to warn his patient about the danger of sudden cessation of therapy. When clonidine must be withdrawn, gradual tapering is preferable. If elective surgery is planned, substitution of an alternative antihypertensive medication is advisable. Therapy of the withdrawal syndrome is similar to that for phaeochromocytoma: combined alpha- and beta-blockade.

Methlydopa

Methyldopa is a centrally acting antihypertensive drug of intermediate potency (Oates et al, 1960). The mechanism of action of the drug is still not completely understood. Because it is metabolised by dopa decarboxylase and dopamine beta-hydroxylase into alpha-methylnoradrenaline (Muscholl and Maitre, 1963; Day and Rand, 1964), it was thought that this 'false neurotransmitter' accounted for the antihypertensive effect. However, alpha-methylnoradrenaline was found to be almost as potent as noradrenaline in its peripheral cardiovascular effects (Sugarman et al, 1968; Altura, 1975). An alternative hypothesis that the alpha-methylnoradrenaline exerted feedback inhibition on tyrosine hydroxylase thus reducing catecholamine formation has not been supported by subsequent experimental data (Haefely, Hürlimann and Thoenen, 1966; Altura, 1975; Lokhandwala, Buckley and Jandhyala, 1975).

The major action of methyldopa is now felt to be on the alpha-receptors in the medulla oblongata which govern sympathetic outflow to the cardiovascular system. Its metabolite alpha-methylnoradrenaline is a powerful stimulator of central alpha-receptors, and its action thus resembles clonidine's. Since concomitant inhibition of dopa decarboxylase and/or dopamine-beta-hydroxylase abolishes the hypotensive effect of methyldopa, it would appear that the alpha-methylnoradrenaline itself is required for effect. That this metabolite acts on central alpha-receptors is supported by the observation that intravenous or intraventricular administration of an alpha-adrenergic blocker will prevent the hypotensive action of the drug (Heise and Kroneberg, 1973).

Following oral administration, absorption is incomplete and variable. The observation that the dextro-rotatory isomer is more poorly absorbed than the usual levo-rotatory form (Lin, Hagihira and Wilson, 1962; Au et al, 1972) suggests the existence of a stereospecific transport system in the gastrointestinal tract. The maximum antihypertensive effect occurs in 3 to 8 h and lasts up to 24 h. The plasma half-life of the drug is only about 1 to 2 h. It is excreted in the urine both as unchanged drug and as sulphate conjugates, but neither hepatic nor renal disease has been reported to alter drug requirement. The intravenous formulation is methyldopate hydrochloride, an ethyl ester of methyldopa. Animal studies suggest that less than half of this ester is actually hydrolysed to methyldopa (Walson et al, 1975).

The administration of methyldopa reduces peripheral vascular resistance and often also heart rate and cardiac output. However, since renal vascular resistance is reduced at least proportionately to blood pressure, the renal fraction of the cardiac output remains the same or increases slightly (Morin, Turmel and Fortier, 1964; Mohammed et al, 1968a,b). The Valsalva overshoot and venoconstrictor reflexes are reduced in some patients but postural hypotension is mild if present at all (Oates et al, 1965). While plasma renin activity is slightly decreased by the drug, the reduction is not sufficient to result in misclassification of a patient's renin status. Although the reduced plasma renin activity may contribute to the action of the drug, it is not a dominant or necessary component of its antihypertensive effect (Halushka and Keiser, 1974; Lowder and Liddle, 1975).

The most common side effects include decreased intellectual drive, drowsiness, forgetfulness, and fatigue. Although depression has been reported, it is far less common than with reserpine. Failure of ejaculation is uncommon but the psychic lassitude occasionally observed can lead to reduced libido and functional impotence. Very rarely extrapyramidal signs have appeared. Dryness of the mouth is less severe than with clonidine. A reversible side effect of lactation in either sex has occurred uncommonly (Horwitz et al, 1967).

Perhaps the most serious and unpredictable forms of toxicity are drug fever and hepatitis. The drug fever can mimic sepsis with shaking chills and temperatures spiking to 105°F (Glontz and Saslaw, 1968). The hepatic dysfunction can be quite varied in its manifestations, but may resemble viral hepatitis. Occasionally massive hepatic necrosis has occurred (Rehman, Keith and Gall, 1973; Toghill et al, 1974; Rodman, Deutsch and Gutman, 1976). Chronic active hepatitis and cholestatic jaundice have been reported. More than 90 per cent of these reactions occur within the first few months of therapy with methyldopa. However, rare instances of jaundice have been reported as late as a year or more, and therefore they must constantly be borne in mind.

Up to 25 per cent of persons on 1 g of methyldopa daily for six months or more develop a positive direct Coombs test (Carstairs et al, 1966). For most of these persons, this causes no problem except that it interferes with blood cross-matching. However, 5 per cent of these patients with a positive direct Coombs test will develop a raised reticulocyte count and one per cent will have frank haemolytic anaemia. Since this reaction does not occur until a patient has been taking methyldopa for three months, it is postulated that methyldopa or one of its metabolites is incorporated into the developing erythrocyte which is then antigenic. The antibody responsible is a gamma-G type which will not react with methyldopa alone. The Coombs test will usually but not always become negative within six months of withdrawal of drug (LoBuglio and Jandl, 1967). In severe haemolysis, steroids in addition to drug discontinuation may be of value. A positive Coombs test does not mean that hepatotoxicity will develop; hepatotoxicity many in fact occur with a persistently negative Coombs reaction.

There are many other drugs whose antihypertensive effects may be in part centrally mediated: reserpine, propranolol, and hydralazine are discussed elsewhere since the central mechanism is not felt to be the most important factor in their antihypertensive effects. In addition certain drugs no longer thought of as antihypertensive medications (e.g. phenobarbital) undoubtedly exert part of their effect centrally, though peripheral effects are also possible (Exley, 1954).

Drugs that block autonomic ganglia

The ganglionic blockers were the first potent antihypertensive agents widely used for therapy of hypertension but their use has declined as agents with fewer side effects became available: today these are used only in certain emergencies.

Drugs that act at postganglionic sympathetic nerve endings

Guanethidine

Guanethidine is a potent antihypertensive agent whose strongly basic guanidine group prevents entry of the drug into the central nervous system so that it lacks many of the central side effects of reserpine. Following administration of the drug, impulses are conducted normally down the adrenergic neuron, but release of noradrenaline from the terminal is blocked. Prolonged administration of guanethidine depletes stores of noradrenaline in most tissues outside the blood–brain barrier (Cass and Spriggs, 1961; Chang et al, 1965; Oates et al, 1971).

The administration of a single large dose of guanethidine somehow interferes with the excitation–depolarisation mechanism prior to major decreases in catecholamine stores and the inhibition of sympathetic function disappears before amine content in storage sites is depleted (Cass and Spriggs, 1961; Sanan and Vogt, 1962). With chronic therapy the drug enters the neurosecretory granule and substitutes as a false neurotransmitter when the granule is released. It seems likely that the excitation–depolarisation inhibition predominates acutely and that the false neurotransmitter mechanism is dominant with chronic therapy.

Guanethidine must enter the adrenergic neuron before it can act. It is normally concentrated at its site of action by the noradrenaline pump. Drugs that interfere with the noradrenaline pump will prevent guanethidine from reaching its site of action and its therapeutic effect will not appear (Brodie, Chang and Costa, 1965; Mitchell and Oates, 1970). Tricyclic antidepressants, phenothiazines, amphetamine, cocaine and probably metaraminol and ephedrine can block uptake of guanethidine into nerve endings (Brodie et al, 1965; Gulati et al, 1966; Mitchell et al, 1970; Janowsky et al, 1972; Woosley et al, 1976). Amphetamine administration to a patient on guanethidine causes a rapid reversal of its antihypertensive effect since it both blocks the noradrenaline pump and releases guanethidine from the nerve ending. The antagonism of the pump by chlorpromazine even in high doses, is rather weak and may be partially overcome by the administration of increased amounts of guanethidine. Tricyclic antidepressants, however, act so powerfully that raising the guanethidine dosage to 150 mg daily will not restore the full therapeutic effect. The effect of the tricyclic antidepressant drugs on guanethidine's antihypertensive effect may persist for several days after the tricyclic drug is discontinued.

Many over-the-counter cold remedies and decongestants contain agents which can antagonise guanethidine's effect. Since the patient on guanethidine suffering from the frequent side effect of nasal stuffiness is especially likely to use one of the preparations it is important to caution the patient about this in advance.

Intravenous guanethidine in man results in a transient elevation of blood pressure that could be life threatening in the patient with phaeochromocytoma and is therefore not used clinically. Following oral administration the initial release of norepinephrine proceeds more slowly and the initial hypertensive response is not likely to occur even with initial doses up to 100 mg (Walter and Nies, 1977).

Chronic therapy with guanethidine will lower blood pressure in almost all patients. By blocking sympathetic reflexes guanethidine reduces venous tone allowing increased venous capacitance (Walter et al, 1975). Heart rate is often slowed and cardiac output decreases. Stroke volume is usually little affected. Renal blood flow and glomerular filtration rate are decreased but these are usually clinically inconsequential (Freis, 1965). Surprisingly plasma renin activity, which is usually correlated with sympathetic activity, is not suppressed but may actually be increased during guanethidine therapy (Ferguson, Rothenberg and Nies, 1976). Patients with low renin hypertension may be misclassified if they are tested while taking guanethidine (Lowder and Liddle, 1975).

Once sympathetic reflexes are inhibited, blood pressure becomes a function of blood volume and posture. In this situation the volume expansion that occurs with chronic guanethidine therapy may result in tolerance to its antihypertensive effect. Thus in patients on chronic therapy with guanethidine a failure in blood pressure control could be due to inadequate drug reaching its site of action in the neuron terminal or to tolerance due to volume expansion. The former might result from poor compliance or suboptimal dosage while the latter might be due to inadequate diuretic therapy. Even in patients careful about compliance, the interindividual variation in required dose is very large; some patients need as little as 10 mg daily while others require more than 100 mg daily.

When an inadequate clinical response to guanethidine occurs, the physician may have difficulty deciding whether the guanethidine should be increased or more diuresis effected (Dustan et al, 1972). A very useful test in such a situation is the venous reflex. Sympatholytic doses of guanethidine strikingly reduce the intensity of the venous reflex. Therefore if the venous reflex is attenuated in an uncontrolled hypertensive patient, this implies that adequate sympatholytic effect of guanethidine has occurred and increased diuresis should be instituted. However, a failure of the venous reflex to be attenuated implies inadequate sympatholysis and guanethidine should be increased (Walter et al, 1975).

An understanding of the pharmacokinetics of guanethidine is essential for rational use of the drug. From 3 to 50 per cent of an oral dose reaches the systemic circulation. Half the drug is excreted unchanged in the urine and half is metabolised. The tubular secretion of the compound accounts for the fact that guanethidine clearance exceeds glomerular filtration rate.

Following intravenous administration the drug is rapidly removed from circulation. There follows a period of slower removal for which a half-life of 20 h can be calculated. Finally a third phase of elimination has a half-life of five days. Pretreatment of a patient with protriptyline (inhibiting uptake of guanethidine into the neuronal pool) results in increased elimination in the early phase 'pools' and decreased elimination in the late phase 'pools'. Furthermore, amphetamine releases drug from the late phase pool (Chang et al, 1965; Shand, Morgan and Oates, 1973). These two observations plus the correlation of the late phase of elimination with therapeutic effect are strong evidence that the five-day elimination phase represents the deposition of the drug in the adrenergic neuron.

The long half-life of guanethidine's late-phase pool approximates the half-life of digitoxin. Therapy with digitoxin is best initiated with a loading dose, if early therapeutic effects are desired. The same applies to guanethidine since therapy with a maintenance dose would require 17 days to achieve 90 per cent of its maximal pharmacologic effect (Rahn and Goldberg, 1969; McMartin et al, 1970; Gibaldi, Levy and Weintraub, 1971, Lukas, 1973). A loading regimen has been developed that takes into account that the maximal effect from a single oral dose is not apparent for 6 h and that patients will differ in the amount of guanethidine they require for loading (Shand et al, 1975). Because of these special considerations, the loading regimen for guanethidine must be more graduated than that for digitoxin. The loading regimen is both effective and safe. It usually leads to control of blood pressure in one to three days. Thus, patients with malignant hypertension whose therapy was initiated with rapidly acting anti-hypertensives can be switched to an effective regimen of guanethidine in this relatively brief time.

The loading regimen is begun with a single oral dose of 75 mg. Excessive reduction in blood pressure has not been seen with this dosage. Following this initial dose, each subsequent dose amounts to 30 per cent of all the previously administered guanethidine; it is given after a 6 h interval. The 6 h interval allows time for the maximal antihypertensive effect to occur, and since this requires blood pressure evaluation in both upright and supine postures, no night-time dose of guanethidine is given. Once the patient's blood pressure begins to fall, longer intervals between doses and smaller percentage increments are employed. When the standing blood pressure is reduced to the desired level, the maintenance dose is estimated as one-seventh of the total loading regimen administered. This amount is given after a 24 h interval and daily thereafter.

The side effects of guanethidine are primarily unwanted aspects of adrenergic blockade. Postural hypotension is more of a problem with guanethidine than with alpha-methyldopa or reserpine. Exercise can lead to more pronounced hypotension. In the sexually active male, erection, a parasympathetic function, is achieved but there may be delayed or retrograde ejaculation. Diarrhoea is commonly seen with guanethidine therapy but its cause has never been adequately explained. Occasionally an increase in bronchial smooth muscle tone is noted and commonly nasal stuffiness can be a problem. No hypersensitivity reactions have been noted.

In spite of these problems, guanethidine's potency as an antihypertensive and its relative freedom from central nervous system side effects have made it a major agent not only for chronic therapy of severe hypertension but also for treatment of mild to moderate hypertensives who do not tolerate the CNS side effects of other drugs (Ferguson et al, 1976).

Bethanidine and debrisoquine
Bethanidine resembles guanethidine in its clinical effects and its probable mechanism of action (Chrysant et al, 1975). Like guanethidine its therapeutic effect is also abolished by inhibitors of the norepinephrine pump (Mitchell et al, 1970).

Bethanidine differs from guanethidine in its pharmacokinetics. The elimination of bethanidine is entirely by the kidney where it is excreted unchanged with a half-life of 7 to 11 h (Shen et al, 1975). Therefore, the drug accumulates in the body more rapidly than guanethidine does; bethanidine reaches plateau concentrations in plasma within two to three days, and the drug must be given several times daily for sustained effect (Gupta and McNay, 1972). The requirement for multiple daily doses constitutes an inconvenience to the patient. A multicentre trial has confirmed that guanethidine is associated with greater overall reduction of blood pressure than bethanidine even though the latter was associated with considerably more postural hypotension (Veterans' Administration, 1977).

Bethanidine's undesirable effects are explained by its pharmacologic action. The only reported difference from guanethidine is that the patient may have less diarrhoea while taking bethanidine but this may not be significant (Bath, Pickering and Turner, 1967; Prichard et al, 1968; Veterans' Administration, 1977).

Debrisoquine is another, shorter acting adrenergic neuron blocking drug which has antihypertensive efficacy and a spectrum of side effects similar to the other drugs of its class (Bauer, 1970). In common with guanethidine, the individual variation in the antihypertensive response to debrisoquine appears to occur largely on the basis of variable bioavailability (Silas et al, 1977).

Reserpine

Reserpine, an antihypertensive drug of intermediate potency, is a rauwolfia alkaoid which depletes the stores of catecholamines and serotonin in many organs including the brain, adrenal medulla and heart (Chidsey et al, 1963; Mason and Braunwald, 1964).

Tolerable doses of reserpine have a modest antihypertensive effect: alone it is usually less potent than a thiazide diuretic. It should usually therefore be given with a diuretic. Clinically, the antihypertensive effect is often associated with a slowing of the pulse, and both peripheral resistance and cardiac output decrease. Venous capacitance is increased and peripheral pooling of blood may lead to fluid retention.

There are several serious side effects associated with reserpine therapy. There is a dose-associated risk of psychotic depression and suicide, so the drug is usually not given in dosages greater than 0.5 mg daily (Gaffney et al, 1969). Although peptic ulceration is uncommon in patients on oral reserpine, almost 50 per cent of patients receiving emergency parenteral reserpine develop gastrointestinal bleeding.

A proposed causal association of reserpine and breast cancer has not been substantiated (Armstrong, Stevens and Doll, 1974; Boston Collaborative Drug Surveillance Program, 1974; Heinonen et al, 1974; Laska et al, 1975; O'Fallon, Labarthe and Kurland, 1975).

Monoamine oxidase inhibitors

Monoamine oxidase inhibitors such as pargyline have now been largely replaced by other antihypertensive agents because of serious side effects. Like guanethidine, postural hypotension is sometimes severe. However in mechanism of action, differences are great. When monoamine oxidase is blocked, the stores of noradrenaline as well as of other amines (e.g. octopamine) increase in the storage granules. These other amines become potential false neurotransmitters in the storage granule where they can compete with norepinephrine for release. Octopamine is probably a key false neurotransmitter during monoamine oxidase inhibition, since its potency is less than 1 per cent that of norepinephrine. The result is that the released norepinephrine is diluted out by the presence of the weaker octopamine. Sympathetic blockade is thus effected (Kopin et al, 1965).

In normal persons, infusion of tyramine results in a transient elevation of blood pressure due to release of norepinephrine from the nerve endings. The effect is brief because monoamine oxidase rapidly destroys the tyramine. During therapy with monoamine oxidase inhibitors, tyramine is protected from destruction. Under these circumstances even the small quantities of tyramine in foods may cause significant hypertension. Reactions have been reported following ingestion of aged cheese, wine, beer, pickled herring, broad beans, and chicken liver (Horwitz et al, 1964; Pettinger and Oates, 1968). Similarly, catecholamines in many over-the-counter remedies can cause severe reactions in subjects on monoamine oxidase inhibitors. Appropriate therapy for such reactions is with alpha-adrenergic blockade.

Adrenergic receptor blocking drugs

Adrenergic receptors are subdivided into alpha and beta subgroups. Alpha-receptor stimulation produces vasoconstriction of arterioles and veins. Beta-receptor stimulation dilates arterioles and arteries, increases the rate and force of contraction of the heart, dilates bronchi, stimulates renin release, and promotes glycogenolysis and lipolysis (Michelakis and McAllister, 1972; Porte, 1967, 1969). The subdivision of the beta effects into beta-1 (cardiac effects) and beta-2 (bronchodilation and vasodilation) arose as more and more selective blocking agents were found. It is not yet certain if renin release is governed by beta-1- or beta-2-receptors (Weber, Stokes and Gain, 1974; Bühler et al, 1975).

Such a classification of catecholamines and their action is only a general guide: in most cases a catecholamine will possess alpha, beta-1, and beta-2 activity to a greater or lesser degree, so that large doses of alpha-stimulators will usually exhibit some beta-stimulation as well. The converse is also true.

Alpha-adrenergic blocking drugs

Phentolamine, indoramin and phenoxybenzamine are alpha-blocking drugs employed in circumstances where hypertension is due to overactivity of the adrenergic system or the overproduction of adrenergic neurotransmitting substances (clonidine withdrawal, guanethidine-induced acute hypertension, pheochromocytoma, tetanus). Phentolamine has a half-life of several hours, while phenoxybenzamine produces blockade for several days.

Phentolamine has been used in hypertensive crisis to determine whether the hypertension was due to catecholamine excess. A significant blood pressure reduction following 0.5 to 5.0 mg of phentolamine points toward catecholamine excess and guanethidine loading, for example, would be contraindicated.

Prazosin, introduced as a vasodilator, appears to act also through alpha-blockade (see below).

Beta-adrenergic blocking drugs

From a study of the individual effects produced by beta-agonists (vasodilation) one might expect that beta-adrenergic blockers would raise blood pressure. In fact, however, propranolol has proved to be an extremely effective antihypertensive agent (Prichard and Gillam, 1964). It acts to reduce cardiac contractility and heart rate. Total peripheral resistance is either unchanged or slightly reduced by acute intravenous administration of the drug, while with chronic therapy, peripheral resistance may decrease (Ulrych et al, 1968; Tarazi and Dustan, 1972; Bühler et al, 1975). Renin release by the kidney is partially under beta-adrenergic control and propranolol therapy reduces plasma renin activity at relatively low doses and particularly attenuates the elevation in renin activity that occurs with standing or exercise (Michelakis and McAllister, 1972). Propranolol is most successful in reducing blood pressure in patients with normal or high levels of plasma renin (Hollifield et al, 1976). It accomplishes this at doses of 80 to 320 mg/day. However, even in patients with very low renin levels, some antihypertensive activity is usually observed if doses in the range 1000 to 2000 mg are administered. There thus appear to be at least two mechanisms of action with different dose–response curves. Among all patients with essential hypertension 90 per cent will eventually respond to propranolol, but in a small minority of patients, blood pressure may actually rise (Drayer et al, 1976).

The mechanism by which propranolol lowers blood pressure is not entirely clear. Suggested mechanisms have been (1) reduced plasma renin activity, (2) reduced cardiac output, (3) peripheral adrenergic neuron blockade, (4) interference with baroreceptor function, and (5) an effect on the cardiovascular control system of the medulla. Different mechanisms may be operative in different patients. The observation that intravenous propranolol lowers plasma renin activity and also cardiac output without lowering blood pressure underscores the fact that mechanisms other than simply renin reduction are involved (Julius and Esler, 1975).

The wide range of doses required in hypertension (10–4000 mg daily) are not explained by the patient's renin status alone (Prichard and Gillam, 1969; Zacharias et al, 1972). Individuals vary considerably in their disposition of the drug. As much as a twenty-fold difference in plasma concentration following an oral dose is observed in different individuals (Shand, 1975). Although the drug is almost completely absorbed from the intestine, there is a significant 'first-pass' metabolism as drug is removed by liver before reaching systemic circulation. Single small oral doses are more completely extracted by the liver than larger doses, suggesting saturation of the extraction process. With chronic administration of the drug in clinical doses at 6 h intervals, the very avid extraction process is chronically saturated but still as much as 40 to 70 per cent of the orally administered drug may be removed in a single pass through the liver. The half-life of the drug is 2.5 h after intravenous administration, 3.3 h after a single oral dose and 4.5 h after stopping a chronic oral regimen. However, the half-life varies depending on the isomeric form of the drug. The d-isomer of propranolol has a shorter half-life than the l-isomer because the l-isomer (but not the d-isomer) reduces hepatic blood flow and thus slows its elimination. The racemate behaves as the l-isomer since the haemodynamic effects are similar. Another factor in individual variation in propranolol levels is binding. Plasma protein binding of propranolol varies between 90 and 95 per cent in normal subjects and the concentration of free drug thus varies two-fold. The pharmacokinetics of propranolol were recently reviewed (Shand, 1974; Nies and Shand, 1975).

Hepatic disease significantly increases the fraction of an oral dose reaching the systemic circulation (Branch and Shand, 1976) and since both clearance and binding are reduced, the half-life is prolonged. In patients with severe renal failure, there appears to be a slightly reduced hepatic extraction of propranolol and a decreased metabolic clearance of the drug (Lowenthal et al, 1974).

Because of the large interindividual variation in dosage required to achieve desired effects, it was hoped that measurement of plasma levels would provide better correlation with pharmacologic effect. This has been partially realised. Plasma concentrations above 50 ng/ml are associated with reduced plasma renin activity in most subjects concentrations above 100 ng/ml at the end of the 6 h dosage interval should achieve a consistently high degree of beta-blockade (Nies and Shand, 1975; Zacest and Koch-Weser, 1972a).

Although propranolol can be used alone to treat hypertension, it is often given with a diuretic or a vasodilator. Propranolol and hydralazine are at least additive in their therapeutic effect and the addition of a diuretic provides further antihypertensive activity (Gilmore, Weil and Chidsey, 1970; Pettinger and Keeton, 1975). Attenuation of the tachycardia, raised cardiac output, and elevated renin activity induced by hydralazine will rarely require doses of propranolol greater than 240 mg daily. Similar doses of propranolol are useful also with diazoxide and minoxidil.

While it would seem that a drug with a half-life of 4.5 h would require that the drug be given four times daily, it has been shown that a twice daily regimen is satisfactory in many patients (Berglund et al, 1973).

The side effects of propranolol therapy include (1) heart failure, (2) worsened asthma, (3) hypoglycaemia, (4) central nervous system disturbances, and (5) certain non-specific effects such as rashes or paresthesias. These side effects have not been as serious in clinical practice as was initially feared (Greenblatt and Koch-Weser, 1973; Simpson, 1974).

In certain patients heart failure has progressed to a point that the sympathetic drive on the heart is essential in avoiding decompensation. Blockade of beta-adrenergic activity in such patients may lead to bradyarrhythmias and severe decompensation. This problem is uncommon in patients without clinical evidence of congestive heart failure before propranolol therapy; it usually appears early in therapy if it is going to occur at all. Digitalis and diuretics may reverse this failure even if propranolol is continued, though the obvious dangers of such a compromise should lead to the choice of an alternate antihypertensive agent in almost all cases. In severe bradyarrhythmias or cardiovascular collapse, such as may occur in compromised patients given intravenous propranolol, acute treatment with atropine, isoproterenol, or glucagon may be required.

If heart failure is due to hypertension, lowering blood pressure with propranolol may actually improve the failure. Such a patient must be approached cautiously when this agent is being used, however.

The abolition of the adrenergic bronchodilator activity in the lung may lead to worsened asthma in patients on propranolol.

The physiological response of the body to severe hypoglycaemia includes adrenal medullary discharge of catecholamines followed by a beta-adrenergic dependent release of glucose from the liver. In diabetic patients on hypoglycaemic agents, propranolol can prevent this metabolic effect of the released catecholamines and mask the usual symptoms of tremor and palpitation. Since propranolol can prevent the development of ketosis, non-ketotic hyperosmolar coma has been observed (Podolsky and Pattavina, 1973).

Propranolol may cause a deterioration in renal function in patients with established renal disease and some sodium retention is commonly seen (Tarazi, Fröhlich and Dustan, 1971; Stokes et al, 1974a; Drayer et al, 1975). These effects may be related to the reduction of renal blood flow and glomerular filtration rate which occur with propranolol (Nies, McNeil and Schrier, 1971; Warren, 1976).

Raynaud's phenomenon, peripheral arterial insufficiency, and exacerbation of myasthenia gravis have been reported. Since the drug crosses the blood–brain barrier, propranolol has occasionally been associated with lack of concentration, lethargy, disturbance of sleep patterns, and vivid nightmares, especially in the morning just before awakening.

Although propranolol is the most widely studied of the beta-blockers and the only one currently available in the United States, other agents such as oxprenolol, alprenolol, sotalol, timolol, pindolol, atenolol and metoprolol have been shown to have beta-blocking activity in man. Beta-blockers differ not only in potency but in relative effect on various receptors. Drugs which are either beta-1-blockers (cardioselective) or non-selective beta-blockers tend to have antihypertensive activity with chronic use. The development of safe cardioselective beta-blockers such as atenolol and metoprolol may provide the physician with a drug capable of lowering blood pressure without the danger of pulmonary complications of therapy. However because the mechanism of the antihypertensive effect of these drugs is unknown, each beta-blocker must be judged individually in clinical studies to determine its efficacy.

The relative merits of the various beta-adrenoceptor blocking drugs as antihypertensives has recently been reviewed at length by Waal-Manning (1976). It is the general consensus that other pharmacological properties, such as membrane stabilisation and intrinsic sympathiomimtic activity, are of little consequence. Indeed intrinsic activity may be associated with the paradoxical increase in blood pressure with large doses of pindolol (Waal-Manning and Simpson, 1975) and practolol (Sundquist, Antilla and Arstila, 1974). The cardioselectivity of metoprolol and atenolol should, however, be of advantage in patients with a tendency to bronchospasm. In comparing the newer agents with propranolol, it should be remembered that they can all lower the blood pressure, but there is a strong suggestion that the ceiling of dosage beyond which no further effect occurs seems lower than propranolol with oxprenolol, pindolol and atenolol (see Waal-Manning, 1976). It is also clear, that despite their relatively short half-lives of 2 to 6 h propranolol, pindolol, metoprolol, alprenolol, and oxprenolol can all be effective on a twice daily dosage regimen. This is true because the duration of a drugs action depends just as much on dosage as on elimination rate. The two drugs with the longest half-lives, sotalol and atenolol, may well be effective following a single oral dose.

All of the available compounds seem to show considerable interindividual variation in their effective dosage. Several factors may be involved, including varied bioavailability and 'severity' of the disease, as well as the possibility that higher levels are required to produce an effect in low-renin essential hypertensives. All of these variables require individual dosage titration.

There has been considerable debate concerning the speed of onset of the antihypertensive effects of these drugs since Prichard and Gillam (1969) first suggested that the full effect might take as long as one to two months to develop in some cases. Certainly acute i.v. administration does not produce a fall in blood pressure, because of reflex alpha-vasoconstrictor. This compensatory mechanism seems to wane quite quickly as several studies have now shown that a significant effect occurs within 24 to 48 h and certainly by the end of the first week, provided an adequate dose is administered (Waal-Manning, 1976).

Labetalol

Labetalol is an investigational drug possessing both alpha- and beta-adrenoceptor blocking properties both in animals and man (Dollery, 1976). It may prove particularly useful because the beta-blockade can block certain side effects of alpha-blockade such as tachycardia and palpitation (Mehta and Cohn, 1977; Richards et al, 1977). In animals the competitive blockade of labetalol is more potent on beta- than on alpha-receptors by an estimated 3 : 1 ratio (Richards, Tuckman and Prichard, 1975).

In patients with moderately severe hypertension, labetalol reduces peripheral resistance without significantly reducing cardiac output (Prichard et al, 1975). A double-blind trial has confirmed that dosages as low as 400 mg/day significantly lower blood pressure (Kane et al, 1976). The major side effect has been postural hypotension. It is still not clear if the melanin-binding property of the drug is of clinical significance or not (Poynter et al, 1976).

Vasodilators

The direct peripheral vasodilators reduce blood pressure by relaxation of the arteriolar smooth muscle. Some dilate veins as well. Recently these drugs have proved to be very useful in hypertensive emergencies and, when combined with a renin-suppressing antihypertensive, in the chronic management of hypertension. These agents differ considerably in potency. Since these drugs lower arterial pressure without blocking the sympathetic nervous system, a reflex stimulation occurs which leads to increased heart rate and contractility, and increased beta-induced output of renin. Those agents which lack intrinsic capacity to dilate veins will thus reflexly cause increased venous tone. The resultant central redistribution of blood increases cardiac output and myocardial work load (Ablad, 1963).

Hydralazine

Hydralazine lowers peripheral vascular resistance causing a fall in blood pressure and an increase in cardiac output by baroreceptor reflex mechanisms. Although it is a monoamine oxidase inhibitor this probably does not contribute to its clinical effect. It directly dilates arterioles by relaxing the arteriolar smooth muscle. The effect of hydralazine on the tone in the venous capacitance system is very much less than in the arteriolar system. The baroreceptor-induced increase in cardiac output occurs through increased stroke volume and heart rate with increased myocardial oxygen requirements. Because tone in venous capacitance vessels is maintained during therapy venous return and pulmonary blood volume are also maintained. Occasional patients will have an increase in pulmonary artery pressure and elevated pulmonary vascular resistance.

The renin-stimulating effect of hydralazine correlates better with the patient's increase in heart rate than his blood pressure reduction. Because of this and the observation that the increase in plasma renin activity with hydralazine did not occur in a renal transplant patient, the renin release is assumed to be the result of reflex sympathetic discharge (Ueda et al, 1970).

Absorption of hydralazine is rapid. More than 50 per cent is metabolised during the first pass through the liver and less than 10 per cent is excreted unchanged in the urine. Peak plasma levels are reached 1 to 2 h after an oral dose.

The metabolism of hydralazine, like that of isoniazid, is under genetic control with the population divided into two groups, one which acetylates the drug rapidly and another which acetylates the drug slowly. Plasma hydralazine levels are higher in the slow acetylators, in spite of similar volumes of distribution. Plasma half-life of the drug has been estimated at 2 to 8 h. There are two phases of elimination, suggesting a 'deep-pool' for hydralazine or one of its metabolites, probably representing persistent vascular tissue binding. Recognition of this prolonged late phase half-life resulted in the suggestion that twice daily therapy might be as effective as four times daily therapy. Clinical studies have verified the adequacy of the twice daily regimen (Zacest and Koch-Weser, 1972b; Reidenberg et al, 1973; Lesser et al, 1974; O'Malley et al, 1975a).

The hypotensive effect of hydralazine is greatly enchanced by the addition of a diuretic. It is further enhanced and some of its side effects reduced by the addition of propranolol. Propranolol, through beta-blockade, diminishes the adrenergically mediated chronotropic and inotropic effects of hydralazine on the heart and renin release from the kidney. The combined regimen has had good patient acceptance, since it avoids the disturbed sexual function and the more severe postural hypotension of many of the sympathetic reflex blockers.

Side effects of hydralazine include headache, palpitation, nausea, and sweating; occasional patients will complain of nasal congestion, tremors and flushing. However the most serious toxicity of hydralazine is the risk of developing lupus erythematosus. This risk is dose dependent and almost never occurs if the dosage is less than 200 mg daily (Alarcon-Segovia et al, 1967). The lupus syndrome occurs almost exclusively in Caucasian slow acetylators and almost never in Caucasian fast acetylators or Blacks regardless of their acetylator phenotype. The lupus syndrome is reversible with cessation of the drug (Perry et al, 1970; Perry, 1973), and its danger has probably been exaggerated. In the largest reported series, patients who developed the lupus syndrome had no worse a long-term prognosis than patients who did not develop such toxicity.

Minoxidil

Minoxidil is an investigational vasodilator that has been effective in patients whose blood pressure could not be controlled on any other oral regimen. The drug appears to have the same mechanism of action as hydralazine but is more potent (Gottlieb, Katz and Chidsey, 1972).

Following oral administration, the peak plasma level of minoxidil is achieved in 1 h. The administration of isotopically labelled minoxidil is followed by the accumulation of radioactivity in vascular tissue, the site of its pharmacologic effect. The half-life of the drug in plasma appears to be about 4 h but, based on the linear decay of pharmacologic effect with time, the effective half-life of the drug at its site of action is 24 h. About 10 per cent of the drug appears in the urine as the parent compound, and a further 85 per cent of the drug is excreted as various metabolites during six days following therapy.

As with hydralazine, minoxidil's lowering of peripheral vascular resistance is associated with reflex heart stimulation and sodium retention (Dormois, Young and Nies, 1975). Pulmonary hypertension has been reported in some minoxidil-treated patients with high output, right-sided heart failure and gross fluid overload but careful studies of pulmonary artery pressures before and after minoxidil have not confirmed drug-induced pulmonary hypertension (Klotman et al, 1977). With minoxidil therapy over one to two weeks, a small increase in renal blood flow with no change in glomerular filtration has been found. Marked sodium retention on the order of 20 to 40 mEq/day has been seen in minoxidil-treated patients who had no renal impairment. This is felt to be mediated by increased reabsorption from the proximal renal tubule. This sodium retention can be controlled by diuretics in patients with unimpaired renal function, but may be refractory even to furosemide in patients with moderate renal failure.

Like hydralazine, minoxidil reflexly stimulates the release of renin and the addition of propranolol to the regimen results in a more potent antihypertensive effect. In such a combination minoxidil often controls blood pressure when all other therapeutic agents have failed (Pettinger and Mitchell, 1973).

Minoxidil has not yet been implicated in causing the lupus syndrome. The major adverse effect so far has been increased hair growth.

The marketing of the drug has been delayed because its use in dogs is associated with a right atrial lesion. No such lesions have been found in any other animal species or in man. If the drug is approved for the market, its use probably should be initially limited to those patients who do not respond to conventional medications.

Diazoxide

Diazoxide is an analogue of the thiazide diuretics which differs considerably from them in its clinical effects. It promotes retention of sodium and water rather than diuresis and it has a powerful direct effect on the vascular smooth muscle to lower peripheral resistance (Thirlwell and Zsoter, 1972). By relaxing uterine smooth muscle as well, the drug can interrupt labour (Landesman et al, 1968) but some have found no difficulty in using diazoxide to treat hypertension associated with labour (Michael, 1972). The action on vascular (and much non-vascular) smooth muscle may be mediated by competitive antagonism of calcium. Responses of vascular smooth muscle to many stimulations including angiotensin and noradrenaline are reduced.

Diazoxide is about 90 per cent protein-bound. The administration of a rapid bolus of the drug has been advocated as a means of transiently achieving a critical fraction of free drug to saturate receptor sites in the vascular wall (Sellers and Koch-Weser, 1969; Mroczek et al, 1971). However, since there is now evidence that the tissue binding of diazoxide is acutely reversible and that the degree of antihypertensive effect observed is proportional to the achieved plasma diazoxide level, the rapid bolus regimen appears to be less critical to blood pressure control than was formerly assumed (Powell et al, 1971; Johnson and Kapur, 1972; Lee et al, 1975; Boerth and Long, 1977). The drug is partly metabolised and partly excreted unchanged. Its half-life is approximately 24 h and its duration of action is 2 to 24 h (Dayton et al, 1975).

In the light of recent information (Nies, 1975) it is unwise to give all patients 300 mg boluses of diazoxide since some will become dangerously hypotensive with this amount. A more cautious approach is to administer 75 mg intravenously (this alone will control blood pressure in some patients), and then give 150 mg at 5-min intervals until control is achieved.

Blood pressure reductions of 15 to 35 per cent in malignant hypertension are often achieved. In patients with less severe hypertension, 300 mg of diazoxide over 10 min reduces blood pressure an average of 16 per cent.

Diazoxide therapy leads to reduction in glomerular filtration rate and renal blood flow (Hamby et al, 1968; Johnson, 1971). Plasma renin activity is stimulated. Because of reduced peripheral vascular resistance in the face of unaltered right atrial pressure, there is an increase in cardiac output, heart rate and myocardial oxygen demand. Thus it should not be used in patients with ischaemic heart disease. Diazoxide also induces hyperglycaemia (with low serum immunoreactive insulin levels) and hyperuricaemia (Updike and Harrington, 1969). A hypertrichosis occurs only when it is given chronically.

Prazosin

Although introduced into therapy as a vasodilator, there is increasing evidence that much of prazosin's pharmacologic effect is through alpha-adrenoceptor blockade (Cavero, Leférre and Roach, 1977). The drug also possesses phosphodiesterase inhibiting activity (Hess, 1974) and appears to have a direct effect on smooth muscle (Constantine et al, 1973). It blocks vasconstrictor effects of norepinephrine and epinephrine (Wood, Phelan and Simpson, 1975).

Prazosin lowers supine and upright blood pressures, but the greater effect is on the upright blood pressure (Bolli, Wood and Simpson, 1976). Fluid retention occurs and may blunt the antihypertensive effect (Koshy et al, 1977). Postural hypotension occurring 1 to 2 h after the first few doses of prazosin has been the major side effect: loss of consciousness has occasionally occurred. Palpitations, headache, drowsiness, nausea, lack of energy, and weakness have also been seen.

The ultimate place of prazosin in antihypertensive therapy remains to be established.

Nitroprusside

Nitroprusside is the most potent and predictably effective parenteral drug available for rapid control of severe hypertension regardless of aetiology. The hypotensive effect is attributed to the nitroso (–NO) group which dilates both arteries and veins. Unlike hydralazine, minoxidil and diazoxide, nitroprusside increases venous capacitance. Thus it reduces preload as well as afterload and heart rate is not substantially increased. Left ventricular and diastolic pressure is reduced and an improvement in left ventricular function occurs in patients in heart failure. Unlike the ganglionic blocker trimethaphan, nitroprusside reduces both preload and afterload without blocking autonomic transmission.

Because of its rapid onset of action and short half-life, nitroprusside can provide minute-to-minute control of blood pressure in hypertensive emergencies. It has also been used in management of aortic aneurysm (usually with beta-blockade), in refractory heart failure, and in ergotamine toxicity. When it is used for controlled hypotension during anesthesia, arterial P_{O_2} may drop, though not usually to dangerous levels (Wildsmith, Drummond and MacRae, 1975). In patients with heart failure, nitroprusside will often increase cardiac output (Guiha et al, 1974) while in subjects without failure the output remains stable or decreases slightly (Schlant, Tsagaris and Robertson, 1962; Bhatia and Fröhlich, 1973).

Renal blood flow and the glomerular filtration rate are maintained, and renin secretion is increased during the use of this drug. Angina is often improved as nitroprusside is given. This effect is in marked contrast to that of other arteriolar vasodilators that do not affect veins.

Nitroprusside is administered by constant intravenous infusion and requires continuous monitoring by a physician or nurse in the setting of an intensive care unit. The patient's blood pressure can be easily titrated to almost any level by altering the rates of infusion.

The drug decays rapidly particularly when exposed to light and the light brown solution will darken as decomposition occurs. The infusion bottle should therefore be covered with opaque wrapping and new solution prepared every 4 h. Usually 50 to 100 mg of the water-soluble sodium nitroprusside is diluted in 500 ml of 5 per cent dextrose in water and therapy initiated at 0.5 μg/kg/min with titration to higher doses according to the blood pressure response. The doses required are variable and average 200 μg/min. Tolerance or unresponsiveness to the drug is rare (Tuzel, 1974). However, sustained administration of doses greater than 10 μg/kg/min may lead to toxicity, particularly if renal failure is present.

The drug is converted into cyanide and thiocyanate in the body. The half-life of thiocyanate is one week in patients with normal renal function. Thus accumulation of thiocynate is a major problem in prolonged therapy with this agent. Thiocyanate toxicity presents as weakness, aphasia, psychoneurosis, slurred speech, muscle twitching, sweating and tinnitus and may progress to stupor. It occurs when serum levels of thiocyanate exceed 10 mg per cent. Hypothyroidism, probably due to thiocyanate, has been described in a patient with renal failure. If nitroprusside therapy must be continued beyond 48 h, daily thiocyanate levels should be obtained. The risk of toxicity is great with plasma levels of 10 to 12 mg per cent and the drug ought to be discontinued at this point. Toxicity has been observed with serum thiocyanate levels as low as 5 mg per cent.

Cyanide toxicity can also occur with high infusion rates ($\leftarrow$ 20 μg/kg/min) resulting in a falling blood pH, a high venous P_{O_2} and elevated lactate/pyruvate ratio. Several deaths due to probable cyanide toxicity have been reported (David et al, 1975; Merrifield and Blundell, 1974; Vesey, Cole and Simpson, 1976).

At the commencement of therapy some patients have had side effects such as diaphoresis, hyperventilation, vomiting, apprehension and yawning. These have been attributed to medullary ischaemia from excessive hypotension and are an indication for reduction or temporary discontinuation of therapy. Blood pressure usually returns to pretreatment levels within 10 min of discontinuation of the drug.

Diuretics

Severe sodium restriction will lower the blood pressure of many but not all hypertensive patients (Kempner, 1948) even as serum noradrenaline levels rise (Robertson et al, 1977). Diuretics probably exert their beneficial effects by altering sodium balance. Acute diuretic therapy usually lowers blood volume and cardiac output, but with chronic therapy, the cardiac output returns to normal, peripheral resistance falls, and there is a persistent small reduction in extracellular water and plasma volume (Leth et al 1970; Tarazi, Dustan and Fröhlich, 1970; Dustan, Poravo and Tarazi, 1973). These changes are similar to those occurring with severe sodium restriction.

The thiazide diuretics and the pharmacologically similar chlorthalidone and quinethazone are antihypertensive agents of intermediate potency. Small doses that have little effect on serum electrolytes (e.g. 25 mg hydrochlorothiazide daily) may have about as much antihypertensive action as huch higher doses (Degnbol, Dorph and Marner, 1973; Bengtsson et al, 1975).

The decreased peripheral resistance induced by thiazide therapy was initially felt to be due both to the diuresis and to a direct action on arteriolar smooth muscle (Peters, 1966; Tobian, 1967). The observation that the non-diuretic analogue diazoxide also had antihypertensive effect strengthened this view. However, diuretics do not produce any effects on haemodynamics in anephric animals (Coleman et al, 1970; Freis, 1976), and it seems likely that for the thiazide diuretics, no clinically significant action on smooth muscle occurs.

None of the available thiazide diuretics is superior to the other in its toxic/therapeutic ratio or antihypertensive effect. However, the 'loop' diuretics are considerably more potent as diuretics. In spite of this, it has not been demonstrated that with equivalent sodium depletion, the antihypertensive potency of the loop diuretics differs from that of thiazide diuretics. The 'loop' diuretics are most useful as antihypertensive adjuncts in situations where there is reduced glomerular filtration.

The side effects of diuretic therapy include hyperuricaemia, hypokalaemia, hyperglycaemia and occasional hypercalcaemia. Diuretic therapy may also be associated with small increases in serum cholesterol and triglycerides (Ames and Hill, 1976). Rare cases of pancreatitis, interstitial nephritis, and allergic reactions have been described with both thiazides and the loop diuretics. The potassium depletion with alkalosis can be corrected by concomitant administration of a potassium-sparing diuretic or with potassium chloride. Other potassium salts will not correct the alkalosis and until alkalosis is corrected potassium repletion will not occur (Schwartz, van Ypersele de Strihou and Kassirer, 1968). Liquid preparations of potassium chloride are preferable in such a situation. Hyperglycaemia is also helped by the potassium supplement (McFarland and Carr, 1977). Since small-bowel ulceration has occurred with the new wax-matrix preparation of potassium chloride, further experience is necessary to determine the magnitude of the risk associated with its use (Farquharson-Roberts, Giddings and Nunn, 1975; Hutcheon, 1976).

The aldosterone antagonist spironolactone and the aldosterone-independent drugs triamterene and amiloride are weak diuretics. Of these spironolactone is most widely used in the treatment of hypertension.

The mineralocorticoids such as aldosterone act on the distal tubule to augment reabsorption of sodium and loss of potassium by an exchange mechanism. Spironolactone blocks this effect presumably by binding the mineralocorticoid receptor sites in the renal tubule without evoking the usual sodium–potassium exchange.

Spironolactone has been especially useful in low renin hypertension. It has been postulated that these patients have low renin levels because of excess mineralocorticoid activity not related to aldosterone (which is normal in such patients). However, hydrochlorothiazide appears to work equally well with fewer side effects (Ferguson, Turek and Rovner, 1977).

Spironolactone is usually given in doses of 100 to 500 mg daily. It is frequently given in four divided doses but twice-a-day or even once-a-day regimens are sufficient in most patients. Plasma renin activity often rises during therapy with spironolactone. When propranolol and spironolactone are used together they are significantly more effective in lowering blood pressure than when they are used alone: the combination is associated with a two-fold mean increase in plasma renin activity levels over control values (Weber et al, 1977).

Because of its potassium-sparing properties, it must be used cautiously in renal failure. Other adverse effects of spironolactone include drowsiness, muscle weakness and occasionally gynaecomastia.

THE INDIVIDUALISATION OF ANTIHYPERTENSIVE THERAPY

During the past half century major advances in antihypertensive therapy have primarily been discoveries of more potent drugs with fewer side effects. Widespread acceptance of a new drug was usually motivated by a desire to minimise the side effects of normalising blood pressure with an older drug.

With the categorisation of essential hypertensive subjects by renin-profiling and 'vasoconstrictor-volume analysis' (Laragh, 1976), attempts are being made to individualise antihypertensive therapy on a more positive basis (Koch-Weser, 1974). Thus patients with volume-dependent hypertension, primarily those with LREH, would be treated initially with diuretics while those with vasoconstriction-dependent hypertension (usually subjects with HREH or NREH) would initially receive propranolol or another drug that either lowers plasma renin activity or reduces sympathetic tone by a central or peripheral effect.

Such an approach constitutes a departure from the trend of the 1960s to begin each hypertensive subject on a diuretic as the first-line drug. Indeed, perhaps only 20 per cent of essential hypertensive subjects would initially receive diuretics if only subjects with LREH are started out on these drugs. The majority of hypertensive subjects would be begun on beta-blockade.

It seems clear that LREH patients respond more readily to diuretics than do HREH subjects, and conversely, that HREH patients respond more readily to propranolol than do LREH subjects. However, it is equally clear that the majority of essential hypertensive subjects will have blood pressure reduction no matter which drug is used. What is still not known is whether HREH subjects whose blood pressure is controlled by diuretics have a less favourable prognosis than those controlled by propranolol and whether LREH subjects whose blood pressure is controlled by propranolol have a less favourable prognosis than those controlled by diuretics. The answers to such questions will require considerably more clinical experience than we presently have, especially since great gaps still exist in our understanding of whom as well as how to treat (Alderman, 1977).

Since there is now a large body of evidence suggesting the validity of vasoconstrictor-volume analysis as defined by renin-sodium profiling, it is probably helpful to consider such data before instituting therapy in the mild to moderate hypertensive patient. However, as an adjunct or as an alternative, considerable attention should be directed to the hypertensive patient's clinical status, for the potential toxicities of the diuretics and propranolol in the individual may, in a substantial proportion of patients suggest the most appropriate initial therapy.

Thus the insulin-dependent diabetic should be started on diuretics since they will not attenuate his perception of hypoglycaemia. The asthmatic or the patient with chronic obstructive pulmonary disease should also receive diuretics initially rather than propranolol. The patient with congestive failure and hypertension again should be a candidate for diuretic therapy, even though many patients with congestive failure will have increased renin levels. On the other hand, the maturity-onset diabetic not yet on insulin may find his serum glucose is more easily controlled when he is on propranolol than when he is on diuretics.

Finally, the use of salt-restriction as an antihypertensive regimen still has much to recommend it (Meneely and Battarbee, 1976) as 'initial' therapy of hypertension.

REFERENCES

Ablad, B. (1963) A study of the mechanism of the haemodynamic effects of hydralazine in man. *Acta pharmacologica et toxicologica*, **20** Suppl. 1, 1–53.

Alarcon-Segovia, D., Wakim, K.G., Worthington, J. W. & Ward, L.E. (1967) Clinical and experimental studies on the hydralazine syndrome and its relationship to system lupus erythematosus. *Medicine*, **46**, 1–33.

Alderman, M. H. (1977) High blood pressure: do we really know whom to treat and how? *New England Journal of Medicine*, **296**, 753–755.

Altura, B. M. (1975) Pharmacological effects of alpha-methyldopa, alpha-methylnorepinephrine, and octopamine on rat arteriolar, arterial and terminal vascular smooth muscle. *Circulation Research*, **36**, Suppl. 1, 223–246.

Amer, M. D. (1975) Cyclic nucleotides in disease: on the biochemical etiology of hypertension. *Life Sciences*, **17**, 1021–1038.

Ames, R. P. & Hill, P. (1976) Elevation of serum lipid levels during diuretic therapy of hypertension. *American Journal of Medicine*, **61**, 748–757.

Anderson, G. H., Streeten, D. H. P. & Dalakos, T. G. (1977) Pressor response to 1-Sar-8-Ala-angiotensin II (saralasin) in hypertensive subjects. *Circulation Research*, **40**, 243–250.

Armstrong, B., Stevens, N. & Doll, R. (1974) Retrospective study of the association between use of rauwolfia derivatives and breast cancer in English women. *Lancet*, ii, 672–675.

Au, W. Y. W., Drig, L. G., Grahame-Smith, D. G., Isaac, P. & Williams, R. T. (1972) The metabolism of ^{14}C-labelled alpha-methyldopa in normal and hypertensive human subjects. *Biochemical Journal*, **129**, 1–10.

Axelrod, J. (1962) Purification and properties of phenylethanolamine-N-methyl transferase. *Journal of Biological Chemistry*, **237**, 1657–1660.

Bath, J., Pickering, D. & Turner, R. (1967) Clinical experience with bethanidine in treatment of hypertension. *British Medical Journal*, **4**, 519–521.

Bauer, G. E. (1970) Debrisoquine, a five year study of a new hypotensive agent. *Medical Journal of Australia*, **2**, 911–916.

Bengtsson, C., Johnsson, G., Sannerstedt, R. & Werko R. (1975) Effect of different doses of chlorthalidone on blood pressure, serum potassium, and serum urate. *British Medical Journal*, i, 197–199.

Berglund, G., Andersson, O., Hansson, L. & Olander, R. (1973) Propranolol given twice daily in hypertension. *Acta medica scandanavica*, **194**, 513–515.

Bhatia, S. K. & Fröhlich, E. D. (1973) Hemodynamic comparison of agents useful in hypertensive emergencies. *American Heart Journal*, 55, 365–373.

Bianchi, G., Campolo, L., Veceto, H., Pietra, V. & Piazza, U. (1970) Value of plasma renin concentration per se, and in relation to plasma and extracellular fluid volume in diagnosis and prognosis of human renovascular hypertension. *Clinical Science*, **39**, 559–576.

Blaine, E. H., David, J. O. & Prewitt, R. L. (1971) Evidence for a renal vascular receptor in control of renin secretion. *American Journal of Physiology*, **220**, 1593–1597.

Boerth, R. C. & Long, W. R. (1977) Dose-response relation of diazoxide in children with hypertension. *Circulation*, **56**, 1062–1066.

Bolli, P., Wood, A. J. & Simpson, F. O. (1976) Effects of prazosin in patients with hypertension. *Clinical Pharmacology and Therapeutics*, **20**, 138–141.

Boston Collaborative Drug Surveillance Program (1974) Reserpine and breast cancer. *Lancet*, ii, 669–671.

Brackett, N. C., Jr, Koppel, M., Randall, R. E. & Nixon, W. P. (1968) Hyperplasia of the juxtaglomerular complex with secondary aldosteronism without hypertension (Bartter's syndrome). *American Journal of Medicine*, **44**, 803–819.

Branch, R. A. & Shand, D. G. (1976) Propranolol disposition in chronic liver disease: a physiological approach. *Clinical Pharmacokinetics*, **1**, 264–276.

Bravo, E. L., Khosla, M. C. & Bumpus, F. M. (1976) The role of angiotensins in aldosterone production. *Circulation Research*, **38**, Suppl. II, 104–107.

Briant, R. H., Reid, J. L. & Dollery, C. T. (1973) Interaction between clonidine and desipramine in man. *British Medical Journal*, i, 522–523.

Brod, J., Horbach, L., Just, H., Rosenthan, J. & Nicolescu, R. (1972) Acute effects of clonidine on central and peripheral haemodynamics and plasma renin activity. *European Journal of Clinical Pharmacology*, **4**, 107–114.

Brodie, B. B., Chang, C. C. & Costa, E. (1965) On the mechanism of action of guanethidine and bretylium. *British Journal of Pharmacology*, **25**, 171–178.

Brown, J. J., Lever, A. F., Robertson, J. I. S. & Schalekamp, M. A. (1974). Renal abnormality of essential hypertension. *Lancet*, ii, 320.

Brunjes, S. (1964) Catecholamine metabolism in essential hypertension. *New England Journal of Medicine*, **271**, 120.

Bucher, T. J., Buckingham, R. E., Finch, L. & Moore, R. A. (1973) Studies on the central hypotensive effects of clonidine. *Journal of Pharmacology and Pharmacokinetics*, **25**, 1398.

Bühler, F. R., Furkart, F., Lütold, B. E., Kung, M., Marbet, G. & Pfisterer, M. (1975) Antihypertensipe beta blocking action as related to renin and age: a pharmacologic tool to identify pathogenetic mechanisms in essential hypertension. *American Journal of Cardiology*, **36**, 653–669.

Bühler, F. R., Laragh, J. H., Vaughan, E. D., Brunner, H. R., Gavras, H. & Baer, L. (1973) Antihypertensive action of propranolol. *American Journal of Cardiology*, **32**, 511.

Burn, J. H. (1975) *The Autonomic Nervous System*. 5th ed, pp. 3–70. Oxford: Blackwell.

Carey, R. M., Douglas, J. G., Schweikert, J. R. & Liddle, G. W. (1972) The syndrome of essential hypertension and suppressed plasma renin activity. *Archives of Internal Medicine*, **130**, 849–854.

Carlsson, A. A. (1966) Pharmacological depletion of catecholamine stores. *Pharmacology Review*, **18**, 541–549.

Carstairs, K. C., Breckenridge, A., Dollery, C. T. & Worlledge, S. M. (1966) Incidence of positive direct Coombs' test in patients on alpha methyldopa. *Lancet*, **ii**, 133–135.

Case, D. G., Wallace, J. M., Keim, H. J., Weber, M. A., Drayer, J. M., White, R. P., Sealey, J. F. & Laragh, J. H. (1976) Estimating renin participation in hypertension: superiority of converting enzyme inhibitor over saralasin. *American Journal of Medicine*, **61**, 790, 796.

Case, D. G., Wallace, J. M., Keim, H. J., Weber, M. A., Sealey, J. E. & Laragh, J. H. (1977) Possible role of renin in hypertension as suggested by renin–sodium profiling and inhibition of converting enzyme. *New England Journal of Medicine*, **296**, 641–646.

Cass, R. & Spriggs, T. L. B. (1961) Tissue amine levels and sympathetic blockade after guanethidine and bretylium. *British Journal of Pharmacology*, **17**, 442–450.

Cavero, I., Leférre, F. & Roach, A. (1977) Further studies on cardiovascular effects of Prazosin (abstract). *Federation Proceedings*, **36** (3), 955.

Chalmers, J. P., Korner, P. I. & White, S. W. (1967) The relative roles of the aortic and carotid sinus nerves in the rabbit in the control of respiration and circulation during arterial hypoxia and hypercapnia. *Journal of Physiology (London)*, **188**, 435.

de Champlain, J., Mueller, R. A. & Axelrod, J. (1969) Subcellular localisation of monoamine oxidase in rat tissue. *Journal of Pharmacology and Experimental Therapeutics*, 339–345.

Chang, C. C., Costa, E. & Brodie, B. B. (1965) Interaction of guanethidine with adrenergic neurons. *Journal of Pharmacology and Experimental Therapeutics*, **147**, 303–312.

Chidsey, C. A., Braunwald, E., Morrow, A. G. & Mason, D. T. (1963) Myocardial norepinephrine concentration in man: effects of reserpine and of congestive heart failure. *New England Journal of Medicine*, **269**, 653–658.

Chrysant, S. G., Nishiyama, K., Adamopoulos, P. N. & Fröhlich, E. D. (1975) Systemic hemodynamic effects of bethanidine in essential hypertension. *Circulation*, **52**, 137–140.

Coleman, T. G., Bower, J. D., Langford, H. G. & Guyton, A. C. (1970) Regulation of arterial pressure in the anephric state. *Circulation*, **42**, 509–514.

Conolly, M. E., Briant, R. H., George, C. F. & Dollery, C. T. (1972) A crossover comparison of clonidine and methyldopa in hypertension. *European Journal of Clinical Pharmacology*, **4**, 222–227.

Constantine, J. W., McShane, W. K., Scriabine, A. & Hess, H. J. (1973) Analysis of the hypotensive action of prazosin. In *Hypertension: Mechanisms and Management*, ed. Onesti, G., Kim, K. E. & Moyer, J.H. pp. 429–444. New York: Grune and Stratton, Inc.

Crout, J. R., Pisano, J. J. & Sjoerdsma, A. (1961) Urinary excretion of catecholamines and their metabolites in pheochromocytoma. *American Heart Journal*, **61**, 375.

Cuche, J-L., Kuchel, O., Barbeau, A., Langlois, Y., Boucher, R. & Genest, J. (1974) autonomic nervous system and benigh essential hypertension in man. *Circulation Research*, **35**, 281–289.

Dahlström, A., Fuxe, K. & Hillarp, N.-A. (1965) Site of action of reserpine. *Acta pharmacologica et toxicologica*, **22**, 277–292.

Davies, D. W., Kadar, D., Steward, D. J. & Munro, I. R. (1975) A sudden death associated with the use of sodium nitroprusside for induction of hypotension during anaesthesia. *Canadian Anaesthetist Society Journal*, **22**, 553–560.

Day, M. D. & Rand, M. J. (1964) Some observations on the pharmacology of alpha-methyldopa. *British Journal of Pharmacology*, **22**, 72–86.

Dayton, P. G., Pruitt, A. W., Faraj, B. A. & Israili, Z. H. (1975) Metabolism and disposition of diazoxide. *Drug Metabolism and Disposition*, **3**, 226–229.

Dean, R. H. & Foster, J. H. (1973) Criteria for the diagnosis of renovascular hypertension. *Surgery*, **74**, 926–930.

Degnbol, B., Dorph, S. & Marner, T. (1973) The effect of different diuretics on elevated blood pressure and serum potassium. *Acta medica scandinavica*, **193**, 407–410.

DeQuattro, V., Campese, V., Miura, Y. & Meijer, D. J. (1976) Increased plasma catecholamines in high renin hypertension. *American Journal of Cardiology*, **38**, 801–804.

Dissman, T. H., Gotzen, R., Muller, B. et al (1967) Plasma and red blood cell volume in incipient essential hypertension. *Verhandlungen der Deutschen Gesellschaft für innere Medizin*, **73**, 604–607.

Dollery, C. T. (1976) Current status of labetalol. *British Journal of Clinical Pharmacology*, **3**, 823–824.

Dollery, C. T., Davies, D. S., Draffan, G. H., Dargie, H. J., Dean, C. R., Reid, J. L., Clare, R. A. & Murray, S. (1976) Clinical pharmacology and pharmacokinetics of clonidine. *Clinical Pharmacology and Therapeutics*, **19**, 11–17.

Dormois, J. C., Young, J. L. & Nies, A. S. (1975) Minoxidil in severe hypertension: value when conventional drugs have failed. *American Heart Journal*, **90**, 360–368.

Drayer, J. I. M., Keim, H. J., Weber, M. A., Case, D. B. & Laragh, J. H. (1976) Unexpected pressor responses to propranolol in essential hypertension. *American Journal of Medicine*, **60**, 897–903.

Drayer, J. I. M., Kloppenberg, P. W. C., Festen, J., Van't Laar, A. & Benraad, T. J. (1975) Inpatient comparison of treatment with chlorthalidone, spironolactone and propranolol in normoreninemic essential hypertension. *American Journal of Cardiology*, **36**, 716–721.

Dustan, H. P., Bravo, E. L. & Tarazi, R. C. (1973) Volume-dependent essential and steroid hypertension. *American Journal of Cardiology*, **31**, 606–615.

Dustan, H. P., Tarazi, R. C. & Bravo, E. L. (1972) Dependence of arterial pressure on intravascular volume in treated hypertensive patients. *New England Journal of Medicine*, **286**, 861–866.

Engelman, K., Portnoy, B. & Sjoerdsma, A. (1970) Plasma catecholamine concentrations in patients with hypertension. *Circulation Research*, **27** Suppl I, 141–145.

Erdös, E. G. (1976) Conversion of angiotensin I to angiotensin II. *American Journal of Medicine*, **60**, 749, 759.

Esler, M., Julius, S., Zweifler, A., Randall, O., Harburg, E., Gardiner, H. & DeQuattro, V. (1977) Mild high-renin essential hypertension: neurogenic human hypotension. *New England Journal of Medicine*, **296**, 405–411.

Von Euler, E. V. & Hillarp, N.Å. (1956) Evidence for the presence of noradrenaline in submicroscopic structures of adrenergic axons. *Nature (London)*, **177**, 44–45.

Exley, K. A. (1954) Depression of autonomic ganglia by barbiturates. *British Journal of Pharmacology and Chemotherapy*, **9**, 170–181.

Farquharson-Roberts, M. A., Giddings, A. E. B. & Nunn, A. J. (1975) Perforation of small bowel due to slow release potassium chloride (Slow-K). *British Medical Journal*, **iii**, 206.

Ferguson, R. K., Rothenberg, R. J. & Nies, A. S. (1976) Patient acceptance of guanethidine as therapy for mild to moderate hypertension. A comparison with reserpine. *Circulation*, **54**, 32–37.

Ferguson, R. K., Turek, D. M. & Rovner, D. R. (1977) Spironolactone and hydrochlorothiazide in normal-renin and low-renin essential hypertension. *Clinical Pharmacology and Therapeutics*, **21**, 62–69.

Freis, E. D. (1965) Guanethidine. *Progress in Cardiovascular Disease*, **8**, 183–193.

Freis, E. D. (1960) Hemodynamics of hypertension. *Physiological Reviews*, **40**, 27–54.

Freis, E. D. (1976) Salt, volume and the prevention of hypertension. *Circulation*, **53**, 589–595.

Frölich, J. C., Hollifield, J. W., Dormois, J. C., Frölich, B. L., Seyberth, H., Michelakis, A. M. & Oates, J. A. (1976) Suppression of plasma renin activity by indomethacin in man. *Circulation Research*, **39**, 447–452.

Gaffney, T. E., Sigell, L. T., Mohammed, S. & Atkinson, A. J., Jr, (1969) The clinical pharmacology of antihypertensive drugs. *Progress in Cardiovascular Disease*, **12**, 52–71.

Gavras, H., Brunner, H. R., Thurston, H. & Laragh, J. H. (1975) Reciprocation of renin dependency with sodium volume dependency in renal hypertension. *Science*, **188**, 1316–1217.

Gavras, H., Ribeiro, A. B., Gavras, I. & Brunner, H. R. (1976) Reciprocal relation between renin dependency and sodium dependency in essential hypertension. *New England Journal of Medicine*, **295**, 1278–1283.

Genest, J. (1968) The value of the angiotensin infusion test in the diagnosis of true renovascular hypertension. *American Heart Journal*, **76**, 443–444.

Gibaldi, M., Levy, G. & Weintraub, H. (1971) Drug distribution and pharmacologic effects. *Clinical Pharmacology and Therapeutics*, **12**, 734–742.

Gilmore, E., Weil, J. & Chidsey, C. (1970) Treatment of essential hypertension with a new vasodilator in combination with beta-adrenergic blockade. *New England Journal of Medicine*, **282**, 521–527.

Gitlow, S. E., Mendlowitz, M., Bertani, L. M., Wilk, E. K. & Glabman, S. (1969) Tritium excretion of normotensive subjects after administration of tritiated norepinephrine. *Journal of Laboratory Clinical Medicine*, **73**, 129.

Glontz, G. E. & Saslaw, S. (1968) Methyldopa fever. *Archives of Internal Medicine*, **122**, 445–447.

Goodfriend, T. L. & Peach, M. J. (1975) Angiotensin III: (Des-aspartic acid[1])-angiotensin II. Evidence and speculation for its role as an important agonist in the renin–angiotensin system. *Circulation Research*, **36**, Suppl. 1, 38–48.

Gottlieb, T. B., Katz, F. H. & Chidsey, C. A. (1972) Combined therapy with vasodilator drugs and beta-adrenergic blockade. A comparative study of minoxidil and hydralazine. *Circulation*, **45**, 571–582.

Greenblatt, D. J. & Koch-Weser, J. (1973) Adverse reactions to propranolol in hospitalised medical patients. *American Heart Journal*, **86**, 478–484.

D

Guiha, N. H., Cohn, J. N., Mikulic, E., Franciosa, J. A. & Limas, C. J. (1974) Treatment of refractory heart failure with infusion of nitroprusside. *New England Journal of Medicine*, **291**, 587–592.

Gulati, O. D., Dave, B. T., Gokhale, S. D. & Shah, K. M. (1966) Antagonism of adrenergic neuron blockade in hypertensive subjects. *Clinical Pharmacology and Therapeutics*, **7**, 510–514.

Gupta, N. & McNay, J. L. (1972) Rapid control of hypertension with oral bethanidine. *European Journal of Clinical Pharmacology*, **4**, 217–221.

Guyton, A. C., Coleman, T. G., Cowley, A. W., Scheel, K. W., Manning, R. D. & Norman, R. A. (1972) Arterial pressure regulation. Overriding dominance of the kidneys in long-term regulation and in hypertension. *American Journal of Medicine*, **52**, 584–594.

Haefely, N., Hürlimann, A. & Thoenen, H. (1966) The effect of stimulation of sympathetic nerves in the cat treated with reserpine, alpha-methyldopa and alpha-methylmetatyrosine. *British Journal of Pharmacology*, **26**, 172–185.

Haeusler, G. (1975) Cardiovascular regulation by central adrenergic mechanisms and its alteration by hypotensive drugs. *Circulation Research*, **37**, Suppl. 1, 223–232.

Halushka, P. V. & Keiser, H. R. (1974) Acute effects of alpha-methyldopa on mean blood pressure and plasma renin activity. *Circulation Research*, **35**, 458–463.

Hamby, W. M., Janowski, G. P., Pouget, J. M., Dunea, G. & Gantt, C. L. (1968) Intravenous use of diazoxide in the treatment of severe hypertension. *Circulation*, **37**, 169–174.

Hamet, P., Kuchel, O. & Genest, J. (1973) Effect of upright posture and isoproterenol infusion on cyclic adenosine monophosphate excretion in control subjects and patients with labile hypertension. *Journal of Endocrinology Metabolism*, **36**, 218–226.

Hansson, L., Hunyor, S. N., Julius, S. & Hoobler, S. W. (1973) Blood pressure crisis following withdrawal of clonidine (Catapres, Catepresan), with special reference to arterial and urinary catecholamine levels, and suggestions for acute management. *American Heart Journal*, **85**, 605–610.

Heinonen, O. P., Shapiro, S., Tuominen, L. & Turunen, M. I. (1974) Reserpine use in relation to breast cancer. *Lancet*, **ii**, 675–677.

Heise, A. & Kroneberg, G. (1973) Central nervous alpha-adrenergic receptors and the mode of action of alpha-methyldopa. *Archives of Pharmacology*, **279**, 285–300.

Hellström, R. (1961) Body build, muscular strength and certain circulatory factors in military personnel. *Acta medica scandinavica*, **170**, Suppl. 371, 1–84.

Hess, H. J. (1974) Biochemistry and structure-activity studies with prazocin. In *Prazocin—Evaluation of a New Antihypertensive Agent*, ed. Cotlon, D. W. K., pp. 3–15. Amsterdam: Excerpta Medica Foundation.

Hökfelt, B., Hedeland, H. & Dymling, J. F. (1970) Studies on catecholamines, renin and aldosterone following Catepresen R (2-(2,6-dichlor-phenylamine)-2-imidazoline hydrochloride) in hypertensive patients. *European Journal of Pharmacology*, **10**, 389–397.

Hoefke, W. & Warnke-Sachs, E. (1974) Influence of desmethylimipramine on the hypotensive effect of clonidine. *Arzneimittel-Forschung (Drug Research)*, **24**, 1046–1047.

Hollifield, J. W. (1976) The incidence of low renin essential hypertension in Davidson County, Tennessee, hypertensives. *Journal of Tennessee Medical Association*, **69**, 102–109.

Hollifield, J. W. (1977) Personal communication.

Hollifield, J. W., Sherman, K., Vander Zwagg, R. & Shand, D. G. (1976) Proposed mechanisms of propranolol's antihypertensive effect in essential hypertension. *New England Journal of Medicine*, **295**, 68–73.

Hollifield, J. W. & Wilson, H. M. (1976) The hypertensive effects of saralasin. *Journal of Tennessee Medical Association*, **69**, 491.

Hoobler, S. W. & Sagastume, E. (1971) Clonidine hydrochloride in the treatment of hypertension. *American Journal of Cardiology*, **28**, 67–73.

Horwitz, D., Pettinger, W. A., Orvis, H. & Sjoerdsma, A. (1967) Effects of methyldopa in fifty hypertensive patients. *Clinical Pharmacology and Therapeutics*, **8**, 224–234.

Horwitz, D., Lovenberg, W., Engelman, K. & Sjoerdsma, A. (1964) Mononoamine oxidase inhibitors, tyramine and cheese. *Journal of the American Medical Association*, **188**, 1108–1110.

Horwitz, D. & Sjoerdsma, A. (1964) Effects of alpha-methyl-metatyrosine intravenously in man. *Life Science*, **3**, 41–48.

Howard, J. & Connor, T. B. (1962) Hypertension produced by unilateral renal disease. *Archives of Internal Medicine (Chicago)*, **109**, 8–17.

Hunt, J. C., Sheps, S. G., Harrison, E. G., Jr, Strong, C. G. & Bernatz, P. E. (1974) Renal and renovascular hypertension. A reasoned approach to diagnosis and management. *Archives of Internal Medicine*, **133**, 988–999.

Hutcheon, D. E. (1976) Benefit–risk factors associated with supplemental potassium therapy. *Journal of Clinical Pharmacology*, **16**, 85–87.

Janowsky, D. S., El-Yousef, M. K., Davis, J. M., Fann, W. E. & Oates, J. A. (1972) Guanethidine antagonism by antipsychotic drugs. *Journal of the Tennessee Medical Association*, **65**, 620–622.

Johnson, B. F. (1971) Diazoxide and renal function in man. *Clinical Pharmacology and Therapeutics*, **12**, 815–824.

Johnson, B. F. & Kapur, M. (1972) The influence of rate of injection upon the effects of diazoxide. *American Journal of Medical Science*, **263**, 418–488.

Julius, S. & Esler, M. (1975) Autonomic nervous cardiovascular regulation in borderline hypertension. *American Journal of Cardiology*, **36**, 685–696.

Julius, S., Randall, O. S., Esler, M. D. et al (1975) Altered cardiac responsiveness and regulation in the normal cardiac output type of borderline hypertension. *Circulation Research*, **36**, (37), Suppl. 1, 199–207.

Kane, J., Gregg, I. & Richards, D. A. (1976) A double blind trial of labetalol. *British Journal of Clinical Pharmacology*, **3**, 737–741.

Kempner, W. (1948) Treatment of hypertensive vascular disease with rice diet. *American Journal of Medicine*, **4**, 545–577.

Klotman, P. E., Grim, C. E., Weinberger, M. H. & Judson, W. F. (1977) The effects of minoxidil on pulmonary and systemic hemodynamics in hypertensive man. *Circulation*, 55, 394–400.

Koch-Weser, J. (1974) Individualisation of antihypertensive drug therapy. *Medical Clinics of North America*, **58**, 1027–1036.

Kobinger, W. & Walland, A. (1972a) Evidence for a central activation of a vagal cardiodepressor reflex by clonidine. *European Journal of Pharmacology*, **19**, 203–209.

Kobinger, W. & Walland, A. (1972b) Facilitation of vagal reflex bradycardia by an action of clonidine on central alpha-receptors. *European Journal of Pharmacology*, **19**, 210–217.

Kopin, I. (1964) Storage and metabolism of catecholamines: the role of monoamine oxidase. *Pharmacology Review*, **16**, 179–191.

Kopin, I., Fischer, J. E., Musacchio, J. M., Horst, W. D. & Weise, V. K. (1965) False neurochemical transmitters and the mechanism of sympathetic blockade by monoamine oxidase inhibitors. *Journal of Pharmacology and Experimental Therapeutics*, **147**, 186–193.

Korner, P. I. (1976) Central control of blood pressure: implications in the pathophysiology of hypertension. In *Regulation of Blood Pressure by the Central Nervous System*, ed. Onesti, G., Fernandes, M. & Kim, K.E. New York: Grune & Stratton.

Koshy, M. C., Mickley, D., Bourgoignie, Jr, & Blaufox, M. D. (1977) Physiologic evaluation of a new antihypertensive agent: Prazosin HC1. *Circulation*, 55, 533–537.

Landesman, R., Coutinho, E. M., Wilson, K. H. & Lopes, A. C. V. (1968) The relaxant effect of diazoxide on non-gravid human myometrium in vivo. *American Journal of Obstetrics and Gynecology*, 102, 1080–1084.

Laragh, J. H. (1976) Modern system for treating high blood pressure based on renin profiling and vasoconstrictor-volume analysis: a primary role for beta blocking drugs such as propranolol. *American Journal of Medicine*, **61**, 797–810.

Laska, E. M., Meisner, M., Siegel, C., Fischer, S. & Wanderling, J. (1975), Matched pairs study of reserpine use and breast cancer. *Lancet*, **ii**, 296–300.

Lee, W. R., Mroczek, W. J., Davidov, M. E. & Finnerty, F. A. (1975) Non-emergency use of slow infusions of diazoxide. *Clinical Pharmacology and Therapeutics*, **18**, 154–157.

Lesser, J. M., Israili, Z. H., Davis, D. C. & Dayton, P. G. (1974) Metabolism and disposition of hydralazine-^{14}C in man and dog. *Drug Metabolism and Disposition*, **2**, 351–360.

Leth, A. (1970) Changes in plasma and extracellular fluid volumes in patients with essential hypertension during long-term treatment with hydrochlorothiazide. *Circulation*, **42**, 479–485.

Liddle, G. W. (1975) Is hypertension essential? *Transactions of the Association of American Physicians*, **88**, 55–69.

Lin, E. C. C., Hagihira, H. & Wilson, T. H. (1962) Specificity of the transport system for neutral amino acids in the hamster intestine. *American Journal of Physiology*, **202**, 919–925.

Linden, R. J. (1963) The control of output of the heart. In *Recent Advances in Physiology*, ed. Creese, R., Ch. 10. London: Churchill.

LoBuglio, A. F. & Jandl, J. H. (1967) Nature of alphamethyldopa red-cell antibody. *New England Journal of Medicine*, **276**, 658–665.

Lokhandwala, M. F., Buckley, J. P. & Jandhyala, B. S. (1975) Effect of methyldopa treatment on peripheral sympathetic nerve function in the dog. *European Journal of Pharmacology*, **32**, 170–178.

Louis, W. J., Doyle, A. E. & Anavekar, S. (1973) Plasma norepinephrine levels in essential hypertension. *New England Journal of Medicine*, **288**, 599–601.

Lowder, S. C., Hamet, P. & Liddle, G. W. (1976) Contrasting effects of hypoglycemia upon plasma renin activity and cyclic AMP in low renin and normal renin hypertension. *Circulation Research*, **38**, 105–108.

Lowder, S. C. & Liddle, G. W. (1975) Effects of guanethidine and methyldopa on a standardised test for renin responsiveness. *Annals of Internal Medicine*, **82**, 757, 760.

Lowenthal, D. T., Briggs, W. A., Gibson, T. P., Nelson, H. & Criksena, W. J. (1974) Pharmacokinetics of oral propranolol in chronic renal disease. *Clinical Pharmacology and Therapeutics*, **16**, 761–769.

Lukas, G. (1973) Metabolism and biochemical pharmacology of guanethidine and related compounds. *Drug Metabolism Research*, **2**, 101–116.

MacDonald, G. J., Boyd, G. W. & Peart, W. S. (1975) Effect of the angiotensin II blocker 1-sar-8-ala-angiotensin II on renal artery clip hypertension in the rat. *Circulation Research*, **37**, 640–646.

Mahomed, F. A. (874) The etiology of Bright's disease and the pre-albuminuric stage. *Medical–Chirurgical Transactions*, **57**, 197.

Mannick, J. A., Huvos, A. & Hollander, W. E. (1969) Post-hydralazine renin release in the diagnosis of renovascular hypertension. *Annals of Surgery*, **170**, 409–415.

Marks, L. S., Maxwell, M. H. & Kaufman, J. J. (1975) Saralasin bolus test. Rapid screening procedure for renin-mediated hypertension. *Lancet*, **ii**, 784–787.

Mason, Dr. & Braunwald, E. (1964) Effects of guanethidine, reserpine and methyldopa on reflex venous and arterial constriction in man. *Journal of Clinical Investigation*, **43**, 1449–1463.

McFarland, K. F. & Carr, A. A. (1977) Changes in the fasting blood sugar after hydrochlorothiazide and potassium supplementation. *Journal of Clinical Pharmacology*, **17**, 13–17.

McMartin, C., Rondel, R. K., Vinter, J., Allan, B. R., Humberstone, P. M., Leishman, A. W. D., Sandler, G. & Thirkettle, J. L. (1970) The fate of guanethidine in two hypertensive patients. *Clinical Pharmacology and Therapeutics*, **11**, 423–431.

Mehta, J. & Cohn, J. N. (1977) Hemodynamic effects of labetalol, an alpha and beta adrenergic blocking agent, in hypertensive subjects. *Circulation*, **55**, 370–375.

Meneely, G. R. & Battarbee, H. B. (1976) High-sodium–low-potassium environment and hypertension. *American Journal of Cardiology*, **38**, 768–785.

Merguet, P., Heimsoth, V., Murata, T. & Bock, K. D. (1968) Experimental study on the circulatory effects of 2-(2,6-dichlorophenylamino)-2-imidazoline-hydrochloride in man. *Pharmacologica clinica*, **1**, 30–37.

Merrifield, A. J. & Blundell, M. D. (1974) Toxicity of sodium nitroprusside. *British Journal of Anaesthesia*, **46**, 324.

Meyer, P. (1976) Summary of current studies on angiotensin induced aldosterone release. *Circulation Research*, **38**, Suppl. II, 127–128.

Michael, C. A. (1972) The control of hypertension in labour. *Australia and New Zealand Journal of Obstetrics and Gynaecology*, **12**, 48–54.

Michelakis, A. M., Caudle, J. & Liddle, G. W. (1969) In vitro stimulation of renin production by epinephrine, norepinephrine, and cyclic AMP. *Proceedings Society of Experimental Biology and Medicine*, **130**, 748–753.

Michelakis, A. M., Foster, J. H., Liddle, G. W., Rhamy, R. K., Kuchel, O. & Gordon, R. D. (1967) Measurement of renin in both renal veins: its use in diagnosis of renovascular hypertension. *Archives of Internal Medicine (Chicago)*, **120**, 444–448.

Michelakis, A. M. & McAllister, R. M. (1972) The effect of chronic adrenergic receptor blockade on plasma renin activity in man. *Journal of Clinical Endocrinology Metabolism*, **34**, 386–394.

Michelakis, A. M. & D. H. Robertson (1970) Plasma renin activity and levodopa in Parkinson's disease. *Journal of the American Medical Association*, **213**, 83–87.

Michelakis, A. M. & Simmons, J. (1969) Effect of posture on renal vein renin activity in hypertension: its implications in the management of patients with renovascular hypertension. *Journal of the American Medical Association*, **208**, 659–662.

Mizukoshi, H. & Michelakis, A. M. (1972) Evidence for the existence of a sensitising factor to pressor agents in the plasma of hypertensive patients. *Journal of Clinical Endocrinology Metabolism*, **34**, 1016–1024.

Mitchell, J. R., Cavanaugh, J. H., Arias, L. & Oates, J. A. (1970) Guanethidine and related agents. III. Antagonism by drugs which inhibit the norepinephrine pump in man. *Journal of Clinical Investigation*, **49**, 1596–1604.

Mitchell, J. R. & Oates, J. A. (1970) Guanethidine and related agents. I. Mechanism of the selective blockade of adrenergic neurons and its antagonism by drugs. *Journal of Pharmacology and Experimental Therapeutics*, **172**, 100–107.

Mohammed, S., Gaffney, T. E., Yard, C. A. & Gomez, H. (1968a) Effect of methyldopa, reserpine and guanethidine on hindleg vascular resistance. *Journal of Pharmacology and Experimental Therapeutics*, **160**, 300–307.

Mohammed, S., Hanenson, I. B., Magenheim, H. G. & Gaffney, T. E. (1968b) The effects of alpha-methyldopa on renal function in hypertensive patients. *American Heart Journal*, **76**, 21–27.

Morin, Y., Turmel, L. & Fortier, J. (1964) Methyldopa: clinical studies in arterial hypertension. *American Journal of Medical Science*, **248**, 633–639.

Mroczek, W. J., Davidov, M. & Finnerty, F. A. (1973) Intravenous clonidine in hypertensive patients. *Clinical Pharmacology and Therapeutics*, **14**, 847–851.

Mroczek, W. J., Leibel, B. A., Davidov, M. & Finnerty, F. A. (1971) The importance of the rapid administration of diazoxide in accelerated hypotension. *New England Journal of Medicine*, **285**, 603–606.

Muscholl, E. & Maitre, L. (1963) Release by sympathetic stimulation of alpha-methylnoradrenaline stored in the heart after administration of alpha-methyldopa. *Experientia*, **19**, 658–659.

Nagatsu, T., Levitt, M. & Udenfriend, S. (1964) Tyrosine hydroxylase: the initial step in norepinephrine biosynthesis, *Journal of Biology and Chemistry*, **239**, 2910–2917.

Nathan, M. A. & Reis, D. J. (1977) Chronic labile hypertension produced by lesions of the nucleus tractus solitarii in the cat. *Circulation Research*, **40**, 72–81.

Nestel, P. J. & Doyle, A. E. (1968) The excretion of free noradrenaline and adrenaline by healthy young subjects and by patients with essential hypertension. *Australian Annals of Medicine*, **17**, 295–299.

Nies, A. S. (1975) Adverse reactions and interactions limiting the use of antihypertensive drugs. *American Journal of Medicine*, **58**, 495–503.

Nies, A. S., McNeil, J. S. & Schrier, R. W. (1971) Mechanism of increased sodiumreabsorption during propranolol administration. *Circulation*, **44**, 596–604.

Nies, A. S. & Shand, D. G. (1975) Clinical pharmacology of propranolol. *Circulation*, **52**, 6–15.

Oates, J. A., Gillespie, L., Udenfriend, S. & Sjoerdsma, A. (1960) Decarboxylase inhibition and blood pressure reduction by alpha-methyl-3,4-dihydroxy-d, 1-phenylalanine. *Science*, **131**, 1890–1891.

Oates, J. A., Mitchell, J. R., Feagin, O. T., Kaufmann, J. S. & Shand, D. G. (1971) Distribution of guanidinium antihypertensives — mechanism of their selective action. *Annals of New York Academy of Sciences*, **179**, 302–308.

Oates, J. A., Seligman, A. W., Clark, M. A., Rousseau, P. & Lee, R. E. (1965) The relative efficacy of guanethidine, methyldopa and pargyline as antihypertensive agents. *New England Journal of Medicine*, **273**, 729–724.

O'Fallon, W. M., Labarthe, D. R. & Kurland, L. T. (1975) Rauwolfia derivatives and breast cancer. *Lancet*, **ii**, 292–296.

O'Malley, K., Segal, J. L., Israili, Z. H., Boles, M., McNay, J. L. & Dayton, P. G. (1975a) Duration of hydralazine action in hypertension. *Clinical Pharmacology and Therapeutics*, **18**, 581–586.

O'Malley, K., Velasco, M., Pruitt, A. & McNay, J. L. (1975b) Decreased plasma protein binding of diazoxide in uremia. *Clinical Pharmacology and Therapeutics*, **18**, 53–58.

Onesti, G., Bock, K. D., Hermsoth, V., Kim, K. E. & Merguet, P. (1971) Clonidine: a new antihypertensive agent. *American Journal of Cardiology*, **28**, 74–83.

Oparil, S. & Haber, E. (1974) The renin–angiotensin system. *New England Journal of Medicine*, **291**, 389–401.

Padfield, P. L., Brown, J. J., Lever, A. F., Schalekamp, M. A. D., Beevers, D. G., Davies, D. L., Robertson, J. I. S., Tree, M. & Titterington, M. (1975) Is low-renin hypertension a stage in the development of essential hypertension or a diagnostic entity. *Lancet*, **i**, 548–550.

Passon, P. G. & Peulor, J. D. (1973) A simplified radiometric assay for plasma norephinephrine and epinephrine. *Analytical Biochemistry*, **51**, 618–631.

Peart, W. S. (1975) Renin–angiotensin system. *New England Journal of Medicine*, **292**, 302–306.

Perry, H. M., Tan, E. M., Carmody, S. & Sakamato, A. (1970) Relationship of acetyl transferase activity to antinuclear antibodies and toxic symptoms in hypertensive patients treated with hydralazine. *Journal of Laboratory and Clinical Medicine*, **76**, 114–125.

Perry, H. M. (1973) Late toxicity to hydralazine resembling systemic lupus erythematosis or rheumatoid arthritis. *American Journal of Medicine*, **54**, 58–72.

Peters, W. G. (1966) Pharmacology of diuretics. In *Antihypertensive Therapy, Principles and Practices*: An International Symposium. ed. Gross, F. pp. 31–57. Berlin: Springer-Verlag.

Pettinger, W. A. (1975) Clonidine, a new antihypertensive drug. *New England Journal of Medicine*, **293**, 1179–1180.

Pettinger, W. A. & Keeton, K. (1975) Altered renin release and propranolol potentiation of vasodilatory drug hypotension. *Journal of Clinical Investigation*, **55**, 236–243.

Pettinger, W. A., Keeton, T. K., Campbell, W. B. & Harper, D. C. (1976) Evidence for a renal alpha-adrenergic receptor inhibitory on renin release. *Circulation Research*, **38**, 338–346.

Pettinger, W. A., Keeton, K. & Tanaka, K. (1975) Radioimmunoassay and pharmacokinetics of saralasin in the rat and hypertensive patients. *Clinical Pharmacology and Therapeutics*, **17**, 146–158.

Pettinger, W. A. & Mitchell, H. C. (1973) Minoxidil—an alternative to nephrectomy for refractory hypertension. *New England Journal of Medicine*, **289**, 161–171.

Pettinger, W. A. & Oates, J. A. (1968) Supersensitivity to tyramine during monoamine oxidase inhibition in man: mechanism at the level of the adrenergic neuron. *Clinical Pharmacology and Therapeutics*, **9**, 341–344.

Podolsky, S. & Pattavina, C. G. (1973) Hyperosmolar non-ketotic diabetic coma: a complication of propranolol therapy. *Metabolism*, **22**, 685–693.

Porte, D., Jr, (1967) A receptor mechanism for the inhibition of insulin release by epinephrine in man. *Journal of Clinical Investigation*, **46**, 86–94.

Porte, D., Jr (1969) Sympathetic regulation of insulin excretion: its relation to diabetes mellitus. *Archives of Internal Medicine*, **123**, 252–260.

Powell, W. J., Green, R. M., Whiting, R. B. & Sanders, C. A. (1971) Action of diazoxide on skeletal muscle vascular resistance. *Circulation Research*, **28**, 167–178.

Poynter, D., Martin, L. E., Harrison, C. & Cook, J. (1976) Affinity of labetalol for ocular melanin. *British Journal of Clinical Pharmacology*, **3**, 711–721.

Prichard, B. N. C. & Gillam, P. M. S. (1964) Use of propranolol in treatment of hypertension. *British Medical Journal*, **ii**, 725.

Prichard, B. N. C. & Gillam, P. M. S. (1969) Treatment of hypertension with propranolol. *British Medical Journal*, **i**, 7–16.

Prichard, B. N. C., Johnstone, A. W., Hill, I. D. & Rosenheim, M. L. (1968) Bethanidine, guanethidine and methyldopa in treatment of hypertension: a within-patient comparison. *British Medical Journal*, **1**, 135–144, 1968.

Prichard, B. N. C., Thompson, F. D., Boakes, A. M. & Joekes, A. M. (1975) Some hemodynamic effects of compound AH 5158 compared with propranolol, propranolol plus hydrallazine and diazoxide: the use of AH 5158 in the treatment of hypertension. *Clinical Science and Molecular Medicine*, **48**, 79s–100s.

Purves, M. J. (1972) *The Physiology of the Cerebral Circulation*. Cambridge: University Press.

Raftos, J., Bauer, G. E., Lewis, R. G., Stokes, G. S., Mitchell, A. S. & Young, A. A. (1973) Clonidine in the treatment of severe hypertension. *Medical Journal of Australia*, **1**, 786–793.

Rahn, K. H. & Goldberg, L. I. (1969) Comparison of antihypertensive efficacy, intestinal absorption, and excretion of guanethidine in hypertensive patients. *Clinical Pharmacology and Therapeutics*, **10**, 858–866.

Rehman, O. U., Keith, T. A. & Gall, E. A. (1973) Methyldopa-induced submassive hepatic necrosis. *Journal of American Medical Association*, **224**, 1390–1392.

Reid, I. A., MacDonald, D. M., Pachnis, B. & Ganong, W. F. (1975) Studies concerning the mechanism of suppression of renin secretion by clonidine. *Journal of Pharmacology and Experimental Therapeutics*, **192**, 1713–1721.

Reid, J. L., Briant, R. H. & Dollery, C. T. (1973) Desmethylimipramine and the hypotensive action of clonidine in the rabbit. *Life Science*, **12**, Part I, 459–467.

Reidenberg, M. M., Drayer, D., DeMarco, A. & Bello, C. T. (1973) Hydralazine elimination in man. *Clinical Pharmacology and Therapeutics*, **14**, 970–977.

Richards, D. A., Tuckman, J. & Prichard, B. N. C. (1975) Assessment of alpha- and beta-adrenoceptor blocking actions of labetalol. *British Journal of Clinical Pharmacology*, **2**, 342–343.

Richards, D. A., Woodings, E. P. & Maconochie, J. G. (1977) Comparison of the effects of labetalol and propranolol in healthy men at rest and during exercise. *British Journal of Clinical Pharmacology*, **4**, 15–21.

Robertson, D. H., Johnson, G. A., Brilis, G. M., Hill, R. E., Watson, J. T. & Oates, J. A. (1977) Salt restriction increases serum catecholamines and urinary normetanephrine excretion (Abstract). *Federation Proceedings*, **36** (3), 956.

Robertson, D. H. & Michelakis, A. M. (1972) Effect of anesthesia and surgery on plasma renin activity in man. *Journal of Clinical Endocrinology and Metabolism*, **34**, 831–836.

Robertson, D. H. & Michelakis, A. M. (1975) The effect of chlorpromazine on plasma renin activity and aldosterone in man. *Journal of Clinical Endocrinology and Metabolism*, **41**, 1166–1171.

Rodman, J. S., Deutsch, D. J. & Gutman, S. I. (1976) Methyldopa hepatitis. *American Journal of Medicine*, **60**, 941–948.

Rowe, G. G., Huston, J. H., Maxwell, G. M., Crosley, A. P., Jr. & Crumpton, C. W. (1955) Hemodynamic effects of 1-hydrazinopthalazine in patients with arterial hypertension. *Journal of Clinical Investigation*, **34**, 115–120.

Safar, M. E., Weiss, Y. A., Levenson, J. A., London, G. M. & Milliez, P. A. (1973) Hemodynamic study of 85 patients with borderline hypertension. *American Journal of Cardiology*, **31**, 315–317.

Sanan, S. & Vogt, M. (1962) Effect of drugs on the noradrenalin content of brain and peripheral tissue and its significance. *British Journal of Pharmacology*, **18**, 109–126.

Schambelan, M., Glickman, M., Stockigt, J. R. & Biglieri, E. C. (1974) Selective renal-vein renin sampling in hypertensive patients with segmental renal lesions. *New England Journal of Medicine*, **290**, 1153–1157.

Schlant, R. C., Tsagaris, T. S. & Robertson, R. J. (1962) Studies on the acute cardiovascular effects of intravenous sodium nitroprusside. *American Journal of Cardiology*, **9**, 51–59.

Schwartz, W. B., van Ypersele de Strihou, C. & Kassirer, J. P. (1968) Role of anions in metabolic alkalosis and potassium deficiency. *New England Journal of Medicine*, **279**, 630–639.

Sellers, E. M. & Koch-Weser, J. (1969) Protein binding and vascular activity of diazoxide. *New England Journal of Medicine*, **281**, 1141–1145.

Sennett, J. A. (1974) Low renin essential hypertension. *Journal of Tennessee Medical Association*, **67**, 212–214.

Shand, D. G. (1974) Pharmacokinetic properties of the beta-adrenergic receptor blocking drugs. *Drugs*, **7**, 39–47.

Shand, D. G. (1975) Drug therapy. Propranolol. *New England Journal of Medicine*, **293**, 280–285.

Shand, D. G., Morgan, D. H. & Oates, J. A. (1973) The release of guanethidine and bethanidine by splenic nerve stimulation: a quantitative evaluation showing dissociation from adrenergic blockade. *Journal of Pharmacology and Experimental Therapeutics*, **184**, 73–80.

Shand, D. G., Nies, A. S., McAllister, R. G. & Oates, J. A. (1975) A loading-maintenance regimen for more rapid initiation of the effect of guanethidine. *Clinical Pharmacology and Therapeutics*, **18**, 139–144.

Shen, D., Gibaldi, M., Throne, M., Bellward, G., Cunningham, R., Israili, Z. & McNay, J. (1975)

Pharmacokinetics of bethanidine in hypertensive patients. *Clinical Pharmacology and Therapeutics*, **17**, 363–373.

Silas, J. F., Lennard, M. S., Tucker, G. T., Smith, A. J., Malcolm, S. L. & Marten, T. R. (1977) Why hypotensive patients vary in their response to oral debrisoquine. *British Medical Journal*, **1**, 422–425.

Simpson, F. O. (1974) Beta-adrenergic receptor blocking drugs in hypertension. *Drugs*, **7**, 85–105.

Sjoerdsma, A. (1961) Relationships between alterations in amine metabolism and blood pressure. *Circulation Research*, **9**, 734–743.

Skeggs, L. T., Kahn, J. R., Dorer, F. E. & Lentz, K. D. (1977) Chronic one-kidney hypertension in rabbits. III. Renopressin, a new hypertensive substance. *Circulation Research*, **40**, 143–149.

Spector, S., Gordon, R., Sjoerdsma, A. & Udenfriend, S. (1967) End-product inhibition of tyrosine hydroxylase as a possible mechanism for regulation of norepinephrine synthesis. *Molecular Pharmacology*, **3**, 549–555.

Spector, S., Tarver, J. H. & Berkowitz, B. A. (1971) Disposition and regulation of norepinephrine in blood vessels. In *Physiology and Pharmacology of the Vascular Neuroeffector System*, ed. Bevan, J. A. et al. New York: Karger.

Stamey, T. A. (1963) *Renovascular Hypertension*, p. 200. Baltimore: Williams and Wilkins, Co.

Stason, W. B. & Weinstein, M. C. (1977) Allocation of resources to manage hypertension. *New England Journal of Medicine*, **296**, 732–739.

Stokes, G. S., Weber, M. A., Thornell, I. R., Stokes, L. M. & Sebel, E. F. (1974a) Effects of acute and chronic administration of propranolol on blood pressure and plasma renin activity in hypertensive patients. *Progress in Biochemistry and Pharmacology*, **9**, 29–44.

Stokes, G. S., Weber, M. A. & Thornell, I. R. (1974b) Beta-blockers and plasma renin activity in hypertension. *British Medical Journal*, **i**, 60–62.

Stott, A. W. & Robinson, R. (1967) Urinary normetanephrine excretion in essential hypertension. *Clinica chimica acta*, **16**, 249.

Strandell, T. (1964) Circulatory studies in healthy old men. *Acta medica scandinavica*, **175**, Suppl. 414, 1–44.

Streeten, D. H. P., Anderson, G. H., Freiberg, J. M. & Dalakos, T. G. (1975) Use of an angiotensin II antagonist (Saralasin) in the recognition of 'angiotensinogenic' hypertension. *New England Journal of Medicine*, **292**, 658–662.

Strong, C. G., Hunt, J. C., Sheps, S. G., Tucker, R. M. & Bernatz, P. E. (1971) Renal venous renin activity. Enhancement of sensitivity of lateralisation by sodium depletion. *American Journal of Cardiology*, **27**, 602–611.

Sugarman, S. R., Margolius, H. S., Gaffney, T. E. & Mohammed, S. (1968) Effect of methyldopa on chronotropic response to cardioaccelerator nerve stimulation in dogs. *Journal of Pharmacology and Experimental Therapeutics*, **162**, 115–120.

Sundquist, H., Antilla, M. & Arstila, M. (1974) Antihypertensive effect of practolol and sotalol. *Clinical Pharmacology and Therapeutics*, **16**, 465–472.

Tarazi, R. C. & Dustan, H. P. (1972) Beta adrenergic blockade in hypertension. *American Journal of Cardiology*, **29**, 633–640.

Tarazi, R. C., Dustan, H. P. & Fröhlich, E. D. (1970) Long term thiazide therapy in essential hypertension. Evidence for persistent alteration in plasma volume and renin activity. *Circulation*, **41**, 709–717.

Tarazi, R. C., Fröhlich, E. D. & Dustan, H. P. (1971) Plasma volume changes with long-term beta-adrenergic blockade. *American Heart Journal*, **82**, 770–776.

Tarazi, R. C., Fröhlich, E. D. & Dustan, H. P. (1973) Contribution of cardiac output to renovascular hypertension in man. Relation to surgical treatment. *American Journal of Cardiology*, **31**, 600–605.

Tarazi, R. C., Ibrahin, M. M., Dustan, H. P. et al (1974) Cardiac factors in hypertension. *Circulation Research*, **34**, (35), Suppl. I, 213–243.

Thirlwell, M. P. & Zsoter, T. T. (1972) The effect of diazoxide on the veins. *American Heart Journal*, **83**, 512–517.

Tobian, L. (1967) Why do thiazide diuretics lower blood pressure in essential hypertension? *Annual Review of Pharmacology*, **7**, 399–408.

Toghill, P. J., Smith, P. G., Benton, P., Brown, R. C. & Matthews, H. L. (1974) Methyldopa liver damage. *British Medical Journal*, **iii**, 545–548.

Tuzel, I. H. (1974) Sodium nitroprusside. A review of its clinical effectiveness as a hypotensive agent. *Journal of Clinical Pharmacology*, **14**, 494–503.

Ueda, H., Kaneko, Y., Takeda, T., Ikeda, T. & Yagi, S. (1970) Observations on the mechanism of renin release by hydralazine in hypertensive patients. *Circulation Research*, **27**, Suppl. 2, 201–206.

Ulrych, M., Fröhlich, E. D., Dustan, H. P. & Page, I. H. (1968) Immediate hemodynamic effects of beta-adrenergic blockade with propranolol in normotensive and hypertensive men. *Circulation*, **37**, 411–416.

Updike, S. J. & Harrington, A. R. (1969) Acute diabetic ketoacidosis—a complication of intravenous diazoxide treatment for refractory hypertension. *New England Journal of Medicine*, **280**, 768.

Vander, A. J. (1965) Effect of catecholamines and the renal nerves on renin secretion in anesthetised dogs. *American Journal of Physiology*, **209**, 659–662.

Van Zweiten, P. A. (1973) The central action of antihypertensive drugs mediated via central alpha-receptors. *Journal of Pharmacy and Pharmacology*, **25**, 89–95.

Vesey, C. J., Cole, P. V. & Simpson, P. J. (1976) Cyanide and thiocyanate concentrations following sodium nitroprusside infusion in man. *British Journal of Anaesthesia*, **48**, 651–660.

Veterans' Administration Cooperative Study Group on Antihypertensive Agents (1967) Effect of treatment of morbidity in hypertension: results in patients with diastolic blood pressures averaging 115 through 129 mmHg. *Journal of American Medical Association*, **202**, 1028–1034.

Veterans' Administration Cooperative Study Group on Antihypertensive Agents (1970) Effect of treatment on morbidity in hypertension. II. Results in patients with diastolic blood pressure averaging 90 through 114 mmHg. *Journal of the American Medical Association*, **213**, 1143–1152.

Veterans' Administration Cooperative Study Group on Antihypertensive Agents (1972) Effect of treatment on morbidity in hypertension. III. Influence of age, diastolic pressure, and prior cardiovascular disease; further analysis of side effects. *Circulation*, **45**, 991–1104.

Veterans' Administration Cooperative Study (1977) Multiclinic controlled trial of bethanidine and guanethidine in severe hypertension. *Circulation*, **55**, 519–525.

Waal-Manning, H. J. (1976) Hypertension: which beta-blocker? *Drugs*, **12**, 412–441.

Waal-Manning, H. J. & Simpson, F. O. (1975) Paradoxical effect of pindolol. *British Medical Journal*, **iii**, 155–156.

Walson, P. D., Marshall, K. S., Forsyth, R. P., Rapoport, R., Melmon, K. L. & Castagnoli, N., Jr (1975) Metabolic disposition and cardiovascular effects of methyldopa in unanesthetised rhesus monkeys. *Journal of Pharmacology and Experimental Therapeutics*, **195**, 151–158.

Walter, I. E., Khandelwal, J., Falkner, F. & Nies, A. S. (1975) The relationship of plasma guanethidine levels to adrenergic blockade. *Clinical Pharmacology and Therapeutics*, **18**, 571–580.

Walter, I. E. & Nies, A. S. (1977) Safety of single large oral doses of guanethidine. *Clinical Pharmacology and Therapeutics* (in press).

Warren, D. J. (1976) Beta-adrenergic receptor blockade and renal function. *American Heart Journal*, **91**, 265–266.

Weber, M. A., Lopez-Ovejero, J. A., Drayer, J. I., Case, D. B. & Laragh, J. H. (1977) Renin reactivity as a determinant of responsiveness to antihypertensive treatment. *Archives of Internal Medicine*, **137**, 284–289.

Weber, M. A., Stokes, G. S. & Gain, J. M. (1974) Comparison of the effects on renin release of beta-adrenergic antagonists with differing properties. *Journal of Clinical Investigation*, **54**, 1413–1417.

Weidmann, P., Hirsch, D., Beretha-Piccoli, C., Reubi, F. C. & Ziegler, W. H. (1977) Interrelations among blood pressure, blood volume, plasma renin activity, and urinary catecholamines in benign essential hypertension. *American Journal of Medicine*, **62**, 209–218.

Weinberger, M. H., Aoi, W. & Henry, D. P. (1975) Direct effects of beta-adrenergic stimulation on renin release by the rat kidney slice in vitro. *Circulation Research*, **37**, 318–324.

Weiner, N., Cloutier, G., Bjur, R. & Pfeffer, R. I. (1972) Modification of non-epinephrine synthesis in intact tissue by drugs and during short term adrenergic nerve stimulation. *Pharmacology Research*, **24**, 203–221, 1972.

Wildsmith, J. A. W., Drummond, G. B. & MacRae, W. R. (1975) Blood–gas changes during induced hypotension with sodium nitroprusside. *British Journal of Anaesthesiology*, **47**, 907–908.

Wolf, R. L. (1971) Norepinephrine and aldosterone metabolism in hypertension. *Bulletin of Postgraduate Community Medicine, University of Sydney*, **26**, 56.

Wolf, R. L., Mendlowitz, M., Roboz, J. & Gitlow, S. E. (1965) Simultaneous urinary assay for the combined metanephrine and 3-methoxy-4-hydroxyphenyl-glycol in patients with pheochromocytoma and primary hypertension. *New England Journal of Medicine*, **273**, 1459.

Wolff, F. W. & Lindeman, R. D. (1966) Effects of treatment in hypertension: results of a controlled study. *Journal of Chronic Diseases*, **19**, 227–240.

Wood, A. J., Phelan, E. L. & Simpson, F. O. (1975) Cardiovascular effects of prazosin in normotensive and genetically hypertensive rats. *Clinical Experimental Pharmacology and Physiology*, **2**, 297–304.

Woods, J. W., Liddle, G. W., Stant, E. G., Jr, Michelakis, A. M. & Brill, A. B. (1969) Effect of an adrenal inhibitor in hypertensive patients with suppressed renin. *Archives of Internal Medicine (Chicago)*, **123**, 366–370.

Woosley, R. A., Walter, I., Oates, J. A. & Nies, A. S. (1976) Antagonism of the antihypertensive and sympathoplegic effects of guanethidine by ephedrine in man. *Clinical Research*, **24**, 259A.

Zacest, R. & Koch-Weser, J. (1972a) Relation of propranolol plasma level to beta-blockade during oral therapy. *Pharmacology*, **7**, 178–184.

Zacest, R. & Koch-Weser, J. (1972b) Relation of hydralazine plasma concentration to dosage and hypertensive action. *Clinical Pharmacology and Therapeutics*, **13**, 420–425.

Zacharias, F. J., Cowen, K. J., Presst, J., Vickers, J. & Wall, B. G. (1972) Propranolol in hypertension. A study of long-term therapy, 1964-1970. *American Heart Journal*, **83**, 755–761.

5. Antiarrhythmic drugs

Raymond L. Woosley   T. Zvonko Rumboldt

Despite a considerable understanding of the genesis of arrhythmias in experimental animal models, our ability to identify the mechanisms of an arrhythmia in individual patients or to predict the electrophysiological effects of therapeutic concentrations of antiarrhythmic drugs remains limited. Consequently, the treatment of arrhythmias, especially those of ventricular origin, is usually empiric and far from ideal. In recent years there have been new developments, which can make the use of established drugs more rational and increase the possibility of therapeutic success. However, because the standard anti-arrhythmic drugs have either limited efficacy or severe toxicity, there have also been attempts to develop new drugs for clinical trials. Most are analogues of the older compounds and offer little advantage, but others seem to be distinct improvements. Analogues of lidocaine or procainamide that have high oral bioavailability and prolonged elimination half-life are now being investigated. Numerous compounds with in vitro beta-blocking activity and possible superiority to propranolol are available commercially in Europe and in various stages of clinical testing in the US.

RECENT ADVANCES WITH ESTABLISHED ANTIARRHYTHMIC DRUGS

Quinidine

Quinidine sulphate continues to be a widely used drug for both atrial and ventricular arrhythmias even though many new drugs have become available. Quinidine is generally a myocardial depressant in that it reduces all phases of the action potential and in high concentrations, often within the usual therapeutic range, can cause depression of myocardial contractility and hypertension. However, the vagolytic effects of the drug are responsible for causing increased conduction through the AV node and can thereby increase the ventricular rate in the patient with atrial tachyarrhythmias.

Improved analytical capabilities in recent years have made it possible to study quinidine metabolism and several metabolites have been identified. One of these has been found to have anti-arrythmic activity (Conn and Luchi, 1964) and may contribute to the total therapeutic effects. One problem that has evolved from improved analytical techniques is that the therapeutic window for quinidine which was established using the non-specific assay (Härtel and Harjanne, 1969) measured active drug, active metabolites and inactive metabolites. The newer double extraction method measures only active drug and a new therapeutic window for this assay must be established. Kessler et al (1974) have determined the therapeutic range for 14 patients using the double extraction method and found it to be 2.3 to 5 μg/ml, considerably lower than with older methods. They also compared the two methods in patients with renal or hepatic failure and determined that non-active fluorescent metabolites accumulate at levels of active drug which are not excessive. Their final conclusion was that quinidine dosage should not be reduced in patients with renal failure.

The effects of congestive heart failure upon quinidine kinetics has been examined after oral (Bellet, Roman and Boza, 1971) and intramuscular administration. Analysis of these data by Crouthamel (1975) indicated that congestive heart failure leads to reduction of the rate of absorption and the volume of distribution of the drug. Therefore patients with heart failure may have higher plasma drug levels at some times during chronic therapy. The rate of elimination was not significantly changed by heart failure.

Drug interactions
Data, Wilkinson and Nies (1976) have recently reported an important drug interaction that can potentially reduce the efficacy of quinidine therapy. These investigators reported an increased elimination rate of quinidine after treatment with phenobarbital or phenytoin, presumably due to induction of hepatic oxidative enzymes. Figure 5.1

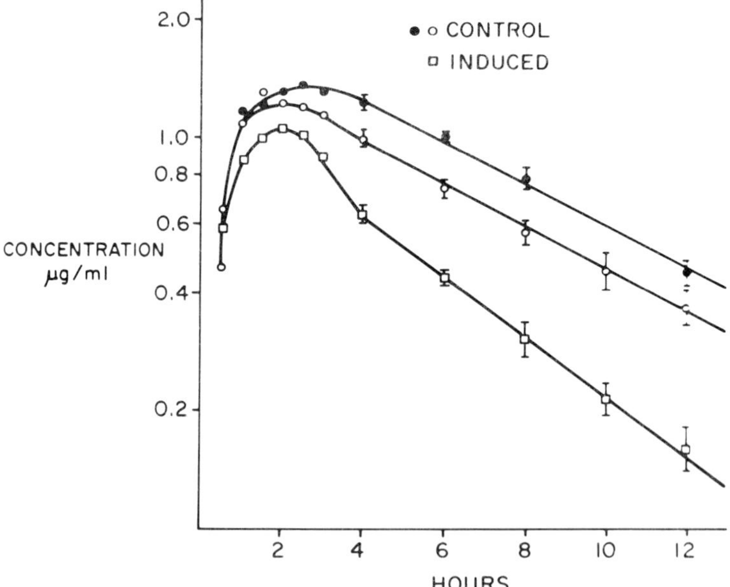

Fig. 5.1 Elimination of quinidine in a normal volunteer before ●, during □, and 2 weeks after ○, administration of phenobarbitone. (Reproduced with permission of the authors, Data et al, 1976)

demonstrates the decrease in elimination half-life in a normal volunteer after treatment with phenobarbital and the return towards normal two weeks after discontinuation of the inducer. Induction of metabolism can change a previously effective dosage to an ineffective one.

Side effects

Diarrhoea usually restricts the usefulness of quinidine and 'quinidine syncope' is not an infrequent adverse effect. Syncope in many cases is most likely due to ventricular tachycardia and can occur with plasma concentrations within or below the usual therapeutic range (Seaton, 1966). Figure 5.2 shows electrocardiographic tracings sampled from continuous recordings of a patient who developed ventricular tachycardia shortly after beginning quinidine therapy for frequent fixed coupled premature ventricular contractions (PVCs). At a plasma concentration of 1.2 μg/ml (below the usual therapeutic range) the patient's ECG showed prolongation of the Q–T interval and

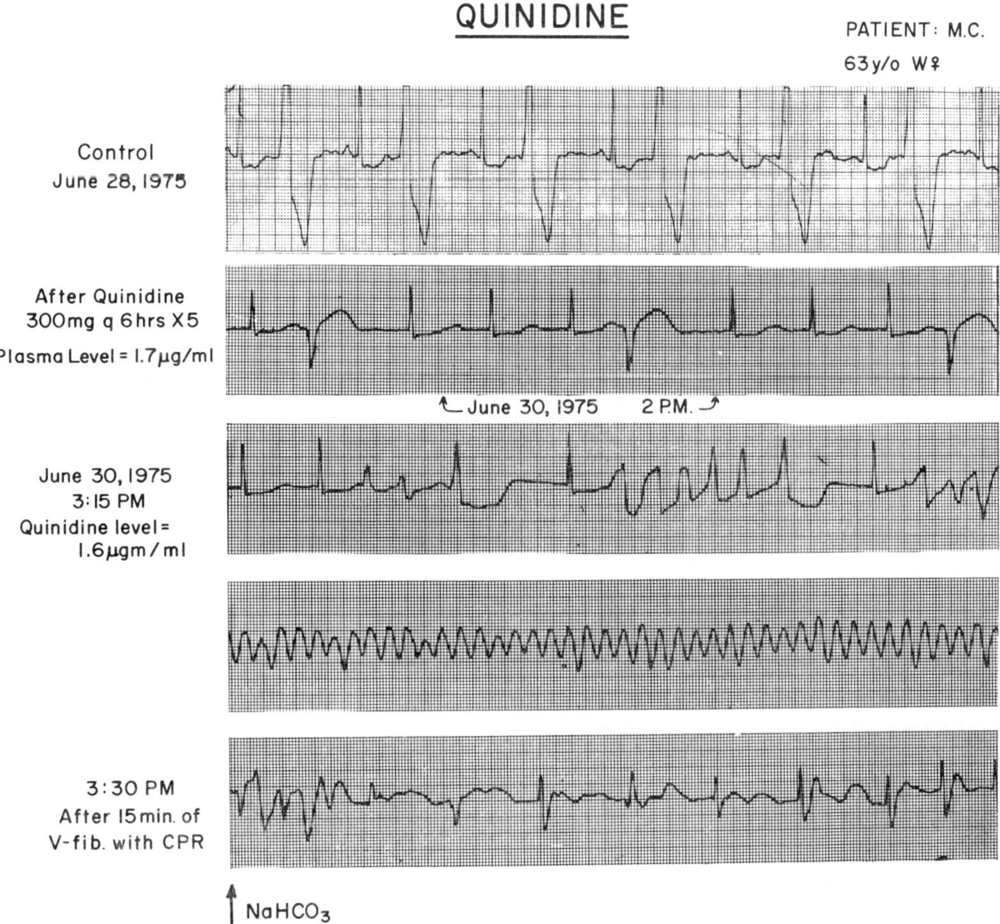

Fig. 5.2   Electrocardiographic tracings selected from continuous recordings of a patient with unifocal PVCs before and after institution of quinidine therapy. (With the permission of the authors and publishers, Woosley et al, 1977a)

development of the R-on-T phenomenon. Seven minutes of alternating ventricular tachycardia and fibrillation followed requiring external cardiac massage. The arrhythmia converted to sinus rhythm after an injection of sodium bicarbonate, an accepted treatment for quinidine toxicity. In the following 18 months this patient continued to have premature ventricular contractions but did not have ventricular tachycardia after quinidine therapy was discontinued. Arrhythmias similar to those seen in this case are probably responsible for most reports of 'quinidine syncope' and could possibly explain the relatively high incidence of sudden death in patients receiving quinidine therapy (Wetherbee, Holzman and Brown, 1952; Seaton, 1966; Reynolds and Vander Ark, 1976).

Procainamide

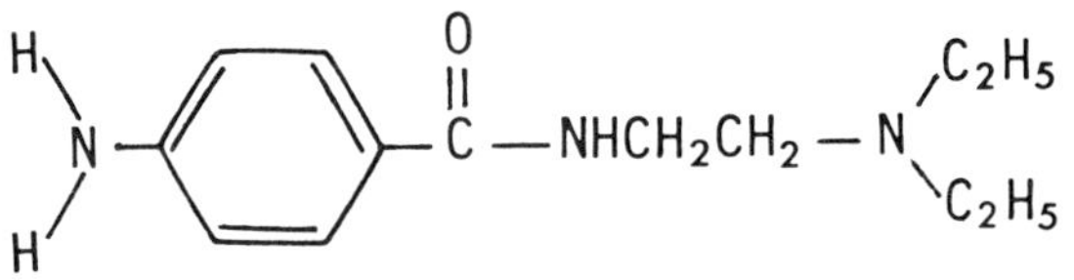

Procainamide is also a very effective drug for control of both ventricular and atrial arrhythmias. Giardina et al (1973) have shown that effective plasma concentrations can be reached rapidly without excessive myocardial depression using a series of small intravenous loading doses followed by a maintenance infusion. They used a loading regimen of 100 mg i.v. given slowly every 5 min until arrhythmia suppression was seen or to a maximum total dose of 1 g. An infusion of 2 to 4 mg/min will usually maintain plasma concentrations in the therapeutic range after such a loading regimen. This infusion rate should be reduced for patients with impaired elimination due to cardiac failure or renal insufficiency (Koch-Weser and Klein, 1971; Weily and Genton, 1972). Blood pressure and the electrocardiogram should be monitored continuously during the loading procedure and regularly during the maintenance infusion. Oral therapy should begin after the infusion has been discontinued for at least 3 h or when the arrhythmias return.

Chronic procainamide therapy frequently leads to a lupus-like syndrome that can be life threatening in some cases and is associated with the development of antinuclear antibodies (Kosowsky et al, 1973; Hope and Bates, 1972; Sunder and Shah, 1975). Like hydralazine, procainamide has been reported to induce the formation of antinuclear antibodies, and perhaps the lupus syndrome, more frequently in patients who are genetically slow acetylators (Henningson et al, 1975; Foad et al, 1977). However, another study found contradictory results regarding the relationship between ANA development and acetylator phenotype (Davies, Beedie and Rawlins, 1975). As shown in Figures 5.3 and 5.4, an increased incidence in slow acetylators in these studies may be an artifact of duration of therapy. Slow acetylators develop antibodies and the lupus syndrome earlier and with a lower total cumulative dose than rapid acetylators (Woosley et al, 1977b). Many patients tolerate procainamide for prolonged periods of time and if other drugs are ineffective, procainamide may be life-saving until alternative therapy becomes available. Since the early symptoms of the lupus syndrome are readily revers-

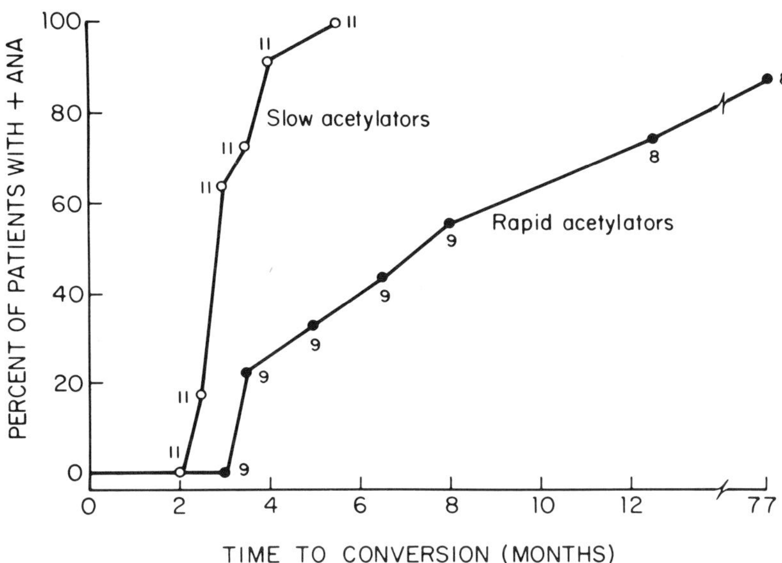

Fig. 5.3 Relationship between acetylator phenotype and the rate of procainamide-induced antinuclear antibodies (ANA). (Reproduced with permission of the authors, Woosley et al, 1977b)

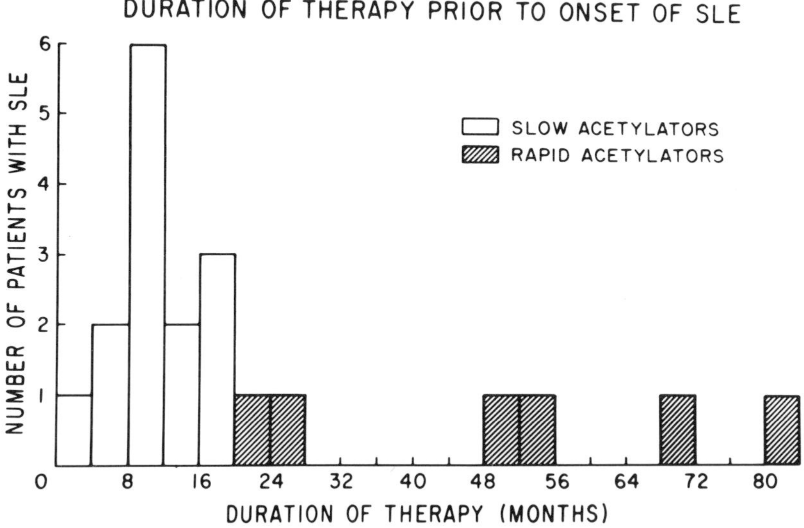

Fig. 5.4 Relationship between acetylator phenotype and the rate of procainamide-induced lupus erythematosus syndrome. (Reproduced with permission of the authors, Woosley et al, 1977b)

ible with discontinuation of therapy, it is important to inform patients of them and to instruct them to report their occurrence.

Accumulation of procainamide in patients with renal insufficiency has been recognised for some time (Weily and Genton, 1972). Recent data has indicated that the pharmacologically active N-acetylated metabolite also depends, almost exclusively, upon the renal route for elimination (see below). Drayer et al (1977) have found extremely high concentrations of N-acetylprocainamide (acecainide) in patients with renal failure who were receiving procainamide chronically. Because acecainide is not measured in the usual spectrophotometric assay (Carr, Woosley and Oates, 1976), the metabolite can accumulate without being detected in the assay. The combination of high concentrations of acecainide and usual concentrations of procainamide was associated with widening of the QRS and hypotension in cases reported by Drayer et al (1977) indicating possible additive toxicity for the two compounds. The degree of acecainide accumulation is dependent upon the patient's acetylator phenotype and the state of renal function. Gibson et al (1976) have recently reported a three-fold variation in haemodialysis clearance of procainamide and acecainide depending upon the type of haemodialysis system utilised. The ranges of clearance for procainamide and acecainide were 37 to 115 ml/min and 28 to 90 ml/min respectively.

Propranolol

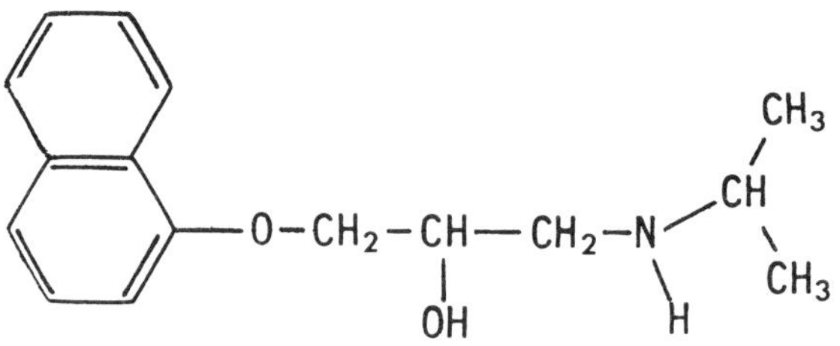

Propranolol was the first beta-adrenergic blocking drug to become clinically available and although many others are now in use in other countries, only propranolol is available in the USA. Propranolol is very useful for treatment of many atrial arrhythmias but has been considered less than optimal treatment for ventricular arrhythmias. Several series have reported that less than 50 per cent of patients with ventricular arrhythmias respond to oral treatment with propranolol at dosages from 40 to 160 mg/day (Winkle et al, 1977; Nagger and Alexander, 1976; Gianelly, Griffin and Harrison, 1967a; Valentine et al, 1974). These studies failed to account for the complex pharmacokinetics and the large interindividual variation in systemic bioavailability of the drug. Evans and Shand (1973) have also shown that only approximately 40 to 50 per cent of patients given these doses will obtain plasma concentrations in the range usually associated with beta-adrenergic blockade. Coltart, Gibson and Shand (1971) have also found that 8 of 12 patients with ventricular arrhythmias respond to intravenous propranolol at plasma concentrations in the range from 40 to 85 ng/ml; that which is generally associated with beta-adrenergic blockade (Coltart and Shand, 1970; Chidsey et al, 1975). However, Woosley et al (1977c) have reported that some ventricular arrhythmias require plasma concentrations between 100 and 1000 ng/ml for suppression; clearly above levels usually associated with beta-adrenergic blockade (Fig. 5.5). The mechanism of action of propranolol in these higher concentrations is unknown but is unlikely to be due to the 'quinidine-like' effects reported from in vitro studies at much higher (ten to thirty-fold) concentrations (Davies and Temte, 1968).

Careful dose ranging and measurement of plasma concentration can decrease the incidence of therapeutic failures with this drug. Because some patients have increased

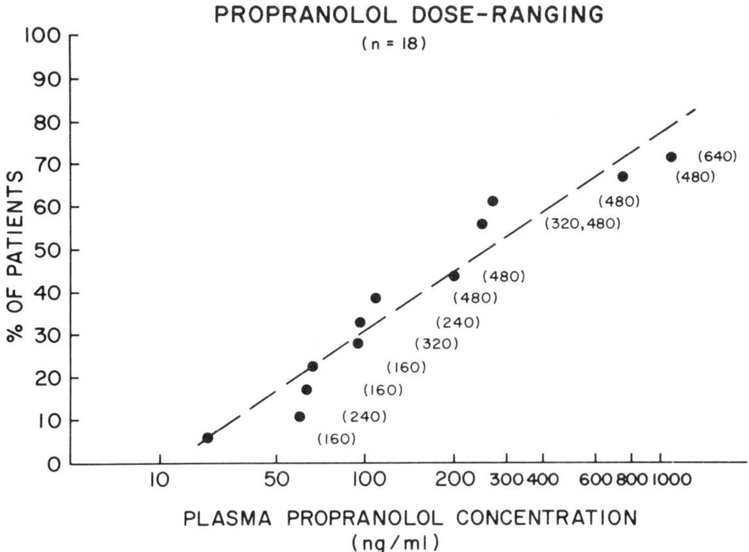

Fig. 5.5   A graded dose–response curve for propranolol therapy of ventricular arrhythmias. Percentage of patients responding versus plasma concentration required for suppression of >80 per cent of PVCs. (Reproduced with permission of the authors, Woosley et al, 1977c)

arrhythmia when treated with increasing doses of propranolol (Woosley et al, 1977c), inadequate documentation of response to therapy may lead one to dose range past the point of maximal arrhythmia suppression. Further definition of the therapeutic plasma concentration range for ventricular arrhythmias is necessary before therapy can be optimised in patients with these arrhythmias. Identification of the precise mechanism of action of propranolol may make it possible to individualise therapy in patients who have arrhythmias of known aetiology or electrophysiological mechanism.

Lignocaine (Lidocaine)

The use of lignocaine for the treatment of ventricular arrhythmias certainly cannot be classified as a recent advance in clinical pharmacology. However, some major therapeutic advances have been made in our understanding of the pharmacokinetics and pharmacodynamics of the drug in normal subjects and in patients with cardiac or renal disease. These findings are of even greater importance since it has been shown that lignocaine can reduce the incidence of, and perhaps eliminate, sudden ventricular fibrillation when given prophylactically to patients during acute myocardial infarction

(Wyman and Hammersmith, 1974; Lie et al, 1974). Because lignocaine has significant and often serious toxicity, it is critical that the drug be administered in a manner that provides maximum benefit and minimum toxicity, especially if large numbers of patients are to receive the drug prophylactically. This can be accomplished if the pharmacokinetics of the drug are considered and the dosage is individualised.

Pharmacokinetics

Because lignocaine has a relatively low therapeutic index (Gianelly et al, 1967b) the proper use of pharmacokinetic principles and individualisation of dosage can facilitate the safe and effective use of the drug. In recent years determination of the pharmacokinetics of lignocaine in normal and diseased states has made it possible to arrive at therapy based upon data instead of on empiricism (Rowland et al, 1971; Stenson, Constantino and Harrison, 1971; Boyes et al, 1971). Lignocaine when administered intravenously behaves according to the kinetics of a linear two-compartment model system (Boyes et al, 1971; Thomson et al, 1969). Dissipation from the central compartment after bolus i.v. administration reflects the combined effects of mixing in the vascular compartment, distribution of the drug to certain tissues such as the heart and brain and to a lesser degree, metabolism. In normal subjects the half-life ($t_{\frac{1}{2}}$) for the central compartment is 8 min and is not altered significantly in diseased states (Thomson et al, 1969). The volume of the central compartment (Vd) in normal subjects ranges from 0.44 to 0.77 litre/kg and decreases to 0.30 litre/kg in patients with heart failure. This smaller volume of the central compartment can cause excessively high levels of lignocaine to occur after rapid injection in patients with heart failure unless a reduced dosage is chosen. After distribution into a peripheral compartment, lignocaine has a second terminal elimination $t_{\frac{1}{2}}$ of approximately 108 min in normal patients that reflects primarily hepatic metabolism and transfer of drug from the peripheral compartment back to the central compartment. The terminal $t_{\frac{1}{2}}$ determines the length of time required to reach steady-state and in normal patients this length of time can be from 6 to 9 h. Because the antiarrhythmic effect of a lignocaine bolus often dissipates as the drug rapidly redistributes to the peripheral compartment, it is a common misconception that lignocaine levels change rapidly under any condition. It is often difficult to convince both clinicians and nurses that the maximum blood level and possible toxic effects of an increased infusion rate can occur as late as 6 to 9 h in normal patients receiving a constant infusion. Patients with congestive heart failure (Stenson, Constantino and Harrison, 1971) or hepatocellular dysfunction (Thomson et al, 1973) have reduced clearance of lignocaine and can accumulate toxic levels of lignocaine if the usual infusion rates are used. Consequently, accumulation to plateau levels will occur in these patients even later than 6 to 9 h required for normal subjects.

Metabolism

The rapid dissipation of drug effect after intravenous injection of lignocaine is primarily due to redistribution in the body (see above) and to hepatic metabolism. The major route of elimination of lignocaine is by hepatic metabolism and at least one of the metabolites, monoethylglycine xylidide (MEGX), has been found to have antiarrhythmic activity (Smith and Duce, 1971). Probably of more importance, another metbolite, glycine xylidide (GX), potentiates the convulsive action of lignocaine and MEGX (Blumer, Strong and Atkinson, 1973). Patients who develop late toxicity during constant lignocaine infusion with low or therapeutic plasma concentrations probably reflects this toxic synergism (Strong, Parkes and Atkinson, 1973).

Haemodynamic effects
Lignocaine has become the drug of choice for acute therapy of ventricular arrhythmias mainly because it can be given intravenously with a very low incidence of adverse effects. Even patients with acute myocardial infarction tolerate rapid intravenous injection in most cases. Dosages from 1 to 2.2 mg/kg given over 0.5 to 1.0 min are tolerated by both normal and cardiac patients without causing depression of ventricular function (Harrison, Sprouse and Morrow, 1963; Binnion et al, 1969; Grossman, Copper and Frieden, 1969; Jewitt, Kishon and Thomas, 1968; Stannard, Sloman and Sangster, 1968). However, excessively rapid intravenous injection has occasionally induced profound bradycardia, sinus arrest, conduction disturbances of hypotension (Jewitt et al, 1968; Lichstein, Chadda and Gupta, 1973; Cheng and Wadhwa, 1973) and the drug should not be given at a rate exceeding 50 mg/min if possible.

Clinical administration
Prior to the availability of pharmacokinetic data, lignocaine was administered in a routine fashion to all patients. Standard orders are often still used for all patients admitted to the coronary care units and usually call for an initial bolus injection of 100 mg for an arrhythmia followed by a 4 mg/min infusion with instructions for the dosage to be tapered by the nursing staff. Tapering is usually based upon the presence or absence of an arrhythmia or toxicity and is subject to variation because of a multitude of factors which might influence the degree of attention available from the nursing staff. There have been several attempts to individualise lignocaine therapy based upon pharmacokinetics principles and data. The most comprehensive protocol has been proposed by Benowitz (1974) and requires a working knowledge of clinical phar-macokinetics. This protocol is most succinctly justified and described by Benowitz in terms readily understandable by even those most averse to mathematics and equations. It involves a series of loading bolus injections designed to initially fill the central compartment and to replace drug as it redistributes to the peripheral compartment. Once loaded the patient can be placed on a maintenance infusion calculated from estimation of his expected clearance and corrected for alterations in clearance due to heart failure or liver disease (see Tables 5.1, 5.2).

Adverse effects upon conduction
The toxic effects of lignocaine upon conduction and automaticity that have been reported have been due to elevated plasma concentration or large doses of the drug in most cases (Lichstein et al, 1973; Cheng and Wadhwa, 1973; Jewitt et al, 1968). Therapeutic levels of lignocaine do not significantly alter A–V conduction or H–V times in most patients with normal (Rosen et al, 1970) or delayed conduction (Bekheit et al, 1973; Kunkel, Rowland and Scheinman, 1974). However, Gupta, Lichstein and Chadda (1974) have reported 4 of 23 patients with bundle branch block who developed complete heart block (2 cases), second degree heart block (1 case) and cardiac standstill (1 case) after 50 to 100 mg of lignocaine. Lignocaine is not felt to be contraindicated in patients with high degrees of intraventricular conduction block but should be used with caution in such patients and the ready availability of a ventricular pacemaker has been recommended (Collingsworth, Kalman and Harrison, 1974; Gupta et al, 1974).

Table 5.1 Protocol to yield plasma lignocaine concentrations of 3 μg/ml

Based on: loading dose = volume of distribution × desired plasma concentration
= 1.32 litres/kg × 3 μg/ml = 3.9 μg/kg

Time (min)	Dose		Normal (μg/kg)	Heart failure (μg/kg)
0	First bolus —	Loads central compartment	1.5	0.9
8	Second bolus —	replaces loss in central compartment in first $t_{1/2}$	0.8	0.4
16	Third bolus —	replaces loss in central compartment in second $t_{1/2}$	0.8	0.4
24	Fourth bolus —	replaces loss in central compartment in third $t_{1/2}$	0.8	0.4
			—	—
		Total body load	3.9	2.1

Table 5.2 Protocol to maintain plasma lignocaine concentration of 3 μg/ml

Based on: dose = desired plasma concentration × clearance
e.g. = 3 μg/ml × 10 ml/min/kg
= 30 μg/kg/min

	Infusion rate (μg/kg/min)
Normal — clearance = 10 ml/min/kg	30
Heart failure — clearance = 6 ml/min/kg	18

Drug interactions

Because lignocaine has a high hepatic extraction ratio, any pharmacological or physiological intervention which alters hepatic blood flow should change dosage requirements for lignocaine. Although drug interactions have not been demonstrated in man to date, animal studies have shown that propranolol (Branch et al, 1973) which decreases cardiac output and hepatic blood flow and noradrenaline (Benowitz, 1974), which reduces hepatic blood flow, decrease lignocaine clearance and increase plasma levels. Other animal studies have shown the lignocaine clearance is increased by phenobarbitone (DiFazio and Brown, 1972), presumably by microsomal enzyme induction and by isoprenaline (Benowitz, 1974) or glucagon (Nies, Shand and Branch, 1973) which increase hepatic blood flow.

Phenytoin

Phenytoin (diphenylhydantoin, Dilantin [R]) is effective for treatment of ventricular arrhythmias in some cases. However, it is rarely effective except in those arrhythmias associated with digitalis toxicity. Phenytoin may have additive or synergistic antiarrhythmic effects when combined with procainamide or propranolol. This would not be predicted from what is known about the electrophysiological effects of these drugs, but Woosley et al (1977a) described 8 of 13 patients whose arrhythmias were not controlled by procainamide or phenytoin alone who responded to the combination with satisfactory arrhythmia suppression. Plasma levels of 10 to 20 μg/ml are considered antiarrhythmic.

NEWER ANTIARRHYTHMIC DRUGS

Tocainide (W-36095)

Lignocaine is an effective antiarrhythmic drug for intravenous usage. However, it has pharmacokinetic characteristics (a high hepatic extraction and thus poor systemic bioavailability and a short half-life) that preclude its effective oral use (Rowland et al, 1971). Two new congeners of lignocaine have been developed and Figure 5.6 shows the structural similarities of the two compounds. In animal studies tocainide was shown to have antiarrhythmic efficacy, good oral bioavailability and a prolonged elimination half-life. McDevitt, Shanks and Prichard, (1976) demonstrated antiarrhythmic effi-

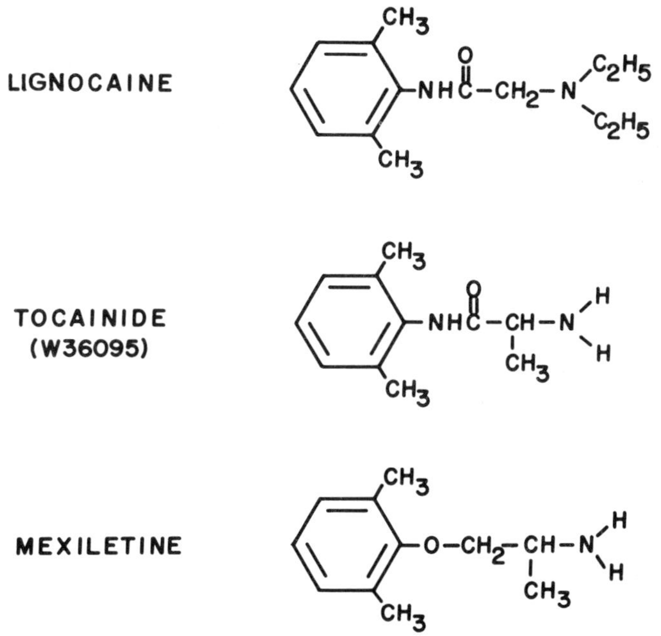

Fig. 5.6   Chemical structure of lignocaine and two of its congeners, tocainide (W36095) and mexiletine

cacy of single doses in patients with premature ventricular contractions. Pharmacokinetic studies have found that the drug has 100 per cent oral bioavailability and a mean elimination half-life of 11 h in normal volunteers (Lalka et al, 1976) and 11 to 22 h in cardiac patients (Winkle et al, 1976; Woosley et al, 1977d). Approximately 40 per cent of the oral dosage is excreted unchanged in the urine. Multiple-dose studies (Winkle et al, 1976; Woosley et al, 1977d) in patients demonstrated suppression of PVCs for 8 to 12 h after dosages of 400 to 1000 mg every 12 h. Antiarrhythmic efficacy was associated with plasma concentrations between 1 and 10 μg/ml. Plasma concentrations between 10 and 15 μg/ml were associated with mild to moderate CNS toxicity. There seems to be a direct association between responsiveness to lignocaine and sensitivity to tocainide. A few patients with life-threatening arrhythmias who could not tolerate or who did not respond to currently available drugs have been treated with tocainide for over a year without evidence of long-term toxicity. However, total experience with the drug is limited at this time and its true clinical utility remains to be determined in studies with larger number of patients of specific arrhythmia aetiology.

Mexiletine (Ko-1173)

Mexiletine is another congener of lignocaine which was found to have local anaesthetic activity and membrane depressant activity in that it reduced the maximum rate of depolarisation of rabbit atrial and ventricular potentials without affecting resting membrane potential or action potential duration (Singh and Vaughan-Williams, 1972a). These same investigators also noted the ability of the drug to suppress experimentally induced ventricular arrhythmias, i.e. those induced by halothane, ouabain, or adrenaline and those after coronary artery ligation (Allen et al, 1970, 1972).

It has near 100 per cent oral bioavailability and a prolonged elimination half-life of 10 to 20 h in cardiac patients. Precise dose-ranging studies have not been performed in large numbers of patients but between 750 and 1000 mg daily in 3 divided doses have been found to suppress ventricular arrhythmias in a variety of patients including those seen after acute myocardial infarction (Talbot et al, 1973; Campbell et al, 1975; Achuff et al, 1976). However 30 to 56 per cent of patients experienced side effects and up to 17 per cent have reported these to be intolerable. When given intravenously, the most serious adverse effects reported were hypotension and bradycardia. Central nervous system side effects were the most common. Unacceptable side effects occurred at plasma concentrations of 3.3 $\pm$ 0.5 μg/ml. CNS side effects occurred at plasma concentrations between 2.25 and 2.75 μg/ml. However, some patients require plasma concentrations approaching 3 μg/ml for antiarrhythmic effects although Campbell et al (1975) estimated the effective plasma concentration to be between 1 and 1.5 μg/ml in 44 patients studied. Therefore the margin between efficacy and toxicity is narrow for mexiletine.

Campbell et al (1975) reported that mexiletine was effective in suppressing arrhythmias previously unresponsive to lignocaine. However, plasma lignocaine concentrations were not measured and, as previously shown by Alderman et al (1974b) lignocaine resistance is often due to subtherapeutic plasma concentrations. Further studies are required to verify this report and to establish the clinical utility of the drug. The high incidence of side effects may limit the usefulness of mexiletine. Mexiletine is available in England and Europe but has not been approved in the US at this time.

Acecainide (N-Acetylprocainamide)

Acecainide was shown to have antiarrhythmic efficacy in animal models (Drayer, Reidenberg and Sevy, 1974; Elson et al, 1975; Bagwell et al, 1976) and recently Lee et al (1976) and Atkinson et al (1977) have demonstrated the ability of acecainide to suppress ventricular ecopic depolarisations in cardiac patients. Because the elimination half-life of acecainide in patients with normal renal function is approximately twice that for procainamide, acecainide may be able to provide sustained antiarrhythmic effect when administered every 6 to 8 h. This would be a distinct advantage over procainamide which must be taken orally every 3 or 4 h by most patients for continuous arrhythmia suppression, an almost impossible regimen.

Because acetylation of procainamide seems to protect against or delay the onset of drug-induced lupus (Woosley et al, 1977b) many have hypothesised that acecainide may not cause this syndrome. Freeman et al (1977) have reported in vitro studies which demonstrate that procainamide is metabolised by mammalian microsomal oxidative enzymes to a highly reactive metabolite which can interact with the DNA of *Salmonella typhimurium* to produce mutations capable of growing in a histidine-free medium. Acecainide or analogues of procainamide without the arylamine group were either less active or inactive in this system. Therefore these data also indicate that acecainide may be less likely to induce the lupus syndrome. However, the final answer will await the results of evaluation of the drug during chronic therapy. Acecainide had recently been approved for testing in the US and the answer may be forthcoming.

Disopyramide

Disopyramide is a chemically unique antiarrhythmic drug which has been found to be effective for suppression of ventricular ectopic contractions and ventricular tachycardia

(Vismara, Mason and Amsterdam, 1974; Danilo and Rosen, 1976; Vismara et al 1977). Electrophysiological studies have found that the drug is similar to quinidine in that it decreased the rate of phase 4 depolarisation, decreased myocardial conduction velocity, prolonged effective and functional refractory periods in the atria, AV node and ventricles (Dean and Ferguson, 1971; Dreifus et al, 1973; Befeler et al, 1975; Yeh, Sung and Scherlag, 1973). However, more recent studies have described other effects which may also be important in disopyramide's antiarrhythmic action. Naylor (1975) found that disopyramide partially inhibited transcellular calcium influx normally occurring during phase 2 of the action potential. Dean (1975) also found that disopyramide has local anaesthetic activity approaching that of lignocaine. Vismara et al (1977) found disopyramide effective for ventricular arrhythmias in patients who had previously been resistant to currently available antiarrhythmic drugs and Danilo and Rosen (1976) found the drug to cause less toxic reactions than quinidine (see below). The drug is considered to be less effective than quinidine for treatment of atrial arrhythmias.

Pharmacokinetics
After i.v. administration the drug rapidly distributes with a $t_{\frac{1}{2}}$ of 3 to 5 min and a $t_{\frac{1}{2}}$ of 5 to 6 h (Karim, 1975). A recent study found the mean $t_{\frac{1}{2}}$ to be 10 h in cardiac patients and increased to 24 h in patients with creatinine clearances <50 ml/min (Rangno et al, 1976). Disopyramide is completely absorbed after oral administration with peak plasma levels obtained at 30 min. The major route of elimination is renal and protein binding is in the range from 21 to 50 per cent (Karim, 1975). The therapeutic range for suppression of ventricular arrhythmias is between 2 and 4 μg/ml (Vismara et al 1974).

Adverse effects
The potential adverse effect of major concern is cardiac depression. Vismara et al (1975) have found that an intravenous injection of disopyramide (2 mg/kg) resulted in a 13 per cent increase in left ventricular end-diastolic pressure and a 12 per cent reduction in cardiac index. Similar results were obtained by Willis (1975) and Vismara et al (1977) who observed dose-related depression of cardiac function in two patients. Therefore, disopyramide, like most antiarrhythmic drugs, must be used with caution in patients with depressed myocardial contractility.

Disopyramide has a prominent anticholinergic action and is reported to increase A–V conduction although it has less effect than quinidine (Mathur, 1972). Mathur (1972) also found that disopyramide did not cause an increase in A–V block even in patients with pre-existing block. Seipel and Breithardt (1976) found an increase in sinus node recovery time in patients with the sick-sinus syndrome and recommended that the drug not be used in patients with this disorder.

The most frequent side effects are due to the anticholinergic side effects of disopyramide. These are not infrequent and consist of nausea, vomiting, urinary retention, blurred vision, dryness of the eyes and mouth (Vismara et al 1977). Urinary retention is common and hypoglyceremia has been noted in patients with liver disease. Danilo and Rosen (1976) compared the incidence of toxicity and adverse effects of disopyramide and quinidine and found these to be less frequent and less severe with disopyramide (9.6 per cent vs. 35.5 per cent for quinidine).

Verapamil

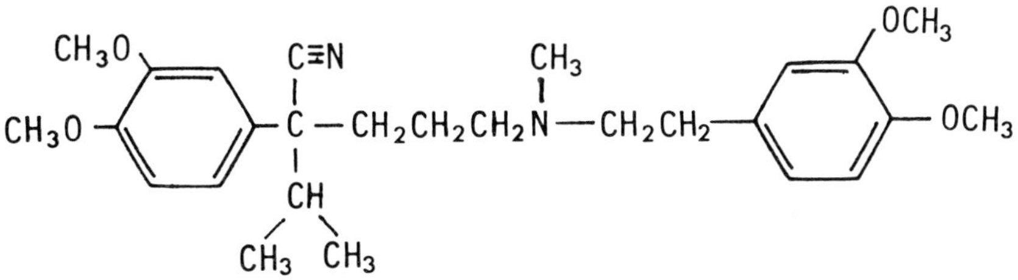

Verapamil is an antiarrhythmic drug with a unique mechanism of action. It is a derivative of papaverine which was initially studied in Europe as an antianginal agent because of its effects as a coronary vasodilator (Haas and Härtfelder, 1962). Controlled trials are not available but because of the tremendous number of patients studied there is little doubt that the drug is also effective in treating and preventing atrial arrhythmias. However, only a few subjects with ventricular arrhythmias have been studied and usually with little success so that proof of efficacy for treatment of ventricular arrhythmias is not currently available (Schamroth, Krikler and Garrett, 1972; Krikler, 1974; Heng et al, 1975). It is possibly effective in abolition of ventricular arrhythmias induced by halothane anesthesia (Brichard, 1971). The mechanism of its antiarrhythmic action is unclear since it does not alter repolarisation or depolarisation in therapeutic concentrations (Singh and Vaughan-Williams, 1972a) as do most antiarrhythmic drugs. However, Fleckenstein, Doring and Kammerneier (1968) have shown that verapamil blocks calcium conductance in myocardial cell membranes and this unique action is probably responisble for its antiarrhythmic effects.

Verapamil has negative inotropic, chronotropic and dromotropic actions as do the beta-adrenergic blocking drugs but it does not antagonise cardiac beta-receptor stimulation or cause bronchoconstriction (Hills, 1970; Naylor, 1974). Verapamil is felt to block the 'slow calcium channels' which determine the speed of conduction in the N region of the A–V node and therefore slows intranodal conduction. This produces a prolongation of the PR interval without altering the QRS duration or QT interval (Heng et al, 1975). Therefore, verapamil slows the ventricular response in patients with atrial fibrillation or flutter although conversion to sinus rhythm is infrequent (Schamroth et al, 1972). Verapamil will slow paroxysmal supraventricular tachycardia and almost always converts junctional tachycardia to sinus rhythm. In the WPW syndrome verapamil has little or no effect on conduction in the anomalous pathway but can be effective by slowing conduction in either direction in the A–V node (Heng et al, 1975). However, controlled studies have not been performed in any of these arrhythmias.

The maximal effect of verapamil upon A–V nodal conduction is seen within 1 to 2 min after intravenous administration of 5 to 10 mg and persists for 15 to 20 min (Roy, Surrell and Sowton, 1974). The half-life of elimination is from 3 to 7 h after i.v. administration. Verapamil is completely absorbed after oral administration but undergoes extensive first pass hepatic metabolism so that oral dosages are usually 10 times the i.v. dosage in order to attain similar plasma levels. However, careful dose-ranging studies to evaluate oral therapy with verapamil have not been performed.

Significant side effects such as hypotension, bradycardia and asystole have been reported and are most commonly seen when beta-adrenergic blockade is present. Many feel that the drug is contraindicated in patients receiving beta-adrenergic blocking drugs. Verapamil is also potentially dangerous in tachyarrhythmias associated with disturbances in impulse conduction and/or generation (A–V block or sick-sinus syndrome) (Heng et al, 1975). In case of excessive depression of A–V nodal conduction, the antidote is either atropine or calcium, or rarely isoprenaline or a pacemaker (Krikler, 1974). Heart failure is another hazard associated with verapamil in some patients who are susceptible to the negative inotropic effects of the drug. Some investigators advocate prophylactic digitalisation in patients at risk (Filias and Zanoni, 1972).

Perhexilene maleate

Perhexilene, as the maleate salt, is a drug that was first found to be effective in the treatment of angina pectoris (Winsor, 1970). Subsequent studies have found that the drug also effectively suppresses ectopic ventricular, and possibly atrial, arrhythmias in cardiac patients during chronic therapy (Drake et al, 1973; Sukerman, 1973). Perhexilene seems to be more effective for suppressing ventricular than atrial arrhythmias.

In vitro electrophysiological studies have shown that perhexilene reduced automaticity of latent pacemakers in canine papillary muscle but not in rabbit atrial tissue (Zakauddin et al, 1975). Clinical studies have found perhexilene to reduce exercise-induced tachycardia without slowing resting heart rate or reducing cardiac output (Winsor, 1970).

Extensive studies of the metabolism and pharmacokinetics of perhexilene have not been performed. Also careful dose-ranging studies to determine the oral dosage or plasma concentration required for the antiarrhythmic or antianginal effects are not currently complete.

Aprindine

Aprindine appears to be an effective drug for suppression of ventricular arrhythmias (Kesteloot, van Meighem and DeGeest, 1973; Kesteloot 1974; Fasola and Carmichael, 1974; Van Durme, 1974a; Bollen and Enderle, 1974). A recent report found it effective for suppression of life-threatening ventricular tachycardia and fibrillation in 23 patients

(Fasola, Noble and Zipes, 1977). It has local anaesthetic properties and electrophysiological in vitro studies have shown it to suppress automaticity, shorten Purkinje fibre action potential duration relatively more than it shortens refractory period duration and to decrease the maximal rate of depolarisation.

Aprindine appears to have high oral bioavailability and is 85 to 95 per cent protein bound. Maximum plasma concentrations occur approximately 2 h after oral administration (Fasola et al, 1977). Adequate pharmacokinetic and pharmacodynamic studies have not been performed to date. However, it is known that the drug has a long elimination half-life (13–58 h; mean = 27.9) (Fasola et al, 1977). Aprindine undergoes hepatic glucuronidation and also relies upon renal function for clearance of the parent compound and metabolites to a significant degree. However, it is not known whether the dosage should be altered for patients with altered hepatic or renal clearance. Careful dose ranging studies are not available. Suppression of ventricular ectopic contractions has been reported to require plasma concentrations from 0.5 to 1.0 μg/ml (Fasola and Carmichael, 1974; Van Durme, Bogaert and Rosseel, 1974b; Van Durme, Rosseel and Bogaert, 1974c).

Adverse effects
Recently fatal agranulocytosis and cholestatic jaundice have been reported during chronic aprindine therapy. The incidence has been estimated to be between 1 in 5000 and 1 in 20,000. These have occurred during the fourth and sixteenth weeks of therapy and in most instances have been reversible (Van Leeuwen and Meyboom, 1976). However, as of July 1977, 7 of 23 patients with agranulocytosis had died, and the drug has been restricted in clinical investigation to use in patients with life-threatening or incapacitating arrhythmias unresponsive to conventional and approved therapeutic agents (personal communication, Armstrong, J. G., Lilly Research Laboratories, USA).

Bretylium

$$\text{Br} \quad \overset{\displaystyle CH_3}{\underset{\displaystyle CH_3}{\overset{|}{\underset{|}{-CH_2-N^+-C_2H_5}}}}$$

Bretylium is a quaternary ammonium compound that is concentrated in postganglionic adrenergic neurons and initially causes release of noradrenaline followed by impairment of neurotransmission (Boura and Green, 1959). It was first tested for its antihypertensive effects but was found to be unsatisfactory because of the frequent development of tolerance (Boura et al, 1959). In 1965 it was found to have antiarrhythmic properties (Leveque, 1965). Possibly of greater importance were the antifibrillatory properties described by Bacaner (1966). This property has been observed in other drugs of the quaternary ammonium class such as pranolium (dimethyl propranolol, UM-272, SC-27761) and QX-572 (Astra, Sweden) (Kniffen, Schuster and Lucchesi, 1973) and may be a unique electopharmacological effect (Rydén et al, 1974).

Clinical studies have shown that bretylium is effective for suppression of ventricular ectopic beats (Romhilt et al, 1972), ventricular tachyarrhythmias (Bacaner, 1968; Bernstein and Koch-Weser, 1972) including those following acute myocardial infarction (Terry et al, 1970; Day and Bacaner, 1971; Cohen et al, 1973) and prosthetic valve insertion (Casteneda and Bacaner, 1970). However, probably because of the drug's complex effects upon adrenergic neurons, there are varied and often unpredictable effects. Bretylium frequently causes initial exacerbation of ventricular arrhythmias and hypertension due to release of catecholamines followed by orthostatic hypotension due to adrenergic nerve block. It is currently in investigation in the US for treatment of ventricular arrhythmias which are life threatening and resistant to currently available antiarrhythmic drugs, (personal communication. Real, M., Arnar-Stone Laboratories, USA).

The recommended initial dosage is 5 mg/kg i.m. or slowly i.v. and repeated every 6 h. If the initial dose is ineffective, it can be repeated every 15 to 30 min to a total dose of 30 mg/kg. Lower doses of bretylium cause peripheral vasodilation but do not have the usual inotropic effects and are more frequently accompanied by hypotension. Adequate pharmacokinetic or pharmacodynamic studies have not been performed but studies in four normal subjects found bretylium to have an elimination half-life of approximately 10 h after i.m. injection. From 70 to 80 per cent of the total dose was excreted unchanged in the urine over the first 24 h after administration.

Bioavailability studies have not been performed with oral therapy although chronic oral therapy at a dosage of 600 mg every 6 h effectively suppressed ventricular arrhythmias in 6 patients for up to 15 months (Bernstein and Koch-Weser, 1972). Quaternary ammonium compounds as a rule have very poor and erratic oral absorption and oral dose-ranging studies are needed.

Chronic therapy with oral bretylium has met with limited success because of lack of information about the oral bioavailability of the drug and the plasma concentration required for antiarrhythmic effect. Because of the adrenergic neuron blocking properties of bretylium, orthostatic hypotension is a universal accompaniment of therapy. Although tolerance often develops to the hypotensive effects of the drug without loss of the antiarrhythmic effects, many patients cannot tolerate the drug because of incapacitating orthostatic hypotension. Several patients have developed painful nonswollen parotid glands during chronic therapy of such severity to necessitate discontinuation of bretylium (Bernstein and Koch-Weser, 1972). Further studies are necessary to determine if chronic oral therapy can be feasible in light of the high incidence of side effects.

NEWER BETA-ADRENERGIC BLOCKING DRUGS

Over 1000 chemicals have been synthesised which have beta-adrenergic blocking activity in in vitro test systems but only 20 have reached clinical testing. Some of the most widely studied and accepted beta-blocking drugs are described in Table 5.3.

Pharmacokinetics

These compounds vary widely in their pharmacokinetic characteristics. Alprenolol and propranolol have a very high first-pass hepatic clearance but this is not the case for oxprenolol, pindolol and practolol. Propranolol is greater than 90 per cent protein bound whereas metoprolol is approximately 12 per cent protein bound. Propranolol is cleared mainly by the liver whereas practolol clearance is determined by renal function. Therefore, the pharmacological actions of each of these drugs is affected differently by these various factors (Johnsson and Regårdh, 1976).

Table 5.3   Properties of beta-adrenoceptor blocking agents [a]

Generic name	Relative potency [b]	ISA [c]	CS [d]	MSA [e]
Acebutolol	0.1	(+)	+	+
Alprenolol	1.0	+	−	+
Atenolol	1.0	−	+	−
Metoprolol	0.1	−	+	(+)
Oxprenolol	2.0	+	−	+
Pindolol	15.0	+	−	(+)
Practolol	0.1	+	+	(+)
Propranolol	1.0	−	−	+
Sotalol	0.1	−	−	(+)
Timolol	10.0	−	−	+
Tolamolol	1.0	?	+	+

[a] Adapted from McDevitt et al (1976b), Johnsson and Regårdh (1976) and Clark (1976)
[b] Based upon the dose which inhibits isoproterenol-induced increases in heart rate of experimental animals
[c] Intrinsic sympathomimetic activity
[d] Cardioselectivity
[e] Membrane-stabilising activity

Cardioselectivity

Most of the actions of these drugs are due exclusively to their ability to block beta-adrenergic receptors and therefore clinically there are few differences in practical terms. Several of the drugs are cardioselective for $beta_1$ cardiac receptors and have less efficacy for blockade of peripheral vascular $beta_2$ receptors. However, those differences are dose-dependent and care must be used in administering any beta-adrenergic blocking drug to a patient with asthma. Practolol was one of the first cardioselective beta-blockers available but it has induced severe side effects (see below) and should not be used in chronic therapy. Atenolol (ICI 66,082) has been administered to patients with labile asthma by Boye and Vale (1977) and compared to propranolol by Astrøm (1976). Single i.v. doses (3 mg) produced a fall in heart rate and systolic blood pressure with only slight alteration of ventilatory function. Astrøm (1976) found less effects upon ventilatory function by atenolol than propranolol and atenolol may succeed practolol for those patients who have pulmonary disease yet require beta-adrenergic blockade. It is important to remember that these drugs are 'cardioselective' and not 'cardiospecific' and in high doses, $beta_2$ receptors will be affected significantly.

Intrinsic sympathomimetic activity (partial agonist activity)

Many of these drugs are partial agonists and when studied in in vitro systems have intrinsic sympathomimetic activity (ISA) although this has not generally been considered an important factor clinically (Tarazi, Dustan and Bravo, 1976). Majid, Saxton and Stoder (1970) have reported that two beta-blockers with ISA, oxprenolol and pindolol, do not increase pulmonary capillary wedge pressure to the same degree as propranolol and have theorised that the beta-blockers with ISA should be less likely to cause heart failure but this is not a clinically apparent difference.

Also Stokes, Weber and Thornell (1974) have observed that large doses of pindolol actually stimulate renin and Bühler et al (1975) have attributed this effect to the drug's ISA. Waal-Manning and Simpson (1975) have reported increased blood pressure in response to pindolol; presumably due to its ISA. McDevitt et al (1977) have found that drugs with ISA have greater flattening of their dose–response curves with exercise compared to drugs without ISA and have suggested that partial agonist activity (ISA) modifies the capacity to block competitively beta-adrenoceptors. This topic is still quite controversial and different opinions are prevalent in the literature. However, many investigators feel that drugs with ISA should be avoided in the management of tachyar-rhythmias associated with hyperthyroidism (Rumboldt, 1974).

Membrane stabilising action

The beta-adrenergic blocking drugs with the exception of atenolol have been found to possess some degree of membrane-stabilising or 'local anaesthetic' effect. There has been a great deal of speculation as to how this effect may contribute to the antiar-rhythmic efficacy of these drugs but no direct evidence. All of the beta-blockers have comparable antiarrhythmic activity regardless of the presence or absence of membrane stabilising activity when administered in corresponding beta-blocking doses (relative potencies are shown in Table 5.3). In the case of propranolol, the local anaesthetic effects have been described only in vitro at concentrations 30 or more times higher than those usually associated with beta-adrenergic blockade and two to three times higher than those obtained even with high oral dosages (Vaughan-Williams, 1966; Davies and Temte, 1968; Coltart and Meldrum, 1971). However, as discussed earlier in this chapter, the plasma concentrations associated with suppression of ventricular arrhyth-mias in many patients is well above that associated with beta-blockade but below the concentrations found to have membrane stabilising activity in in vitro studies.

Prophylaxis of sudden death

A great deal of evidence has accumulated indicating that during acute myocardial infarction (AMI) there is a burst of adrenergic stimulation which may be at least partially responsible for some of the arrhythmias seen in patients with AMI (Wit et al, 1975). Propranolol (Lemberg, Castellamos and Arcebal, 1970) and practolol (Jewitt et al, 1969) have been found effective for reduction of PVCs and the incidence of paroxysmal ventricular tachycardia in patients with AMI but therapy has been limited by their negative inotropic action. However, recent studies have indicated that chronic beta-adrenergic blockade in patients who have had a previous myocardial infarction might be able to protect from reinfarction and or subsequent sudden cardiac death. Wilhelmsson et al (1974) treated 330 patients with either alprenolol (400 mg/day) or placebo during the first two years after AMI and found that the treated group had a significantly lower incidence of sudden death. Ahlmark, Saetre and Korsgren (1974) obtained similar results and also noted a lower incidence of reinfarction in the alprenolol treated group. Additionally, a double-blind multicentre study involving 3038 patients with prior AMI found that the group with a previous anterior wall myocardial infarction treated with practolol appeared to suffer less sudden death. These drugs, alprenolol and practolol, have not been approved for marketing in the United States; similar studies are being conducted with propranolol in that country. Many people have extrapolated the data with alprenolol and practolol to conclude that, unless specific contraindication exists, patients with previous AMI should receive chronic beta-adrenergic blocking treatment (Kortmann, Remme and Roelandt, 1976).

Withdrawal phenomenon

Although chronic beta-blocking therapy may protect against sudden death, it has also been shown that sudden withdrawal of therapy in patients with severe angina is associated with a high incidence of sudden death, myocardial infarction or exacerbation of anginal symptoms (Alderman, Kerber and Harrison, 1974a; Diaz, Somberg and Freeman, 1973; Miller et al, 1975). The exact aetiology of the phenomenon is not understood although it has been theorised that a rebound increase in sympathetic stimulation may be responsible (Miller et al, 1975). Boudoulas et al (1977) have reported hypersensitivity to isoprenaline infusion 24 to 36 h after propranolol withdrawal in normal subjects. However, Patano and Lee (1976) administered propranolol to normal volunteers for 2 weeks and failed to observe evidence of a rebound phenomenon by measuring systolic time intervals and vanillylmandelic acid (VMA) excretion. Whatever the cause, it is felt that beta-adrenergic blocking therapy should be tapered over at least a two-week period in patients with suspected coronary disease (Shand, 1975; Danilevicius, 1977).

Toxicity

The undesired and toxic effects of beta-adrenergic blocking drugs are extensive and have been reviewed quite completely by Hagemeijer (1976). One very impressive and potentially lethal adverse effect has been attributed to chronic practolol therapy but has not been reported to date with other beta-adrenergic blocking drugs. The syndrome of sclerosing peritonitis has been reported after prolonged oral therapy and presents with non-specific complaints, weight loss, anorexia, and sometimes vomiting. A non-tender abdominal mass held suspect for malignancy or intestinal obstruction usually leads to laparotomy. At laparotomy the peritoneum is thickened and retracted and causes mechanical obstruction of the small intestine. Occasionally the entire small bowel is a fibrotic mass. Sixteen patients with this syndrome were recently described by Marshall et al (1977) and in these, complications were frequently seen and three died. Ocular and skin involvement was present in over half of the patients (see below). The skin changes usually improved after discontinuing therapy but the ocular changes did not and the onset of abdominal symptoms was delayed and occurred eight months after practolol therapy had been discontinued. Because of the severity of this adverse reaction, practolol is only recommended for short-term therapy.

Practolol, like several other drugs such as procainamide and hydralazine, has been reported to induce a systemic lupus erythematosus syndrome (Raftery and Denman, 1973; Raftery, 1974). Although the exact incidence of the practolol-induced LE syndrome is not known, the reported incidence of antinuclear antibody development during chronic practolol therapy is 11 to 24 per cent (Raftery, 1974; Jachuck et al, 1977). Like other drug-induced LE syndromes, ocular complications, psoriaform and other cutaneous lesions and antinuclear antibodies have been reported in the same patient. Jachuck et al (1977) found the occurrence of these to be unrelated. The skin and eye changes have been seen together with such frequency that reports have referred to these as an oculocutaneous syndrome. This has only been seen with practolol (Jachuck et al, 1977) to date.

MISCELLANEOUS ANTIARRHYTHMIC DRUGS

Carbamazepine

Carbamazepine is a drug of proven efficacy for control of epileptic seizures or trigeminal neuralgia. Carbamazepine has the same electrophysiological effects as phenytoin (Benaim and Chiche, 1973) and they may have the same mechanism of action in suppressing arrhythmias (Steiner et al, 1970). Sanabria, Croquer and Monsalve (1976) reported that the drug effectively controlled ventricular extrasystoles in patients with Chagas's myocarditis. Further evaluation is necessary to document the antiarrhythmic effects of carbamazepine and to determine the plasma concentration range necessary for such effects.

Antazoline

Antazoline is an antihistaminic drug that has been known since 1948 and was first reported to have antiarrhythmic properties in 1962 (Kline et al, 1962). Although controlled clinical trials have not been conducted, it has been reported to suppress atrial and ventricular extrasystoles, atrial tachycardia and ventricular tachycardia (Kline et al, 1962; Stock and Williams, 1974). No significant side effects have been reported except for sedation. However, the efficacy of the drug has not been proved in large-scale studies and it may have yet undiscovered toxicity.

Propafenon

Propafenon is a newer agent available in Europe for treatment of ventricular and supraventricular arrhythmias. It is effective after both oral or intravenous administration (Aldor and Heeger, 1976). Rapid antiarrhythmic action was seen for approximately 1.5 h after an intravenous dose of 1.0 to 1.5 mg/kg but was associated with P–R prolongation and QRS widening. Side effects were related to the GI tract, heart rate, and depression of A–V and intraventricular conduction. Chronic arrhythmia suppression was seen in 21 patients given a loading dose of 900 mg followed by 300 mg every 8 h.

Ajmaline

Ajmaline was first discovered among the Rauwolfia alkaloids in 1931 and has been clinically available in Europe since 1958 (Forster and Holzmann, 1967a). It has both structural and pharmacological similarities with quinidine. Electrophysiological studies have shown that it reduces the V_{max} of depolarisation without altering resting membrane potential (Petter and Engelmann, 1974). Administration of ajmaline to patients has caused prolongation of the P–R and QT intervals and QRS duration. Also, ajmaline has produced depression of intraventricular conduction in some patients. Ajmaline has little effect upon intraventricular conduction in normal subjects but bundle branch block can readily be elicited in the presence of a diseased system. Because of this effect, ajmaline has been used in the diagnosis of latent or inapparent conduction disturbances (Chaile et al, 1977). It has also been found effective for treatment of patients with the WPW syndrome because of its ability to depress conduction in the anomalous pathway without altering normal conduction (Chaile et al, 1977).

The drug is unpredictably absorbed after oral administration and is metabolised largely by the liver. It is rapidly cleared after intravenous administration (Petter and Engelmann, 1974) and only 0.5 per cent of a dose is present in the serum 30 min after administration.

Controlled studies are not available but case reports indicate that ajmaline by slow intravenous injection is effective for the treatment of atrial or ventricular arrhythmias except for long-standing atrial fibrillation or flutter (Forster and Holzmann, 1967a).

Although it is proposed to be less toxic than quinidine and is widely used in Europe, it still has considerable toxicity especially in patients with acute myocardial infarction (Forster and Holzmann, 1967b). Like quinidine, asystole, ventricular fibrillation, and circulatory collapse have been reported after rapid i.v. administration (Forster and Holzmann, 1967b). Several cases of intrahepatic cholestasis and one report of biliary cirrhosis have also complicated therapy (Einarsson, Hellstrom and Kallner, 1973). Controlled trials are needed to determine if the drug is effective and can be given without excess toxicity.

SUMMARY

Many drugs are now under investigation to supplant the few currently available antiarrhythmic agents that are usually found inadequate because of ineffectiveness or toxicity. Many of these are structual analogues of procainamide or lignocaine and are improvements in some respects. Several beta-adrenergic blocking drugs are becoming available and may have advantages over propranolol, but little comparative data is available.

The major advances in antiarrhythmic drug therapy have generally been from studies of the pharmacokinetics and pharmacodynamics of the older and newer drugs. Recent trends in the investigation of antiarrhythmic drugs have emphasised the importance of pharmacokinetics, dose-ranging, individualisation of therapy and computerised assessment of antiarrhythmic efficacy using ambulatory (Holter) monitoring techniques.

Although the ideal antiarrhythmic drug does not seem to be on the horizon, investigators are learning more about the characteristics deemed necessary for such a drug. Knowledge of the genesis of arrhythmias and a better understanding of the mechanism of action of the current drugs will make it possible to develop far better agents in the future.

REFERENCES

Achuff, S. C. et al (1976) Mexiletine in the prevention of ventricular dysrhythmias in acute myocardial infarction. *American Journal of Cardiology*, **37**, 115.

Ahlmark, G., Saetre, H. & Korsgren, M. (1974) Reduction of sudden death after myocardial infarction. *Lancet*, **ii**, 1563.

Alderman, E. L., Coltart, D. J., Wettach, G. E. & Harrison, D. C. (1974a) Coronary artery syndromes after propranolol withdrawal. *Annals of Internal Medicine*, **81**, 625–627.

Alderman, E. L., Kerber, R. E. & Harrison, D. C. (1974b) Evaluation of lidocaine resistance in man using intermittent large-dose infusion techniques. *American Journal of Cardiology*, **34**, 342–349.

Aldor, E. & Heeger, H. (1976) Propafen ein neues antiarrhythmikum. *Deutsche Medicinische Wochenschrift*, **101**, 1318.

Allen, J. D. et al (1972) Effect of KÖ-1173, a new anticonvulsant agent, on experimental cardiac arrhythmias. *British Journal of Pharmacology*, **45**, 561–573.

Allen, J. D., Kofi Ekue, J. M., Shanks, R. G. & Zadi, S. A. (1970) The effects on experimental cardiac arrhythmias of a new anticonvulsant agent, KÖ-1173, and its comparison with phenytoin and procainamide. *British Journal of Pharmacology*, **39**, 183–184.

Astrøm, H. (1976) Comparison of the effects on airway conductance of a new selective beta-adrenergic blocking drug, atenolol and propranolol in asthmatic subjects. *Scandinavian Journal of Respiratory Diseases*, **56**, 292–296.

Atkinson, A. J., Lee, W. K., Quinn, M. L., Kushner, W., Nevin, M. J. & Strong, J. M. (1977) Dose-ranging trail of N-acetylprocainamide in patients with premature ventricular contractions. *Clinical Pharmacology and Therapeutics*, **21** (5), 575–587.

Bacaner, M. B. (1966) Bretylium tosylate for suppression of induced ventricular fibrillation. *American Journal of Cardiology*, **17**, 528.

Bacaner, M. B. (1968) Treatment of ventricular fibrillation and other acute arrhythmias with bretylium tosylate. *American Journal of Cardiology*, **21**, 530.

Bagwell, E. E., Walle, T., Drayer, D. E., Reidenberg, M. M. & Pruett, J. K. (1976) Correlation of electrophysiological and antiarrhythmic properties of the N-acetyl metabolite of procainamide with plasma and tissue drug concentrations in the dog. *Journal of Pharmacology and Experimental Therapeutics*, **197**, 38–48.

Befeler, B., Castellanos, A. Jr, Wells, D. E., Vaguero, M. C. & Yeh, B. K. (1975) Electrophysiologic effects of the antiarrhythmic agent disopyramide phosphate. *American Journal of Cardiology*, **35**, 282–287.

Bekheit, S., Murtagh, J. G., Morton, P. & Fletcher, E. (1973) Effect of lignocaine on conducting system of human heart. *British Heart Journal*, **35**, 305–311.

Bellet, S., Roman, L. R. & Boza, A. (1971) Relation between serum quinidine levels and renal function. *American Journal of Cardiology*, **27**, 368.

Benaim, R. & Chiche, P. (1973) Les effets anti-arrhythmiques de la carbamazepine. *An. Cardiol. Angeiol.*, **22**, 243–246.

Benowitz, N. (1974) Clinical applications of the pharmacokinetics of lidocaine. In *Cardiovascular Drug Therapy*, ed. Melmon, K. pp. 77–101. Philadelphia: Davis.

Bernstein, J. G. & Koch-Weser, J. (1972) Effectiveness of bretylium tosylate against refractory ventricular arrhythmias. *Circulation*, **45**, 1024–1034.

Binnion, P. F., Murtagh, G., Pollock, A. M. & Fletcher, E. (1969) Relation between plasma lignocaine levels and induced haemodynamic changes. *British Medical Journal*, **iii**, 390.

Blumer, J., Strong, J. M. & Atkinson, A. J. (1973) The convulsant potency of lidocaine and its N-dealkylated metabolites. *Journal of Pharmacology and Experimental Therapeutics*, **186**, 31–36.

Bollen, G. & Enderle, J. (1974) Preliminary experience in the treatment of cardiac arrhythmias with aprindine. *Acta cardiolagica (Bruxelles)*, **18**, Suppl., 355–361.

Boudoulas, H., Lewis, R. P., Kates, R. E. & Dalamangas, G. (1977) Hypersensitivity to adrenergic stimulation after propranolol withdrawal in normal subjects. *Annals of Internal Medicine*, **87**, 433–436.
Boura, A. L. A. & Green, A. F. (1959) The actions of bretylium: adrenergic neurone blocking and other effects. *British Journal of Pharmacology*, **14**, 536.
Boura, A. L., Green, A. F., McCoubrey, A., Lawerence, D. R., Moulton, R. & Rosenheim, M. L. (1959) Darenthin: hypotensive agent of a new type. *Lancet*, **ii**, 17.
Boye, N. P. & Vale, J. R. (1977) Effect in bronchial asthma of a new beta-adrenergic blocking drug, Atenolol (ICI 66,082). *European Journal of Clinical Pharmacology*, **11**, 11–14.
Boyes, R. N., Scott, D. B., Jebson, P. J., Godman, M. J. & Julian, D. G. (1971) Pharmacokinetics of lidocaine in man. *Clinical Pharmacology and Therapeutics*, **12**, 105–116.
Branch, R. A., Shand, D. G., Wilkinson, G. R. et al (1973) The reduction of lidocaine clearance by dl-propranolol: an example of a hemo-dynamic drug interaction. *Journal of Pharmacology and Experimental Therapeutics*, **184**, 515–519.
Brichard, G. (1971) The action of Isoptin on cardiac arrhythmias in anesthesia. *Ars. Med. Gand.*, 31–46.
Bühler, F. R., Burkart, F., Lüfold, B. E., Küng, M., Marbet, G. & Pfisterer, N. (1975) Antihypertensive beta-blocking action as related to renin and age: a pharacologic tool to identify pathogenetic mechanisms in essential hypertension. *American Journal of Cardiology*, **36**, 653–659.
Campbell, R. W. F., Dolder, M. A., Prescott, L. F. et al (1975) Comparison of procainamide and mexiletine in prevention of ventricular arrhythmias after acute myocardial infarction. *Lancet*, Vol. No. 1257–1260.
Carr, K., Woosley, R. L. & Oates, J. A. (1976) Simultaneous determination of procainamide and N-acetylprocainamide in plasma. *Journal of Chromatography*, **129**, 363–368.
Casteneda, A. R. & Bacaner, M. B. (1970) Effect of bretylium tosylate on the prevention and treatment of postoperative arrhythmias. *American Journal of Cardiology*, **25**, 461–466.
Chaile, P. A., Przybylski, J., Halpern, M. S., Lazarri, J. O., Elizari, M. V. & Rosenbaum, M. B. (1977) Comparative effects of ajmaline on intermittent bundle branch block and the Wolff–Parkinson–White syndrome. *American Journal of Cardiology*, **39**, 651–657.
Cheng, T. O. & Wadhwa, K (1973) Sinus standstill following intravenous lidocaine administration. *Journal of the American Medical Association*, **223**, 790.
Chidsey, C., Zanchetti, A., Morselli, P. & Leonetti, G. (1975) Pharmacokinetic and pharmacodynamic studies of propranolol in hypertension. *Recent Advances in Hypertension*. International Symposium, Monte Carlo.
Clark, B. J. (1976) Pharmacology of beta-adrenoceptor blocking agents. *Beta-adrenoceptor Blocking Agents*, ed. Saxena, P. R. & Forsyth, R.P., pp. 45–76. Amsterdam–Oxford: North-Holland Publishing Co.
Cohen, H. C., Gozo, E. G., Langendorf, R., Kaplan, B. M., Chan, A., Pick, A. & Glick, G. (1973) Response of resistant ventricular tachycardia to bretylium. *Circulation*, **47**, 331–340.
Collingsworth, K. A., Kalman, S. M. & Harrison, D. M. (1974) The clinical pharmacology of lidocaine as an antiarrhythmiac drug. *Circulation*, **50**, 1217–1230.
Coltart, D. J., Gibson, D. G. & Shand, D. G. (1971) Plasma propranolol levels associated with suppression of ventricular ectopic beats. *British Medical Journal*, **i**, 490–491.
Coltart, D. J. & Meldrum, S. J. (1971) The effects of racemic propranolol, dextro-propranolol and racemic practolol on the human and canine cardiac transmembrane action potential. *Archives of International Pharmacodynamics*, **192**, 188.
Coltart, D. J. & Shand, D. G. (1970) Plasma propranolol levels in the quantitative assessment of beta-adrenergic blockade in man. *British Medical Journal*, **iii**, 731–735.
Conn, H. L. & Luchi, R. J. (1964) Some cellular and metabolic considerations relating to the action of quinidine as a prototype antiarrhythmic agent. *American Journal of Medicine*, **37**, 685–699.
Crouthamel, W. G. (1975) The effect of congestive heart failure on quinidine pharmacokinetics. *American Heart Journal*, **90** (3), 335–339.
Danilevicius, Z. (1977) Caution in propranolol withdrawal. *Journal of the American Medical Association*, **237** (1), 53.
Danilo, P. & Rosen, M. R. (1976) Cardiac effects of disopyramide. *American Heart Journal*, **92**, 532–536.
Data, J. L., Wilkinson, G. R. & Nies, A. S. (1976) Interaction of quinidine with anticonvulsive drugs. *New England Journal of Medicine*, **13**, 699–702.
Davies, D. M., Beedie, M. A. & Rawlins, M. D. (1975) Antinuclear antibodies during procainamide treatment and drug acetylation. *British Medical Journal*, **iii**, 682 683.
Davies, L. D. & Temte, J. V. (1968) Effects of propranolol on the transmembrane potential of ventricular muscle and Purkinje fibers of the dog. *Circulation Research*, **22**, 661–677.
Day, H. W. & Bacaner, M. (1971) The use of bretylium tosylate in the management of acute myocardial infarction. *American Journal of Cardiology*, **27**, 117–189.
Dean, R. R. (1975) Myocardiol metabolism of disopyramide. *Disopyramide Symposium*, p. 20. London: Royal College of Physicians.

Dean, R. R. & Ferguson, D. M. (1971) Effects of disopyramide on the A–V conduction system. *Archives of International Pharmacodynamics and Therapeutics*, **190**, 183–186.

Diaz, R. G., Somberg, J. C. & Freeman, E. (1973) Withdrawal of propranolol in myocardial infarction. *Lancet*, **i**, 1068.

DiFazio, C. A. & Brown, R. F. (1972) Lidocaine metabolism in normal and phenobarbital-pretreated dogs. *Anesthesiology*, **36** (3), 238–243.

Ditlefsen, E. L. (1957) Quinidine concentration in blood and excretion in urine following parenteral administration as related to congestive heart failure. *Acta medica scandinavica*, **159**, 105–109.

Drake, F. T., Singer, D. H., Haring, O. & Dirnberger, G. (1973) Evaluation of the antiarrhythmic efficacy of perhexilene maleate in ambulatory patients by Holter monitoring. *Postgraduate Medical Journal*, **49** Suppl. 3, 52–63.

Drayer, D., Reidenberg, M. M. & Sevy, R. W. (1974) N-acetylprocainamide: an active metabolite of procainamide. *Proceedings of the Society for Experimental Biology and Medicine*, **146**, 358–363.

Drayer, D. E., Lowenthal, D. T., Woosley, R. L., Nies, A. S., Schwartz, A. & Reidenberg, M. M. (1977) Cumulation of N-acetylprocainamide, an active metabolite of procainamide, in patients with impaired renal function. *Clinical Pharmacology and Therapeutics*, **22** (1), 63–69.

Dreifus, L. S., Filip, Z., Sexton, S. M. et al (1973) Electrophysiological and clinical effects of the new antiarrhythmic agent: disopyramide. *American Journal of Cardiology*, **31**, 129.

Einarsson, K., Hellstrom, K. & Kallner, M. (1973) Liver damage in connection with ajmaline treatment. *Lakartidningen*, **70**, 1288.

Elson, J., Strong, J. M., Lee, W. K. & Atkinson, A. J. (1975) Antiarrhythmic potency of N-acetylprocainamide. *Clinical Pharmacology and Therapeutics*, **17**, 134–140.

Evans, G. H. & Shand, D. G. (1973) Disposition of propranolol V. Drug accumulation and steady-state concentrations during chronic oral administration in man. *Clinical Pharmacology Therapeutics*, **14** (4), Part 1, 487–493.

Fasola, A. F., Noble, R. J. & Zipes, D. P. (1977) Treatment of recurrent ventricular tachycardia and fibrillation with aprindine. *American Journal of Cardiology*, **39**, 903–909.

Fasola, A. F. & Carmichael, R. (1974) The pharmacology and clinical evaluation of aprindine, a new antiarrhythmic agent. *Acta cardiologica (Bruxelles)*, **18**, Suppl., 317–335.

Filias, N. & Zanoni, G. (1972) Klinische analyse der antiarrhythmischen Wirkung des Verapamils. *Schweizetische Medizinische Wochenschrift*, **102**, 406.

Fleckenstein, A., Doring, H. J. & Kammerneier, H. (1968) Einfluss von Beta-rezeptorblockern und verwandten substanzen auf Erregung, Kontraktion und Energiestoffhsel der Myocardfasern. *Klinische Wochenschrift*, **46**, 343.

Foad, B., Litwin, A., Zimmer, H. & Hess, E. V. (1977) Acetylator phenotype in systemic clupus erythematosus. *Arthritis and Rheumatism*, **20** (3), 815–818.

Forster, G. & Holzmann, M. (1967a) Zur Ajmalintherapie von herzrhythmusstörungen I. *Schweizerische Medizinische Wochenschrift*, **97**, 185.

Forster, G. & Holzmann, M. (1967b) Zur Ajmalintherapie von herzrhythmusstörungen II. *Schweizerische Medizinische Wochenschrift*, **97**, 216.

Freeman, R., Harbison, R., Woosley, R. & Oates, J. A. (1977) A proposed reactive metabolite of procainamide and procainamide-induced systemic lupus erythematosus. *Federation Proceedings*, **36** (3), 971.

Gianelly, R., Griffin, J. R. & Harrison, D. C. (1967a) Propranolol in the treatment and prevention of cardiac arrhythmias. *Annals of Internal Medicine*, **66** (4), 667–676.

Gianelly, R. E., Von Der Groeben, J. O., Spivack, A. P. & Harrison, D. C. (1967b) Effects of lidocaine on ventricular arrhythmias in patients with coronary heart disease. *New England Journal of Medicine*, **277**, 1215–1219.

Giardina, E. V., Heissenbuttel, R. H. & Bigger, J. T. (1973) Intermittent intravenous procainamide to treat ventricular arrhythmias. *Annals of Internal Medicine*, **78** (2), 183–193.

Gibson, T. P., Matusid, E., Nelson, L. D. & Briggs, W. A. (1976) Artificial kidneys and clearance calculations. *Clinical Pharmacology and Therapeutics*, **20** (6), 720–726.

Green, K. G. (1975) Improvement in prognosis of myocardial infarction by long-term beta-adrenoceptor blockade using practolol: a multi-centre international trial. *British Medical Journal*, **iii**, 735–740.

Grossman, J. I., Copper, J. A. & Frieden, J. (1969) Cardiovascular effects of infusion of lidocaine in patients with heart disease. *American Journal of Cardiology*, **24**, 191.

Gupta, P. K., Lichstein, E. & Chadda, K. D. (1974) Lidocaine-induced heart block in patients with bundle branch block. *American Journal of Cardiology*, **33**, 487–492.

Haas, H. & Härtfelder, G. (1962) Alpha-Isoprapyl-alpha[(N-methyl-N- homoveratry) y-amino-propyl]-3,4-di-methozyphenly acetonitrile eine substanz mit Koronarge fässer weiternden Eingesehaften. *Arzneimittel-Forschung*, **12**, 549.

Hagemeijer, F. (1976) Undesired and toxic effects of beta-blocking agents. In *Beta-adrenoceptor Blocking Agents*, ed. Saxena, P. R. & Forsyth, R. P., pp. 273–289. Amsterdam–Oxford: North-Holland Publishing Co.

Harrison, D. C., Sprouse, J. H. & Morrow, A. G. (1963) The antiarrhythmic properties of lidocaine and procainamide. *Circulation*, **28**, 486–491.

Härtel, G. & Harjanne, A. (1969) Comparison of two methods for quinidine determination and chromatographic analysis of the difference. *Clinica chimica acta*, **23**, 289–294.

Heng, M. K., Singh, B. N., Roche, A. H. G., Norris, R. M. & Mercer, C. J. (1975) Effects of intravenous verapamil on cardiac arrhythmias and on the electrocardiogram. *American Heart Journal*, **90**, 487–489.

Henningsen, N. C., Cederberg, A. & Hanson, A. et al (1975) Effects of long-term treatment with procainamide. *Acta medica scandinavica*, **198**, 475–482.

Hills, E. A. (1970) Effects of verapamil on airway resistance in patients with bronchial asthma. *British Journal of Clinical Practice*, **24**, 116.

Hope, R. R. & Bates, L. A. (1972) The frequency of procainamide-induced systemic lupus erythematosus. *Medical Journal of Australia*, **2**, 298–303.

Jachuck, S. J., Stephenson, J., Bird, T., Jackson, F. S. & Clark, F. (1977) Practolol-induced autoantibodies and their relation to oculocutaneous complications. *Postgraduate Medical Journal*, **53**, 75–77.

Jewitt, D. E., Mercer, C. J. & Shillingford, J. P. (1969) Practolol in the treatment of cardiac dysrhythmias due to acute myocardial infarction. *Lancet*, **ii**, 227–230.

Jewitt, D. E., Kishon, Y. & Thomas, M. (1968) Lidocaine in the management of arrhythmias after myocardial infarction. *Lancet*, **i**, 266.

Johnsson, G. & Regårdh, C. G. (1976) Clinical pharmacokinetics of beta-adrenoreceptor blocking drugs. *Clinical Pharmacokinetics*, **1**, 233–263.

Karim, A. (1975) The pharmacokinetics of norpac. *Angiology*, **26**, Part 2, 85.

Kessler, K. M., Lowenthal, D. T., Warner, H., Gibson, T., Briggs, W. & Reidenberg, M. M. (1974) Quinidine elimination in patients with congestive heart failure or poor renal function. *New England Journal of Medicine*, **290**, 706–709.

Kesteloot, H., van Meighem, W. & DeGeest, H. (1973) Aprindine (AC 1802) a new antiarrhythmic drug. *Acta cardiologica*, **28**, 145–165.

Kesteloot, H. (1974) General aspects of antiarrhythmic treatment with aprindine. *Acta cardiologica (Bruxelles)*, **18**, Suppl., 303–317.

Klive, S. R., Dreifus, L. S., Watanabe, Y., McGarry, T. F. & Likoff, W. (1962) An evaluation of the antiarrhythmic properties of antazoline. *American Journal of Cardiology*, **9**, 564–567.

Kniffen, F. J., Schuster, D. P. & Lucchesi, B. R. (1973) Antiarrhythmic and electrophysiologic properties of UM-272, dimethyl quaternary propranolol, in the canine heart. *Journal of Pharmacology and Experimental Therapeutics*, **187**, 260.

Koch-Weser, J. & Klein, S. W. (1971) Procainamide dosage schedules, plasma concentrations, and clinical effects. *Journal of the American Medical Association*, **215** (9), 1454–1460.

Kortmann, H., Remme, W. & Roelandt, J. (1976) The use of beta-blocking agents in the treatment of cardiac arrhythmias. In *Beta-adrenoceptor Blocking Agents*, ed. Saxena, P. R. & Forsyth, R. P., pp. 143–154. Amsterdam: North-Holland Publishing Co.

Kosowsky, B. D., Taylor, J., Lown, B. & Ritchie, R. F. (1973) Long-term use of procaine amide following acute myocardial infarction. *Circulation*, **47**, 1204–1210.

Krikler, D. (1974) Verapamil in cardiology. *European Journal of Cardiology*, **2**, 3–10.

Kunkel, F., Rowland, M. & Scheinman, M. M. (1974) The electrophysiologic effects of lidocaine in patients with intraventricular conduction defects. *Circulation*, **49**, 894–899.

Lalka, D., Meyer, M. B., Duce, B. R. & Elvin, A. T. (1976) Kinetics of the oral antiarrhythmic lidocaine congener, Tocainide. *Clinical Pharmacology and Therapeutics*, **19** (6), 757–766.

Lee, W.-K., Strong, J. M., Kehoe, R. F., Dutcher, J. S. & Atkinson, A. J. (1976) Antiarrhythmic efficacy of N-acetylprocainamide in patients with premature ventricular contractions. *Clinical Pharmacology and Therapeutics*, **19** (5), 508–514.

Lemberg, L., Castellanos, A. & Arcebal, A. G. (1970) The use of propanolol in arrhythmias complicating acute myocardial infarction. *American Heart Journal*, **80**, 479–487.

Leveque, P. E. (1965) Antiarrhythmic action of bretylium. *Nature*, **207**, 203.

Lichstein, E., Chadda, K. D. & Gupta, P. K. (1973) Atrioventricular block with lidocaine therapy. *American Journal of Cardiology*, **31**, 277.

Lie, K. I., Wellens, H. J., van Capelle, F. J. & Durrer, D. (1974) Lidocaine in the prevention of primary ventricular fibrillation. *New England Journal of Medicine*, **291**, 1324–1326.

Majid, P. A., Saxton, C. & Stoder, J. B. (1970) Comparison of the hemodynamic effects of acute intravenous and oral therapy with propranolol and oxprenolol in hypertensive patients. *Cardiological Research*, **6**, 208.

Marshall, A. J., Baddeley, H., Barritt, D. W., Davies, J. D., Lee, R. E. J., Low-beer, T. S. & Read, A. E. (1977) Practolol peritonitis. *Quarterly Journal of Medicine*, **46** (181), 135–149.

Mathur, P. (1972) Cardiovascular effects of a newer antiarrhythmic agent, disopyramide phosphate. *American Heart Journal*, **84**, 764–770.

McDevitt, D. G., Shanks, R. G. & Prichard, B. N. C. (1976) The clinical pharmacology of beta-adrenergic blockers. *Journal of the Royal College of Physicians*, **11**, 21.

McDevitt, D. G., Nies, A. S., Wilkinson, G. R., Smith, R. F., Woosley, R. L. & Oates, J. A. (1976) Antiarrhythmic effects of a lidocaine congener, tocainide, 2-amino-2',6'-propionoxylidide, in man. *Clinical Pharmacology and Therapeutics*, **19** (4), 396–402.

McDevitt, D. G., Brown, H. C., Carruthers, S. G. & Shanks, R. G. (1977) Influence of intrinsic sympathomimetic activity and cardioselectivity on beta-adrenoceptor blockade. *Clinical Pharmacology and Therapeutics*, **21** (5), 556–566.

Miller, R. R., Olson, H. G., Amsterdam, E. A. & Mason, D. T. (1975) Propranolol withdrawal rebound phenomenon. *New England Journal of Medicine*, **293**, 416–418.

Naggar, C. Z. & Alexander, S. (1976) Propranolol treatment of VPBs. *New England Journal of Medicine*, **294**, 903–904.

Naylor, W. G. (1974) Verapamil and the myocardium. *Postgraduate Medical Journal*, **50**, 441.

Naylor, W. G. (1975) Pharmacology of disopyramide. In *Disopyramide symposium*, p. 1. London: Royal College of Physicians.

Nies, A. S., Shand, D. G. & Branch, R. A. (1973) Flow dependent hepatic drug elimination. The basis for hemodynamic drug interaction (Abstract). *Clinical Research*, **21**, 471.

Panatano, J. A. & Lee, Y.-C. (1976) Abrupt propranolol withdrawal and myocardial contractibility. *Archives of Internal Medicine*, **136**, 867–871.

Petter, A. & Engelmann, K. (1974) Zur antiarrhythmischen herzwirkung von ajmalin. *Arzneimittel-Forschung*, **24**, 876.

Raftery, E. B. (1974) Cutaneous and ocular reactions to practolol. *British Medical Journal*, **iv**, 653.

Raftery, E. B. & Denman, A. M. (1973) Systemic lupus erythematosus syndrome induced by practolol. *British Medical Journal*, **ii**, 452–455.

Rangno, R. E., Warnica, W., Kreeft, J. & Ogilvie, R. I. (1976) Disopyramide efficacy and kinetics in ventricular tachyarrhythmia. *American Journal of Cardiology*, **37**, 164.

Reynolds, E. W. & Vander Ark, C. R. (1976) Quinidine syncope and the delayed repolarisation syndromes. *Modern Concepts of Cardiovascular Disease*, **45** (8), 117–122.

Romhilt, D. W., Bloomfield, S. S., Lipicky, R. J., Welch, R. M. & Fowler, N. O. (1972) Evaluation of bretylium tosylate for the treatment of premature ventricular contractions. *Circulation*, **45**, 800–807.

Rosen, K., Lau, S., Weiss, M. & Damato, A. (1970) The effect of lidocaine on atrioventricular conduction in man. *American Journal of Cardiology*, **25**, 1–5.

Rowland, M., Thomson, P. D., Gruchard, A. et al (1971) Disposition kinetics of lidocaine in normal subjects. *Annals of the New York Academy of Sciences*, **179**, 383–398.

Roy, R. R., Surrell, R. A. J. & Sowton, E. (1974) The effects of verapamil on the conduction system in man. *Postgraduate Medical Journal*, **50**, 270.

Rumboldt, Z. (1974) Personal communication.

Rydén, L., Hjalmarson, Å., Wisar, H. & Werkö, L. (1974) Effects of a long-acting antiarrhythmic agent-QX-572-on therapy resistant ventricular tachyarrhythmias. *British Heart Journal*, **36**, 811–821.

Sanabria, A., Croquer, F. J. & Monsalve, P. (1976) Effet antiarrhythmique de la carbamazepine. *Nouvelle Presse Medicale*, **5**, 431–432.

Schamroth, L., Krikler, D. M. & Garrett, C. (1972) Immediate effect of intravenous verapamil in cardiac arrhythmias. *British Medical Journal*, **i**, 660.

Seaton, A. (1966) Quinidine-induced paroxysmal ventricular fibrillation treated with propranolol. *British Medical Journal*, **i**, 1522–1523.

Seipel, L. & Breithardt, G. (1976) Sinus recovery time after disopyramide phosphate. *American Journal of Cardiology*, **37**, 1118.

Shand, D. G. (1975) Propranolol withdrawal. *New England Journal of Medicine*, **293**, 449–450.

Singh, B. N. & Vaughan-Williams, E. M. (1972a) A 4th class of anti-dysrhythmic action? Effect of verapamil on ouabain toxicity, on atrial and ventricular intracellular potentials and on other features of cardiac function. *Cardiovascular Research*, **6**, 109.

Singh, B. N. & Vaughan-Williams, E. M. (1972b) Investigations of the mode of action of a new antidysrthmic drug KÖ 1173. *British Journal of Pharmacology*, **44**, 1–9.

Smith, E. R. & Duce, B. R. (1971) The acute antiarrhythmic and toxic effects in mice and dogs of 2-ethylamino-2'6'-acetoxylidine (L-86), a metabolite of lidocaine. *Journal of Pharmacology and Experimental Therapeutics*, **179**, 580.

Stannard, M., Sloman, G. & Sangster, L. (1968) Haemodynamic effects of lignocaine in acute myocardial infarction. *British Medical Journal*, **ii**, 468.

Steiner, C., Wit, A. L., Weiss, M. B. & Domato, A. N. (1970) The antiarrhythmic actions of carbamazepine (Tegretol). *Journal of Pharmacology and Experimental Therapeutics*, **173**, 323–335.

Stenson, R. E., Constantino, R. T. & Harrison, D. C. (1971a) Interrelationships of hepatic blood flow, cardiac output, and blood levels of lidocaine in man. *Circulation*, 43, 205.

Stock, J. P. P. & Williams, D. O. (1974) *Diagnosis and Treatment of Cardiac Arrhythmias*, 3rd edn, p. 190. London: Butterworths.

Stokes, G. S., Weber, M. A. & Thornell, I. R. (1974) Beta-blockers and plasma renin activity in hypertension. *British Medical Journal*, i, 60–62.

Strong, J. M., Parker, M. & Atkinson, A. J. (1973) Identification of glycinexylidide in patients treated with intravenous lidocaine. *Clinical Pharmacology and Therapeutics*, 14, 67–72.

Sukerman, M. (1973) Clinical evaluation of perhexilene moleate in the treatment of chronic cardiac arrhythmias of patients with coronary heart disease. *Postgraduate Medical Journal*, 49 Suppl. 3, 46–52.

Sunder, S. K. & Shah, A. (1975) Constrictive pericarditis in procainamide-induced lupus erythematosus syndrome. *American Journal of Cardiology*, 36, 960–962.

Talbot, R. G. et al (1973) Treatment of ventricular arrhythmias with mexiletine (KÖ-1173) *Lancet*, ii, 399–404.

Tarazi, R. C., Dustan, H. P. & Bravo, E. L. (1976) Hemodynamic effects of propranolol and hypertension: a review. *Postgraduate Medical Journal*, 52, Suppl. 4, 92–100.

Terry, G., Vellani, C. W., Higgins, M. R. & Doig, A. (1970) Bretylium tosylate and treatment of refractory ventricular arrhythmias complicating myocardial infarction. *British Heart Journal*, 32, 21–25.

Thomson, P. D., Melmon, K. L., Richardson, J. A. et al (1973) Lidocaine pharmacokinetics in advanced heart failure, liver disease, and renal failure in humans. *Annals of Internal Medicine*, 78, 499.

Thomson, P. et al (1969) Clinical differences in the pharmacokinetics of lidocaine between normal and congestive heart failure patients (Abstract). *Clinical Research*, 17, 140.

Valentine, P. A., Frew, J. L., Mashford, M. L. & Sloman, J. G. (1974) Lidocaine in the prevention of sudden death in the pre-hospital phase of acute infarction. *New England Journal of Medicine*, 291 (25), 1327–1331.

Van Durme, J. P., Rousseau, M. & Mbuyamba, P. (1974a) Treatment of chronic ventricular dysrhythmias with a new drug: Aprindine (AC-1802). *Acta cardiologica (Bruxelles)*, 18, Suppl., 335–341.

Van Durme, J. P., Bogaert, M. G. & Rosseel, M. T. (1974b) Therapeutic effectiveness and plasma levels of aprinidine, a new antidysrhythmic drug. *European Journal of Clinical Pharmacology*, 7, 343–346.

Van Durme, J. P., Rosseel, M. T. & Bogaert, M. (1974c) Therapeutic effectiveness and plasma levels of a new antidysrhythmic drug: aprindine. *Acta cardiologica (Bruxelles)*, 18, Suppl., 233–235.

Van Leeuwen, R. & Meyboom, R. H. B. (1976) Agranulocytosus with aprindine. *Lancet*, ii, 1137.

Vaughan-Williams, E. M. (1966) Mode of action of beta-receptor antagonists on cardiac muscle. *American Journal of Cardiology*, 18, 399.

Vismara, L. A., Mason, D. T. & Amsterdam, E. A. (1974) Disopyramide phosphate: clinical efficacy of a new oral antiarrhythmic drug. *Clinical Pharmacology and Therapeutics*, 16, 330–335.

Vismara, L. A., Vera, Z., Miller, R. R. & Mason, D. T. (1977) Efficacy of disopyramide phosphate in the treatment of refractory ventricular tachycardia. *American Journal of Cardiology*, 39, 1027–1034.

Vismara, L. A., DeMaria, A. N., Miller, R. R. et al (1975) Effects of intravenous disopyramide phosphate on cardiac function and peripheral circulation in eschemic heart disease. *Clinical Research*, 23, 87a.

Waal-Manning, H. J. & Simpson, F. O. (1975) Paradoxical effect of pindolol. *British Medical Journal*, iii, 155–156.

Weily, H. S. & Genton, E. (1972) Pharmacokinetics of procainamide. *Archives of Internal Medicine*, 130, 366–369.

Wetherbee, D. G., Holzman, D. & Brown, M. G. (1952) Ventricular tachycardia following the administration of quinidine. *American Heart Journal*, 43, 89–96.

Wilhelmsson, C., Vedin, J. A., Wilhelmsson, L. & Tibblem, G. (1974) Reduction of sudden death after myocardial infarction by treatment with alprenolol. *Lancet*, ii, 1157–1160.

Willis, P. W. (1975) The hemodynamic effects of Norpace. *Angiology*, 26, Suppl. 1. Part 2, 102.

Winkle, R. A., Meffin, B. J., Fitzgerald, J. W. & Harrison, D. C. (1976) Clinical efficacy and pharmacokinetics of a new orally effective antiarrhythmic, tocainide. *Circulation*, 54 (6), 884–889.

Winkle, R. A., Lopes, M. G., Goodman, D. J., Fitzgerald, J. W., Schroeder, J. S. & Harrison, D. C. (1977) Propranolol for patients with mitral valve prolapse. *American Heart Journal*, 93 (4), 422–427.

Winsor, T. (1970) Clinical evaluation of perhexilene maleate. *Clinical Pharmacology and Therapeutics*, 11, 85–59.

Wit, A. L., Hoffman, B. F. & Rosen, M. R. (1975) Electrophysiology and pharmacology of cardiac arrhythmias, IX. Cardiac electrophysiology effects of beta-adrenergic receptor stimulation and blockade, Part C. *American Heart Journal*, 90 (6), 795–803.

Woosley, R. L., Kornhauser, D. M. & Smith, R. F. (1977a) Quinidine-induced ventricular tachycardia. *Journal of the American Medical Association*, (submitted).

Woosley, R. L., Nies, A. S., Drayer, D., Reidenberg, M. & Oates, J. A. (1977b) Acetylator phenotype as a factor in procainamide-induced lupus erythematosus. *Clinical Research*, 25 (3), 279a.

Woosley, R. L., Shand, D. G., Kornhauser, D. M., Nies, A. S. & Oates, J. A. (1977c) Relation of plasma concentration and dose of propranolol to its effect on resistant ventricular arrhythmias. *Clinical Research*, **25** (3), 262A.

Woosley, R. L., Reele, S., Kornhauser, D., Price, A. & Oates, J. A. (1978a) Antiarrhythmic therapy with a combination of procainamide and phenytoin. *Circulation*, (submitted).

Woosley, R. L. et al (1977d) Suppression of ventricular ectopic depolarisation by tocainide. *Circulation*, **56**, 980–984.

Wyman, M. G. & Hammersmith, L. (1974) Comprehensive treatment plan for the prevention of primary ventricular fibrillation. *American Journal of Cardiology*, **33**, 661–667.

Yeh, B. K., Sung, P. K. & Scherlag, B. J. (1973) The effects of disopyramide on the electrophysiological and mechanical properties of the heart. *Journal of Pharmacological Science*, **62**, 1924–1929.

Zakauddin, V., Gray, D. R., Harter, K. W., Janzen, D. A., Massumi, R. A. & Mason, D. T. (1975) Electrophysiologic properties of perhexilene. *Clinical Pharmacology and Therapeutics*, **18** (5), 623–628.

6. Drug therapy of shock[*]

W. Leigh Thompson [†]

Shock is an acute syndrome of inadequate perfusion of the essential viscera. It is recognised and its severity gauged most readily from functions of such essential organs as the brain, heart, and kidney, whose visible outputs are modulated closely by perfusion adequacy. Early signs of shock are hyperventilation, anxiety, confusion, and oliguria. Hypoperfusion may be accompanied by hypotension or vasoconstriction, producing the classical thready pulse in cold blue limbs, especially after hypovolaemia or myocardial infarction, but in shock with sepsis or trauma total cardiac output is often greater than normal with only mild hypotension, yet the essential viscera are still ischaemic due to inappropriate distribution of blood flow.

Stages of therapy

Initially mild hypoperfusion evokes many protective mechanisms, such as augmentation of sympathetic nervous system activity, which tends to restore normal perfusion. Early drug therapy is usually directed at complementing such negative feedback systems. Thus one may give fluids to augment the usual transcapillary refill of hypovolaemia or use inotropic catecholamines to complement the increased secretion of noradrenaline and adrenaline. As shock progresses, however, the intracellular metabolic sequelae of ischaemia begin to 'wreck the machinery', altering the response to usual therapies and initiating a self-reinforcing (positive feedback) cycle. At this stage drug therapy must be directed at attenuating the destructive responses (vasoconstriction, excess tachycardia, acidosis, etc.) as well as reinforcing the protective responses so that the overall balance returns to healthy stable equilibria. Thus in severe shock alpha-adrenergic antagonists may be used to counteract excessive vasoconstriction, or some of the endogenous noradrenaline may be replaced by exogenous dopamine that more effectively and safely maintains essential visceral perfusion. The major focus of drug therapy in shock has been 'haemodynamic', to restore optimal blood volumes, pressures and flows. With increasing appreciation of the metabolic consequences of ischaemia, however, attention is now turning to additional therapy directed more specifically at the intracellular milieu rather than the blood pressure cuff. The 'haemodynamic' and 'metabolic' therapies are complementary, and the challenge of future research in drug treatment of shock is to learn how to optimise doses of each to improve maximally the probability of patient survival.

Constant re-evaluation

The patient in shock must be evaluated again and again to discover defects that will respond to specific therapy. If the patient has a perinephric abscess or cardiac tam-

[*] Supported in part by USPHS NIH grants GM07022 and GM21727.
[†] Burroughs Wellcome Scholar in Clinical Pharmacology.

ponade or perforated colon, no combination of haemodynamic and metabolic therapies will be successful until specific intervention is accomplished. Symptomatic management of shock has improved so that more patients are kept alive long enough for discovery and specific treatment of inciting events. But as survival is prolonged, death now results commonly not from the precipitating event itself but from such causes as the myocardial infarction during hypotension, sepsis from catheters left in place too long, or pulmonary sequelae of shock and its therapy. The key to good therapy in shock is — re-evaluation by the physician and the critical care nurse to adjust continually the dosage of each drug and to detect early the intercurrent catastrophe.

Resuscitation

In the emergency setting of severe shock with diminished carotid and femoral pulses, where profound hypotension may cause irreversible cardiac or cerebral damage in minutes, immediate therapy with an inotropic vasoconstrictor (dopamine 200–2000 μg/min or noradrenaline or adrenaline 2–10 μg/min) should be given for a few minutes until adequate intravenous routes can be established and the patient evaluated briefly. Such drugs act in seconds to constrict veins, increasing cardiac preload, and constrict arteries, increasing central perfusion pressures. These actions, as well as the inotropic effects, increase myocardial oxygen consumption and in the initial resuscitation of the profoundly hypotensive patient one should use continuous intravenous infusion of the minimal doses of these drugs to just establish viable central pulses and avoid excessive cardiac stimulation.

BLOOD VOLUME IN SHOCK

The first focus of therapy of shock is usually the blood volume. Replacement of shed blood is obviously advantageous, but in many patients with shock, a 'normal' blood volume may be inadequate and increasing ventricular diastolic filling may, by the Frank–Starling law of the heart, increase cardiac output and overall perfusion. In a mixed population of patients with shock after surgery, Shoemaker (1976a) found the average 'optimal' blood volume to be 200 to 500 ml greater than 'normal'. In these patients the survivors and non-survivors had equivalent central venous pressures (4 mmHg) and pulmonary artery occlusive pressures (6 mmHg) before 0.5 litre *whole blood transfusions* that increased filling pressures an average of 3 mmHg in both groups. After transfusion, the increase in right ventricular stroke work was equivalent (50 per cent) in both groups, but left ventricular stroke work in non-survivors was three-fifths of that in survivors, although the absolute response to transfusion was equal in both groups (Shoemaker, 1976a). The average pretransfusion haemoglobin concentration in Shoemaker's patients was 9.25 g/dl, at which point erythrocytes may be required, but many patients have adequate haemoglobin and respond well to acellular fluid therapy with an increase in oxygen transport. In a comparable group of patients with initial central venous pressures of 3.3 mmHg, Shoemaker (1976b) found that 500 ml of whole blood increased arterial oxygen transport and oxygen consumption 25 per cent, but that 500 ml of acellular albumin or dextran solutions increased oxygen consumption to exactly the same extent with an even greater (29 per cent) increase in arterial oxygen transport.

Crystalloids

Acellular fluids for use in shock may be divided into crystalloids and colloids. Glucose solutions may have metabolic value in shock, as discussed below, but contribute little to increase intravascular volume. Isomolar solutions of sodium salts are often used, both to increase intravascular volume and to replace any deficiency in interstitial space. The distribution of saline between intravascular and interstitial spaces is determined by the relative hydrostatic and effective colloidal osmotic pressures inside and outside the capillaries. Normally the interstitial space is 3.3 times larger than the plasma volume (McNeill, Dixon and Moore, 1963), but this does not mean than 25 per cent of the injected saline will remain in the plasma volume. In critically ill patients give 1000 ml of Ringer's lactate or dextrose 50 g/litre, there was an increase in central venous pressure from 3.6 to 5.6 mmHg, but no increase in cardiac output, arterial oxygen transport or oxygen consumption and only 9 per cent of the infused volume of saline remained in the plasma volume (Shoemaker, 1976b). Excessive infusion of saline in many forms of shock may be inappropriate, because during and after shock resuscitation many patients are found to have interstitial spaces greater than normal despite small plasma volumes (Shoemaker et al, 1973a, 1973b; Shoemaker, 1976b).

In *burn shock* excessive crystalloid infusion is a particular problem in management as the volume of fluids required to maintain intravascular volume in burned patients may be prodigious. Three to four days post-burn, much of this fluid returns to the blood volume from the extravascular spaces, causing pulmonary congestion. A newer form of therapy of burns is use of hypertonic saline solutions, administering the same quantity of sodium but at concentrations of 200 to 300 mEq/litre. Although the acute haemodynamic effects of hypertonic saline solutions are equal to those of larger volumes of isomolar solutions, hypertonic fluids do not cause post-burn hypervolaemia or many of the pulmonary complications (Shimazaki et al, 1977). This therapy appears relatively safe if serum sodium is maintained below 160 mEq/litre with serum osmolality less than 320 mmol/litre.

Heart filling pressures

The efficacy and safety of fluid therapy in shock may be gauged more accurately by pulmonary artery occlusive (wedge) pressures than central venous pressures. In patients with septic shock that had a pulmonary artery occlusive pressure (mean 6 mmHg) less than central venous pressure (9 mmHg), administration of 5 litres of fluid in 24 h increased pulmonary artery occlusive pressure to 10 mmHg (while decreasing central venous pressure) with improved arterial pressures, cardiac output and urine flow and unaltered lung compliance and oxygenation (Krausz, 1977). In contrast, in those patients with a pulmonary artery occlusive pressure (14 mmHg) greater than central venous pressure (8 mmHg), smaller volumes of intravenous fluids (3 litres in 24 h) led to exactly the same filling pressures after 24 h, but in this case right preload increased while left preload decreased and cardiac output was unchanged. If pulmonary artery occlusive pressures cannot be measured, pulmonary artery diastolic pressures, that average 5 mmHg greater, may be employed carefully (Figueras and Weil, 1976). Maximal cardiac output is achieved with pulmonary artery occlusive pressures of 14 to 18 mmHg (Crexalls et al, 1973b), after left ventricular myocardial infarction, and for most patients in shock blood volume should be augmented until filling pressures reach this level.

Filling pressures cannot be augmented without risk, both of increasing myocardial oxygen demand and of pulmonary oedema. The risk of pulmonary oedema is a function of *pulmonary capillary hydrostatic pressure, capillary permeability*, and *plasma colloidal osmotic pressure*. Capillary permeability may be increased especially in opiate (hypoxic) pulmonary oedema, in which sputum protein content equals that of plasma. Sepsis also increases permeability. Brigham et al (1974) found that Pseudomonas sepsis in sheep increased lung lymph flow at all pulmonary capillary pressures. Increasing pulmonary capillary pressures after Pseudomonas sepsis caused particularly severe pulmonary oedema. Although this increased permeability may decrease effectiveness of endogenous or injected albumin, by increasing its leakage into interstitial spaces, it is still the plasma colloids that tend to prevent pulmonary oedema.

Plasma colloidal osmotic pressure

Plasma colloidal osmotic pressure is the major factor preventing pulmonary oedema in patients with elevated hydrostatic pressures. In the normal dog, pulmonary oedema occurs only at left atrial pressures of 24 mmHg, but when plasma proteins are diluted with crystalloid to half their usual concentration, oedema occurs at left atrial pressures of 11 mmHg (Guyton and Lindsey, 1959). da Luz et al (1975) compared 14 patients with pulmonary oedema after myocardial infarction with 12 patients with equivalent arterial pressures and cardiac outputs who did not have pulmonary oedema. Pulmonary artery occlusive pressures averaged 16 mmHg in those with oedema and 11 in those without; plasma colloidal osmotic pressures averaged 17 mmHg in those with pulmonary oedema and 21 mmHg in those without. The gradient (osmotic minus hydrostatic pressure) was less than 8 mmHg in all patients with pulmonary oedema and was more than 8 mmHg in 9 of 12 patients without oedema. During the resolution of pulmonary oedema the gradient increases (da Luz et al, 1975), but colloidal osmotic pressure (and total protein and haematocrit) actually decrease slightly during resolution of pulmonary oedema (Figueras and Weil, 1977). Colloidal osmotic pressure alone, therefore, is no more reliable a guide to pulmonary oedema than hydrostatic pressure alone, but the combination of these two values is particularly powerful and implementation of routine bedside colloidal osmometry (Weil et al, 1974) must be considered as important as the Swan–Ganz balloon-tipped flow-directed thermodilution pulmonary arterial catheter (Swan et al, 1970). Although healthy controls have plasma colloidal osmotic pressures of 25 mmHg, they averaged only 19 ± s.d. 4 mmHg in patients admitted to a medical critical care unit (Weil et al, 1974). Plasma colloidal osmotic pressure do not correlate well with plasma albumin or total protein contents, but it is an excellent prognostic indicator in shock. None of 21 patients having plasma colloidal osmotic pressures less than 10.5 mmHg survived; 85 per cent of 13 patients with pressures greater than 18.5 mmHg survived (Morissette, Weil and Shubin 1975). The median survival point was a colloidal osmotic pressure of 14.4 mmHg and knowledge of colloidal osmotic pressure alone predicted outcome correctly in 80 per cent of patients.

Not only is colloidal osmotic pressure reduced in critically ill patients on admission to hospital, but it decreases in sepsis or septic shock (Deysine, Lieblich and Aufuses, 1973) and on dilution with crystalloid solutions. In most cases, patients with essentially normal plasma albumin concentrations may be given initially saline solutions, but if hypoalbuminaemia, pulmonary congestion, or high pulmonary artery occlusive pressures are expected, colloidal solutions are preferred.

Colloid solutions

Four colloidal solutions are available for use in shock. *Human serum albumin* is an excellent colloid with infrequent side reactions. It is available as 250 g/litre solutions that may be diluted with sodium bicarbonate, saline or other appropriate diluent or, in the oedematous hypovolaemic patient, it may be given in its concentrated 'salt-poor' form. Albumin does have one toxicity — its cost. At University Hospitals of Cleveland it is the most expensive drug in the pharmacy budget, amounting to $104 000 per year or 7 per cent of total drug costs. Albumin now costs $2.71/g, $68/0.5 litre of 50 g/litre solutions, $300 per quarter-pound of protein, and $800 for the albumin content of a healthy patient.

Purified protein derivatives (pasteurised plasma) contain up to 18 per cent globulins in addition to albumin, and their cost is greater per gram of albumin. Although these products do not transmit hepatitis, they do contain vasoactive principles, possibly kinins, that cause hypotensive reactions (Bland, Laver and Lowenstein, 1973). In addition, purified protein fractions are available only in saline, but for many patients other diluents would be preferred.

Dextrans are glucose polymers produced by streptococci. They resist hydrolysis by amylases because the glucose units are joined by alpha-1,6-glucosidic bonds instead of the usual alpha-1,4-glucosidic bonds in glycogen or starch. Native dextrans of several million molecular weight are hydrolysed to dextran-70 and dextran-40 with weight average molecular weights of 70 000 and 40 000. Dextran-70 expands blood volume by 130 per cent of the injected volume, and 30 per cent of the volume remains intravascularly after 24 h (Metcalf et al, 1962), but the effect of dextran-40 is dissipated in 90 min (Gelin, Solvell and Zederfeldt, 1961). Three major toxicities limit dextran use. First, dextrans cause bleeding, probably by interference with platelet function and possibly the von Willebrand component of factor VIII (Alexander et al, 1975a). Dextran-40 causes renal failure by increasing urine viscosity, especially when renal perfusion pressure decreases after it is given (Gelin, 1962; Morgan, Little and Evans, 1966; Yanchick, 1966; Mailloux et al, 1967; Swartz et al, 1967, 1968; Diomi et al, 1969; Thompson, Bloxham and Rudnick, 1977b, 1977d; Thompson et al, 1977c; Thompson, 1977c). Most importantly, dextrans are antigenic (Maurer, 1953; Kabat and Bezer, 1958; Salvaggio, Kayman and Leskowitz, 1966) and cause anaphylactoid shock, including death. In the last three decades 11 studies have carefully observed 2612 patients given dextran-70 or dextran-40, of whom 138 (5.3 per cent) experienced anaphylactoid reactions, most of which were mild (Turner et al, 1949; Craig, Gray and Lundy, 1951; Maycock, 1952; Bowman, 1953; Tarrow and Pulaski, 1953; Wilkinson and Storey, 1953; Tarrow, 1955; Brisman, Parks and Haller, 1968; Michelson, 1968; Strebel and Siegler, 1968; Schöning and Koch, 1975). This reaction rate has remained relatively constant — in the four studies reported in the last decade the rate has been 7 per cent. In one recent study of dextran use without consistently close patient observation, death due to dextran anaphylactoid reactions occurred in 2 of 85 882 patients (Ring and Messmer, 1977).

Hydroxyethyl starches are also glucose polymers, but unlike the long linear molecules of dextrans (that are unstable in solution), these starches are made from amylopectin that is a highly branched thornbush-like polysaccharide similar to glycogen and quite stable in solution (Thompson, 1975, 1977c). Native starches are hydrolysed by amylases with a half-time in vivo of 13 min, but the rate of metabolism can be decreased

100-fold by selectively adding hydroxyethyl groups to the starch molecule. The first hydroxyethyl starch tested in man, hetastarch, has a weight-average molecular weight of 450 000—heavier than the linear dextrans due to its compact highly branched structure. Hetastarch has three-quarters as many hydroxyethyl groups as glucose units, increasing its intravascular half-time to 17 h (Thompson, Britton and Walton, 1962). This is an important difference between hydroxyethyl starches and dextrans—the rates of elimination of dextrans and most other volaemic colloids are controlled solely by molecular size, but with starch it is controlled also by the degree of hydroxyethylation. Hetastarch causes the same increase in plasma volume as dextran-70, but the effect lasts about twice as long (Thompson et al, 1962, 1970; Thompson, 1963). The toxicity of hydroxyethyl starches is distinctly less than that of dextrans. Hydroxyethyl starch does not cause histamine-release reactions in animals (Walton, Richardson and Thompson, 1959; Thompson and Walton, 1964; Silk, 1966; Walton, Hauck and Herman, 1966) or patients (Lorenz et al, 1975, 1976). Hydroxyethyl starch is non-allergenic (Brickman et al, 1966; Maurer and Berardinelli, 1968), and in the clinical use of about 1 000 000 doses in 5 years there have been only infrequent anaphylactoid reactions and no deaths (Ring and Messmer, 1977). Acute renal failure due to hyperviscosity does not occur with hydroxyethyl starches (Thompson, 1975, 1977c; Thompson, Bloxham and Rudnick, 1977e), and it increases bleeding only one-fifth to one-eighth as much as dextrans (Karlson et al, 1967).

In addition to hetastarch, a lower molecular weight (254 000) and less completely substituted (0.43 hydroxyethyl groups per glucose unit) hydroxyethyl starch (HES-S) has been studied in dogs (Thompson et al, 1977b, 1977d, 1977e). HES-S is similar to dextran-40 in maximum effect, increasing plasma volume 25 to 29 ml/g of intravascular polymer. HES-S is eliminated more rapidly than dextran-40 with 69 per cent of the hydroxyethyl starch but only 49 per cent of the dextran appearing in urine during the first 7 h after injection, partly due to severe hyperviscosity oliguria for 2 h after dextran-40. Clinical trials of HES-S are now being conducted, and this product may have special value in safe short-term intravascular volume expansion, just as hetastarch is of value in more prolonged blood volume expansion.

In management of the patient in shock, heart filling pressures are evaluated first and, if low or normal, they are increased by the administration of crystalloids, in patients without hypoproteinaemia or pulmonary congestion, and albumin or hetastarch in patients with low colloidal osmotic pressures, high pulmonary artery occlusive pressures, pulmonary congestion, or in those requiring large volumes of fluids.

INOTROPIC DRUGS

When heart filling pressures are maximal, and shock persists, the next modality of therapy to consider is to increase perfusion by increasing heart force. Many inotropic drugs are available. Glucagon increases heart force by augmenting adenyl cyclase activity without activating the beta$_1$-adrenergic receptor, but its maximal inotropic action is weak and in heart failure its action is attenuated. Glucagon has been used in shock patients who have been given large doses of beta-adrenergic antagonists, but in most patients a larger dose of a catecholamine overcomes this adrenergic blockade. Digoxin increases heart force within 1 h, but its maximal inotropic effect is less than that of catecholamines and its effect is minimal when catecholamines are given in large doses. Digoxin may be of value in treatment of supraventricular tachydysrhythmias in shock, but it is used infrequently in shock for its inotropic action alone.

Catecholamines

Inotropic drugs used frequently in shock are the catecholamines: dopamine, noradrenaline, adrenaline, isoprenaline, and dobutamine. These drugs have similar effects on the beta$_1$-adrenergic receptors increasing heart force, but quite different actions on other receptors.

Heart force is increased by direct action of noradrenaline, adrenaline, isoprenaline and dobutamine on the beta$_1$-adrenergic receptors (Tuttle and Mills, 1975), but dopamine has in addition an indirect effect attributed to release of noradrenaline in adrenergic nerve terminals (Goldberg, 1972; Endoh, 1975).

Heart rate effect of these drugs varies with the preparation employed. Dopamine increases heart rate in isolated (Chiba, 1975) but much less in intact preparations (Alousi et al, 1975). In isolated dog sinus node and papillary muscle preparations, dopamine causes the same increase in heart force as noradrenaline (at 50 times the dose by weight), but at each level of inotropic effect the increase in sinus node rate is about two-thirds as great with dopamine as noradrenaline (Endoh, 1975). In the denervated dog heart, isoprenaline causes a greater increase in heart rate than noradrenaline (Furnival, Linden and Snow, 1971). Isoprenaline also has greater chronotropic action, per unit of inotropic effect, than dobutamine on isolated tissues (Tuttle and Mills, 1975).

In the intact dog, however, dopamine (Alousi et al, 1975; Endoh, 1075; Furukawa et al, 1976) and dobutamine (Vatner, McRitchie and Braunwald, 1974; Hinds and Hawthorne, 1975) cause much less tachycardia than other catecholamines. When compared directly in anaesthetised dogs, dobutamine caused slightly more tachycardia than dopamine per unit of inotropic response (Robie and Goldberg, 1975). Dopamine also decreases the tachycardia in response to the baroreceptor reflex by inhibiting transmission in the postganglionic adrenergic cardioaccelerator nerves (Ilhan and Long, 1975).

Coronary vessels in the intact animal are most responsive to the metabolic demands of the heart, and all inotropic drugs increase total coronary blood flow. Dopamine has at least two other actions on coronary vessels. It causes a dose-dependent coronary vasodilation, the mechanism of which is not certain, and a coronary vasoconstriction that is antagonised by large doses of phenoxybenzamine (Toda and Goldberg, 1975; Toda et al, 1975). In patients with coronary artery disease, dopamine (10 μg/kg/min) increased cardiac output 35 per cent without changing coronary sinus oxygen content or myocardial lactate extraction (Crexalls, Bourassa and Biron, 1973a). Any drug increasing heart force or rate (and oxygen demand) including dopamine (Reid, Pitt and Kelly, 1973; Lekven and Semb, 1974), dobutamine (Loeb et al, 1975; Vasu et al, 1975; Willerson et al, 1976) and digoxin, may worsen myocardial ischaemia, precipitate angina pectoris, initiate dysrhythmias or extend myocardial infarction, especially when used in excessive doses (Maroko et al, 1972).

In the healthy heart, autoregulation normally maintains coronary blood flow constant over a wide range of mean arterial pressures. In the patient with shock and myocardial infarction, however, coronary flow becomes a linear function of mean arterial pressure in the range of 45 to 100 mmHg (Mueller, 1977). Diastolic aortic (coronary perfusion) pressures should be maximised while heart oxygen demands are minimised. Catecholamines, all of which increase myocardial oxygen consumption, may improve oxygen supply to ischaemic myocardium, especially if diastolic aortic pressures increase and heart rates are not increased. With isoprenaline in cardiogenic shock heart rate increases 25 beats/min, diastolic and mean arterial pressures are unchanged and myocardial lactate *production* increases three-fold (Mueller, 1977). With noradrenaline heart rate is unchanged, diastolic and mean arterial pressures increase, and whole heart lactate production reverts to the normal 13 per cent myocardial lactate extraction, despite an increase of myocardial oxygen consumption three times greater than that with isoprenaline. In shock after myocardial infarction catecholamines with these haemodynamic effects (dopamine, dobutamine or noradrenaline) are to be preferred to isoprenaline.

Systemic vascular effects of catecholamines are complex. Noradrenaline and adrenaline are direct alpha-adrenergic vasoconstrictors. Dopamine in large doses also constricts veins (Marino, Romagnoli and Keats, 1975) and arteries in most vascular beds and this effect is inhibited by the alpha-adrenergic antagonists phentolamine and phenoxybenzamine, but only in doses higher than those needed to antagonise other alpha-adrenergic agonists (Goldberg, 1972; Goldberg, Hsieh and Resnekov, 1977). In isolated dog blood vessels, dopamine but not noradrenaline vasoconstriction is attenuated by cyproheptadine, a serotonin antagonist (Gilbert and Goldberg, 1975). Dobutamine also constricts systemic vessels by an alpha-adrenergic effect and is about 6 per cent as active as noradrenaline on constriction of the dog femoral arterial vessels (Robie, Nutter and Moddy, 1974b). In patients with arterial insufficiency and severe shock who require large, vasoconstricting doses of dopamine, gangrene may occur in many organs and is most readily recognised in the feet (Alexander, Sako and Mikulic, 1975b; Greene and Smith, 1976).

The beta$_2$-adrenergic vasodilating effects of dopamine (McNay and Goldberg, 1966) and dobutamine (Robie et al, 1974b) are much less than those of isoprenaline. Dopamine relaxation of some isolated dog arteries is not affected by propranolol in concentrations that antagonise isoprenaline relaxation (Goldberg and Toda, 1975).

Dopaminergic vasodilation
Of particular interest in shock is the predominant direct vasodilation by dopamine of renal and mesenteric vessels (Goldberg, 1972; Goldberg et al, 1977). This effect is shared by several rigid dopamine analogues, including apomorphine (Goldberg, Sonneville and McNay, 1968), 6-propylnorapomorphine, and 2-amino-6,7-dihydroxy-1,2,3,4-tetrahydronaphthalene (Crumly, Hinshaw and Goldberg, 1976), the most potent agonist. These studies indicate that the preferred dopamine configuration for interaction with the receptor causing vasodilation is the fully extended transoid conformer. Such 'dopaminergic' vasodilation is antagonised by butyrophenones, such as haloperidol, bulbocapnine (Goldberg, 1975), phenothiazines such as chlorpromazine, and metoclopramide (Day and Blower, 1975), and is likely caused by a peripheral vascular dopamine receptor similar to the central nervous system dopamine receptors (Goldberg, 1975). Isolated dog renal arteries contain adenylate cyclase that is stimulated by dopamine, and this effect is antagonised selectively by haloperidol but not propranolol. In the femoral artery, where dopamine vasodilation is minimal, the adenylate cyclase effects of dopamine and isoprenaline are antagonised by

propranolol (Murthy et al, 1976). One consequence of the flexibility of the dopamine molecule, that has 6 conformers, is that it interacts with the apomorphine central emetic receptor and causes nausea and vomiting in a few patients, especially those not in shock (Goldberg, 1972; Hollenberg et al, 1973).

Renal vasodilation by dopamine is manifest at doses of 2 to 20 ug/kg/min with increased renal cortical blood flow in man (Hollenberg et al, 1973) and dog (Hardaker and Wechsler, 1973; Nagakawa et al, 1976). In patients with congestive heart failure, dopamine in doses of 1.3 to 10 μg/kg/min causes diuresis and increases glomerular filtration rate by one-third, p-aminohippurate clearance slightly more, and sodium clearance four- to five-fold (McDonald et al, 1964; Rosenblum, Tai and Lawson, 1972; Ramdohr et al, 1973; Beregovich et al, 1974). In chronic renal failure dopamine, 2.5 to 3.5 μg/kg/min, increases glomerular filtration 19 per cent, p-aminohippurate clearance 29 per cent and sodium excretion 199 per cent with a 251 per cent increase in urine flow (Vlachoyannis, Weismüller, and Schoeppe, 1976).

In the oliguria of shock, dopamine is much more effective than isoprenaline or noradrenaline in restoring urine flow, but in patients with refractory shock, much larger doses of all catecholamines may be required. In 156 patients with severe cardiogenic shock, median optimal dopamine doses to maintain mean arterial pressures 20 mmHg less than usual healthy levels were 23.5 μg/kg/min. Overall survival for two days after recovery from shock was 33 per cent; survival was dose-dependent being 49 per cent in patients requiring less than the median dose and 10 per cent in those requiring more (Thompson et al, 1975, 1977a, 1977c; Thompson, 1977a). In 113 patients with severe septic shock, the median optimal dose was 26.5 μg/kg/min, survival for two days after shock was 31 per cent, and it was not dose-dependent, being 43 per cent for patients requiring low doses and 29 per cent for those needing higher than median doses for maintenance of mean arterial pressures 10 mmHg less than usual healthy levels (Thompson, 1976).

Mesenteric vasodilation is especially prominent after dopamine. Mesenteric arterial blood flow is increased twice as much by dopamine as isoprenaline in the anaesthetised dog, but portal venous flow is increased to about the same extent with minimal changes in portal venous pressures (Hirsch, Ayabe and Glick, 1976). Portal venous pressure is increased only 1.6 mmHg in the healthy dog given dopamine in doses that increase mesenteric arterial blood flow 205 per cent, but effects of catecholamines on portal venous pressure in cirrhotic patients have not been defined (Hirsch et al, 1976).

Dopamine increases *pulmonary blood flow*, but not pulmonary vascular resistance in intact dogs (Harrison et al, 1969), healthy men (Holloway, Polumbo and Harrison, 1975), patients with heart failure (Beregovich et al, 1974) and patients with pulmonary hypertension (Holloway et al, 1975). In the isolated perfused dog lung, however, dopamine increases pulmonary vascular resistance during ventilation with normal or reduced oxygen tensions (Mentzer, Alegre and Nolan, 1976), a response that is antagonised by phentolamine. Isoprenaline decreases pulmonary vascular resistance and abolishes pulmonary vasoconstriction in hypoxaemia, a response antagonised by propranolol (Mentzer et al, 1976). In patients with left heart failure, dopamine increases slightly the ventilation/perfusion imbalance, with an increase of venoarterial admixture from 8.2 to 11.6 per cent of cardiac output and a decrease in arterial Po₂ during room air breathing from 76 to 66 mmHg (Huckauf, Ramdohr and Schröder, 1976). *Cerebral vessels* may be dilated by 'dopaminergic' effects (Toda, 1976), but in some preparations dopamine causes cerebral vasospasm (Beregovich et al, 1975).

Dobutamine

Dopamine and dobutamine have been compared in anaesthetised intact dogs (Robie and Goldberg, 1975). Dopamine increases cardiac output progressively to a maximum of +60 per cent at doses of 20 μg/kg/min. Systemic vascular resistance decreased at low doses and then increased so that mean arterial pressures were increased at doses >10 μg/kg/min. Dobutamine, however, decreased systemic vascular resistance at all doses, increasing cardiac output 93 per cent with minimal changes in mean arterial pressures. Dopamine redistributed cardiac output to mesenteric and renal vessels, with maximum visceral vasodilation at doses of 5 to 10 μg/kg/min, but dobutamine predominantly dilated femoral (non-visceral) vessels, with a reduction in the fraction of cardiac output distributed to the kidney and gut (Vatner et al, 1974; Robie and Goldberg, 1975).

The effects of dobutamine resemble closely those of isoprenaline in heart failure (Akhtar et al, 1975; Beregovich et al, 1975) and post-operative hypoperfusion (Jewitt et al, 1974; Kersting et al, 1976; Loeb et al, 1976; Tinker et al, 1976) except tachycardia is less prominent. In heart failure, dopamine (6.2 μg/kg/min) in 10 patients increased cardiac output and heart rate the same as dobutamine (10.4 μg/kg/min), but dobutamine decreased arterial and left ventricular end-diastolic pressures whereas these increased with dopamine (Loeb et al, 1976).

Cardiogenic shock

In dogs with infarction of 23 per cent of the left ventricle by acute occlusion of the left anterior descending coronary artery, dopamine in doses of 5 and 10 μg/kg/min increased cardiac output 20 and 45 per cent, reduced systemic vascular resistance 10 and 27 per cent, and increased renal blood flow 28 and 12 per cent. Aortic diastolic pressures and heart rates were unchanged at 5 μg/kg/min, but heart rate increased 16 per cent at 10 μg/kg/min. If the dose of dopamine was increased excessively to 20 μg/kg/min, it caused increases in systemic vascular resistance, heart rate, and aortic diastolic pressure with dysrhythmias in many dogs (Takeuchi, 1975). In patients with shock after even more severe infarction of left ventricle, dopamine has similar haemodynamic effects at appropriate doses. In one series the maximum increment in stroke volume occurred at doses of 5 μg/kg/min and maximal urine flow at 7.5 μg/kg/min, but at 10 μg/kg/min there were supraventricular tachycardias or conduction defects in some patients (Levine et al, 1975).

In 156 patients with cardiogenic shock we (Thompson et al, 1977a, 1977c) compared dopamine with isoprenaline, noradrenaline or no catecholamine. At doses that maintained mean arterial pressures 20 mmHg below previous healthy levels, cardiac outputs were equal on dopamine and isoprenaline and twice those during noradrenaline, but inulin clearances and urine flows were greatest on dopamine. Although short-term haemodynamic benefits in shock after myocardial infarction may be produced by dopamine, or other catecholamines, survival is quite limited (Karliner, 1975) and no controlled studies have compared survival of patients treated with various catecholamines, counterpulsation or other therapies.

Septic shock

In patients with shock in association with bacterial sepsis, dopamine (400–1300 μg/min) supported mean arterial pressures at levels intermediate between those during isoprenaline (1.5–18 μg/min) or noradrenaline (3–180 μg/min) (Winslow et al, 1973).

Cardiac output was greater during dopamine than noradrenaline, and equal during dopamine and isoprenaline. Systemic vascular resistance increased 41 per cent with noradrenaline, decreased 24 per cent with isoprenaline, and was unchanged with dopamine. Stroke volume increased 13 per cent with noradrenaline, 22 per cent with isoprenaline and 30 per cent with dopamine at doses that produced comparable changes (+83 per cent) in left ventricular stroke work (Winslow et al, 1973).

In 20 other patients with shock in association with bacterial sepsis, dopamine in doses of 2 to 28 μg/kg/min caused an average 38 per cent increase in mean arterial pressure, a 4 per cent increase in heart rate, 28 per cent increase in cardiac output, 91 per cent increase in left ventricular stroke work, and essentially no change in systemic or pulmonary vascular resistances (Wilson, Sibbald and Jaanimagi, 1976). At doses less than 21 μg/kg/min pulmonary occlusive pressures were unchanged, but increased 5 mmHg at doses of 21 to 28 μg/kg/min (Wilson et al, 1976).

In our studies of 113 patients with shock in association with infection, (Thompson et al, 1976, 1977c) mean arterial pressures were maintained 10 mmHg less than previous healthy values with dopamine, isoprenaline, or noradrenaline. Cardiac outputs were equal on isoprenaline or dopamine, heart rates were slower during dopamine, inulin clearances were equivalent on isoprenaline or dopamine but urine flows were twice as great on dopamine.

VASODILATORS

In addition to catecholamines, other vasoactive drugs are of value in shock. Vasodilators such as phentolamine, nitroprusside and nitroglycerine are used in heart failure after acute myocardial infarction. When heart rate and left ventricular end diastolic pressures are constant, vasodilators improve mechanical performance of ischaemic myocardium without extension of infarction (Wyatt et al, 1977), but if coronary perfusion pressure is reduced and reflex cardioacceleration also limits coronary blood flow, ischaemia may be worsened. da Luz, Shubin and Weil (1973) compared responses to phentolamine in 20 patients with shock of various aetiologies and found improved systemic perfusion in patients with cardiogenic shock who had high heart filling pressures and systemic vascular resistances, but little beneficial effects when phentolamine was used alone in patients with hypovolaemia or shock with infection. The combination of vasodilators with inotropic drugs is particularly effective in controlling preload, afterload, arterial pressures, cardiac output and perfusion distribution. When dopamine is given in large doses that cause venoconstriction (increased preload) and arterial vasoconstriction (increased afterload), renal blood flow and general essential visceral perfusion can be maintained by addition of prostaglandin A_1 (Robie, Goetter and Goldberg, 1974a; Vincenti and Goldberg, 1977), alpha-adrenergic antagonists (MacCannell et al, 1966) or nitroprusside (Goldberg et al, 1977). Direct, controlled comparisons among these vasodilators in shock have not been reported, and criteria for selecting patients for use of catecholamines alone, vasodilators alone, or the combination are uncertain.

Other vasoactive drugs
In dogs with shock after bleeding and retransfusion, prostaglandin E_1 increases cardiac output, decreases total systemic vascular resistance and increases survival duration

(Machiedo et al, 1976). The distribution of blood flow during treatment with prostaglandin E_1 in shock has not been reported. Selective vasomotor actions are important in shock; Altura (1976) has studied the effects of 2-phenylalanine-8-ornithine-vasopressin in rats with shock due to bleeding or bowel ischaemia. This new vasopressin analogue corrects hypotension, dilates constricted small arterioles and constricts dilated venules in which blood is sequestered, thereby restoring normal-appearing microcirculatory flow. Research on shock must focus on such distribution of nutritive perfusion in the microvasculature, especially within ischaemic areas of organs, as the total cardiac output and total systemic vascular resistance may not reflect critical local vascular effects.

MECHANICAL CIRCULATORY SUPPORT

Mechanical assistance of the infarcted left ventricle has theoretical merit. Intra-aortic balloon counter pulsation (IACP), external counterpulsation (ECP) (compressing the lower body during diastole), and drug therapy were compared by Mueller (1977). IACP and ECP increased cardiac output and diastolic arterial pressure, but only the sudden deflation of the IACP balloon reduced cardiac afterload. Coronary blood flow increased more with IACP than ECP. Although both IACP and noradrenaline changed myocardial lactate production to the normal lactate extraction, coronary blood oxygen extraction was reduced to normal only by IACP. Only IACP reduced myocardial oxygen consumption, and accomplished this at the same time it increased cardiac output. ECP increased slightly cardiac output and coronary blood flow, but it did not normalise myocardial oxygen extraction or lactate production and did not stabilise the patient.

Survival after shock with myocardial infarction is infrequent and brief. In Mueller's study comparing drug and mechanical therapy, 2 of 15 patients treated only with noradrenaline and 3 of 15 treated only with IACP survived to leave the hospital. In another series of 16 patients with shock after myocardial infarction treated with IACP, five survived hospitalisation (31 per cent) (Ehrich et al, 1977). In the largest series of 120 patients treated with IACP only 34 survived (28 per cent), 13 who did not require surgery (11 per cent) and 21 who survived cardiac surgery (Mueller, 1977). Of 24 patients with shock and myocardial infarction treated with IACP, eight (33 per cent) survived a month but only five (21 per cent) survived 13 to 31 months, two of whom had successful coronary revascularisation in addition to IACP (Bardet et al, 1977). In a parallel series of 18 patients with myocardial infarction and shock complicated by rupture of the interventricular septum or posterior papillary muscle, 12 survived definitive surgery for one month and eight (44 per cent) for one year (Bardet et al, 1977). Thus IACP may be of particular value in those few patients for whom a definitive surgical procedure corrects the fundamental cardiac lesion. IACP is much more successful in short-term haemodynamic support of patients after cardiac surgery who do not have acute myocardial infarction—more than half such patients survive (Kveim et al, 1976).

Each patient in shock is a new experiment. Some will respond best to dopamine, others to dobutamine. Some should have vascular resistances reduced with vasodilators. The only thing certain is that there is no single optimal therapy—each patient must be treated individually with constant adjustment of the dose of the primary inotropic drug, and adjuvant therapy with vasodilators and machines.

METABOLIC THERAPY IN SHOCK

Hypoxia vs. shock

Shock is manifest by inadequate perfusion to essential viscera, but this should not be equated with inadequate oxygen delivery alone (Mela et al, 1973). Holden et al (1965) showed that morphological changes in hypoxaemic rats were much less severe than those with hypovolaemic shock. Chaudry, Sayeed and Baue (1976a) compared rats made hypoxaemic for 2 h ($F_{IO_2} = 0.05$, arterial $P_{O_2} = 18$ mmHg) with rats bled to mean arterial pressures of 40 mmHg for 2 h. In hypoxaemia, the average 43 per cent decrease in liver and kidney ATP concentration was accompanied by a concomitant increase in ADP, and recovered promptly after hypoxaemia. Rats in shock, however, had decreased ADP, greater decreases in ATP (Chaudry, Sayeed and Baue, 1974a), and did not recover after 2 h of shock (Chaudry, Sayeed and Baue, 1974b). Similar changes were observed in working muscle (diaphragm) in shocked rats in which ATP and creatinine phosphate concentrations decreased 53 and 85 per cent after 1 h of shock, but in inactive soleus muscle such changes occurred only after 2 h of shock (Chaudry, Sayeed and Baue, 1976b). Soleus muscles excised from such rats after 2 h of shock take up ATP from an incubation medium three times more rapidly than normal (Chaudry, Sayeed and Baue, 1975). Infusions of ATP *before* shock increase survival of bled rats (Talaat, Massion and Shilling, 1964). Infusion of ATP-MgCl₂ before, during or after shock increases survival of rats (Chaudry et al, 1974b).

Intracellular electrolytes

As much as half of the body's total energy expenditure is needed for the sodium–potassium ATPase at the cell membrane that maintains normal intracellular electrolyte composition and cell membrane potential (Ismail-Beigi and Edelman, 1970, 1971). In shock, transport of sodium and potassium is impaired (Sayeed and Baue, 1973), sodium and water enter the cell, potassium leaves the cell, and the transmembrane potential is reduced by one-third (Shires, Carrico and Canizaro, 1973). As the cell membrane is damaged, calcium is not excluded and intracellular calcium concentrations increase (Schumer, 1976)—in shock mitochondrial uptake of calcium is diminished even earlier than ATP synthesis (Mela, 1977). Morphologically these changes are accompanied by bleb-formation on the cell membrane, shrinking then swelling of mitochondria, and the irreversible changes of disintegration of lysosomes, mitochondria and the cell membrane (Trump, 1975).

Reductosis

Inhibition of aerobic glycolysis and the mitochondrial electron transport to oxygen leads to an accumulation of the reduced forms of oxidation-reduction 'buffers' such as the pyridine nucleotides of which NADH is the reduced and NAD the oxidinised form. In rats after 2 h of hypotension, NAD concentrations decreased 39 per cent and NAD/NADH ratios decreased 54 per cent reflecting the 'reductosis'. In rats subjected to *hypoxaemia* for 2 h (Chaudry et al, 1976a), however, NADH concentrations in liver and kidney *decreased*, with a 30 per cent increase in the ratio of NAD to NADH. Correction of this intracellular reductosis may not increase survival in shock. In rats bled to mean arterial pressures of 40 mmHg for 90 min, injection of NAD, nicotinamide or nicotinic acid increased liver and kidney NAD concentrations to greater than control levels and NAD/NADH ratios *increased* to twice the levels in unbled controls (Chaudry et al, 1976c). The decrease of NADH concentrations following infusion of nicotinamide suggests that NADH was oxidised to NAD via the mitochondrial electron transport chain resulting in formation of ATP from ADP; however, in these rats liver and kidney ATP concentrations were not increased by this therapy and none of treatments enhanced survival even when given before shock (Chaudry et al, 1976c).

Lactic acidosis

The consequences of inhibition of electron transport within the cell are acidosis and reductosis, often termed 'lactic acidosis' because of increased plasma lactate and hydrogen ion concentrations. Although correction of acidosis may increase responsiveness to catecholamines (Thompson and Schwarz, 1969), simply decreasing hydrogen ion concentration does not itself lead to increased survival in shock. Lactate concentrations are more predictive of patient survival than arterial pH (Shubin et al, 1974). In patients admitted to critical care units in whom blood lactate concentrations are increased from normal (1 mM) to 4.5 mM, overall survival is 50 per cent—at lactate concentrations > 12 mM, survival is only 5 per cent (Weil and Afifi, 1970). Measurement of lactate concentrations as prognostic indices in shock must be interpreted carefully because hyperventilation, bicarbonate infusion, and 'wash out' of lactate from hypoperfused tissues during initial effective treatment may increase blood lactate concentrations without such dire consequences.

Hypoglycaemia

Although the primary energy substrate, glucose, may be increased early in shock in response to sympathetic nervous system activation, prolonged shock is marked by glycogen depletion (Schumer et al, 1970), hypoglycaemia (Schuler, Erve and Schumer, 1976) and insulin resistance (Ryan, George and Egdahl, 1974). When rabbits are bled slowly to mean arterial pressures of 48 mmHg for 60 min and treated for 24 h with 24 ml/kg of fluid containing 48 mg/kg of albumin, 1.8 mEq/kg of NaCl and 1.3 g/kg of glucose, 3-day survival is 38 per cent (Whitten and Egdahl, 1976). When the fluid contains an additional 9.6 g/kg glucose with 1.3 mEq/kg KCl and 3.4 units/kg of insulin, survival is increased to 79 per cent ($P<0.025$). The mechanism of improved survival with this 'GIK' therapy is not clear, but greater attention must be paid to such 'metabolic' treatments of shock.

Lysosomes

Intracellular acidosis and reductosis affect not only cytoplasmic anaerobic glycolysis and the mitochondrial oxygen-dependent electron transport respiratory chain but also lysosomes. Lysosomes are packages of hydrolytic enzymes, mostly with acidic pH optima, that are surrounded by membranes impermeable both to their enzymes and to the external substrates (Goldstein, 1975). Normally lysosomes become parts of vacuoles containing cellular debris or foreign material that enters the cell; after digestion of this incorporated material lysosomes persist as residual bodies or are extruded from the cell. In shock, lysosomal membranes become fragile, lysosomal hydrolases are released within the cell, and especially from liver and gut these enzymes leak into plasma (Courtice et al, 1974; Shannon, Adams and Courtice, 1974). Release of lysosomal enzymes from human polymorphonuclear leulcocytes is also stimulated by complement component C5a, that is also an anaphylatoxin, and this is activated by endotoxin via the alternate pathway (Goldstein et al, 1973). Soluble active lysosomal acid hydrolyases do not circulate harmlessly in blood—they may digest normal cell proteins, producing vasoactive and cardiotoxic peptides that perpetuate the shock syndrome.

ADRENAL CORTICOSTEROIDS IN SHOCK

Glucocorticoids in high doses may stabilise lysosomal mitochondrial and cell membranes, possibly antagonising cell damage (Clermont, Williams and Adams, 1974). Beneficial effects of glucocorticoids can be demonstrated readily in cardiogenic shock in dogs (Dietzman, Shatney and Lillehei, 1973), endotoxin shock in rats (Erve, Earnest and Schumer, 1975) and primates (Schuler et al, 1976), haemorrhagic shock in dogs (Spath, Gorczynski and Lefer, 1973) and septic shock in rats (Raflo, Jones and Wangensteen, 1975). Large doses must be employed. In rats given a 100 per cent lethal dose of endotoxin, dexamethasone sodium phosphate 4.7 mg/kg) alone increases survival only 6 per cent, but when methylprednisolone sodium succinate (125 mg/kg) or aldosterone (1 mg/kg) are added in doses that do not alone afford protection, survival increases to 43 and 31 per cent, possibly by slowing of dexamethasone degradation. When the dose of these glucocorticoids is increased 15-fold, survival of rats increases to 60 per cent (Erve et al, 1975).

Endotoxin shock

In monkeys given endotoxin, dexamethasone sodium phosphate (5 mg/kg) during or after endotoxin increases survival from 30 to 93 per cent (Schuler et al, 1976). In monkeys not treated with glucocorticoid, there is a significant decrease in hepatic cell concentrations of ATP, ADP, glycogen, glucose-6-phosphate, fructose-6-phosphate and phosphoenolpyruvate but increased concentrations of lactate and fructose-1-,6-diphosphate. Normally ATP inhibits pyruvate kinase, phosphofructokinase and hexokinase and improves the efficiency of gluconeogenesis (Schuler et al, 1976). Endotoxin by increasing fructose-1,6-diphosphate (Williamson, Refino, and LaNoue, 1970) overcomes ATP-inhibition of pyruvate kinase decreasing glucose production, increasing ATP consumption, and depleting phosphoenolpyruvate. Decreased glucose formation from lactate is manifest in these monkeys by the high concentrations of lactate with hypoglycaemia. Glucocorticoids in these monkeys reverses the metabolic changes, possibly by antagonising the endotoxin inhibition of or by increasing synthesis (Berry and Rippe, 1973) of phosphoenolpyruvate carboxykinase (Rippe and Berry, 1972), fructose-1,6-diphosphatase or glucose-6-phosphatase (McCallum and Berry, 1972).

Haemorrhagic shock

In haemorrhagic shock steroids are less effective (Replogle et al, 1971; Raflo et al, 1975). In dogs bled to mean arterial pressures of 40 mmHg for 4 h or until 20 per cent re-uptake of shed blood, 48 per cent of control dogs were normotensive for 5 h after infusion of all shed blood and when two doses of glucocorticoids were given before and after bleeding, stabilisation of haemodynamics occurred in only 42 per cent of dogs given methylprednisolone (15–120 mg/kg) or dexamethasone (4–30 mg/kg) (Vargish et al, 1977).

Controlled clinical trials

Despite many uncontrolled clinical trials, controversy regarding glucocorticoids efficacy in shock persists, and will not be dispelled by two recent controlled studies with opposite results (Schumer, 1976; Thompson et al, 1976). Surgical patients with positive blood cultures and declining blood pressures were allocated randomly to treatment with saline, dexamethasone 3 mg/kg or methylprednisolone 30 mg/kg given immediately and repeated once at 4 h if required (Schumer, 1976). In 86 saline-treated patients 38 per cent died of septic shock—in 86 glucocorticoid-treated patients 10.4 per cent died of septic shock (with no difference between the two steroids used). In a retrospective review of 328 patients with septic shock in the same hospital, 14 per cent of glucocorticoid-treated patients died of septic shock as compared with 42 per cent of those not given glucocorticoids. In both series when comparisons were restricted to the 130 patients that had shock of more than 4 h duration with acidosis and cardiopulmonary complications, deaths due to septic shock occurred in 33 per cent of patients given glucocorticoids and 74 per cent of those not receiving glucocorticoids. In a smaller prospective double-blind study (Thompson et al, 1976), 60 patients with severe septic shock who had not responded to initial fluid therapy and who required catecholamines for life support were allocated randomly to treatment with placebo or to methylprednisolone 30 mg/kg given immediately and at 2, 8 and 24 h if the patient remained in shock. Deaths during shock or in the subsequent 2 days were 56 and 64 per cent in placebo- and glucocorticoid-treated patients and 22 and 21 per cent left the hospital alive. In this latter study the patients were more seriously ill and there was an average delay of 9 h between the time shock first began, as determined retrospectively, and the first dose of glucocorticoids. Side reactions to therapy, including hyperosmolality, psychosis, and gastrointestinal haemorrhage, were infrequent and occurred equally in patients treated with glucocorticoids or alternative therapy in both studies.

PROGNOSTIC FACTORS IN SHOCK

Shock is a complex syndrome. We understand it poorly. Many variables are measured to determine if the patient has shock, and how severe it is, but the variables of value vary in each type of shock. Both 'haemodynamic' and 'metabolic' variables may be useful. In a group of 98 patients with shock in association with major surgery, 31 non-survivors were distinguished early by having greater pulmonary vascular resistances (>500 dyn/s/cm^5/m^2), systemic vascular resistances (>3500 dyn/s/cm^5/m^2), and arterovenous oxygen extractions (>40 per cent) with lower cardiac indices (<1.8 litre/min/m^2), blood volumes, arterial oxygen tensions (<60 mmHg), arterial pHs (<7.34) and arterial CO_2 tensions (<25 mmHg) (Shoemaker et al, 1974a, 1974b). Metabolic parameters often reflect the status of the patient earlier, and even in shock with haemorrhage the metabolic parameters return to normal almost 1 h earlier than haemodynamic parameters (Schumer, Erve and Miller, 1975). Thus survival of patients with haemorrhagic shock is greatest when they have high concentrations of arterial oxygen and carbon dioxide and low concentrations of blood lactate, phosphate and amino acids (Schumer et al, 1975). Shubin et al (1974) examined 38 variables in 113 patients with shock in association with myocardial infarction (24 per cent survival), drug overdose (65 per cent survival), and sepsis (38 per cent survival). In *shock with sepsis* the combination of high central blood volume, arterial pH and cardiac work predicted patient survival with 89 per cent reliability and the most important single variables were central blood volume >1.6 litres, cardiac work > 4465 g/m, cardiac index >2.95 litre/min/m², and oxygen consumption>193 ml/min. In *shock with drug ingestion* a combination of high systolic arterial pressure and arterial pH with low central venous pressure predicted survival with 76 per cent reliability. In *cardiogenic shock* the combination of a low blood lactate and high arterial pH and P_{CO_2} predicted survival with 82 per cent reliability. When single variables are considered, the most reliable signs early in cardiogenic shock are blood lactate<3.4 m M, mean arterial pressure<67 mmHg, diastolic arterial pressure>55 mmHg and arterial pH>7.38 (Shubin et al, 1974).

In evaluating the patient in shock we must use both haemodynamic and metabolic variables. Many different kinds of haemodynamic derangements may cause hypoperfusion of essential viscera, and we cannot use arterial pressures, cardiac outputs, or vascular resistances alone as indicators of the presence or severity of shock. In some organs ischaemia leads to prompt alterations in visible function. Thus oliguria and anxiety are common early in shock. In other organs the ischaemia may be detected by signs such as altered electrocardiographic ST-segments. The 'metabolic' signs, such as increased concentrations of lactate and hydrogen ions, are influenced predominantly by liver, gut and skeletal muscles and the appearance of these signs may be delayed significantly. In managing the patient in shock at this time we must move swiftly to optimise the haemodynamic state, always protecting the myocardium and other essential viscera from ischaemia, and use the metabolic signs as indicators of the success of our therapy. Improved haemodynamics causes better perfusion of all essential viscera, hopefully reversing intracellular ischaemia before irreversible cell damage has occurred. In the future we may have 'metabolic' treatments that will correct more directly ischaemic damage and achieve more effective rescue of the patient in shock.

Acknowledgements

Ms Camille Duer, Ms in Ls, coordinated the literature review and Ms Elizabeth Hickle supervised manuscript preparation, which the author appreciates deeply.

REFERENCES

Akhtar, N., Mikulic, E., Cohn, J. N. & Chaudhry, M. H. (1975) Hemodynamic effects of dobutamine in patients with severe heart failure. *American Journal of Cardiology*, **36**, 202–205.

Alexander, B., Odake, K., Lawlor, D. & Swanger, M. (1975a) Coagulation, hemostasis, and plasma expanders: a quarter century enigma. *Federation Proceedings*, **34**, 1429–1440.

Alexander, C. S., Sako, Y. & Mikulic, E. (1975b) Pedal gangrene associated with the use of dopamine. *New England Journal of Medicine*, **293**, 591.

Alousi, A. A., O'Connor, W., Fort, D., Santabarbara, L. & Sturdy, M. J. (1975) Cardiovascular effects of dopamine in the normal and failing heart of experimental animals. In *Recent Advances in Studies on Cardiac Structure and Metabolism*, ed. Fleckenstein, A. & Rona, G., Vol. 6. Baltimore: University Park Press.

Altura, B. M. (1976) Microcirculatory approach to the treatment of circulatory shock with a new analog of vasopressin (2-phenylalanine, 8-ornithine) vasopressin. *Journal of Pharmacology and Experimental Therapeutics*, **198**, 187–196.

Bardet, J., Masquet, C., Kahn, J.-C., Gourgon, R., Bourdarias, J.-P., Mathivat, A. & Bouvrain, Y. (1977) Clinical and hemodynamic results of intra-aortic balloon counterpulsation and surgery for cardiogenic shock. *American Heart Journal*, **93**, 280–288.

Beregovich, J., Bianchi, C., Rubler, S., Lomnitz, E., Cagin, N. & Levitt, B. (1974) Dose-related hemodynamic and renal effects of dopamine in congestive heart failure. *American Heart Journal*, **87**, 550–557.

Beregovich, J., Bianchi, C., D'Angelo, R., Diaz, R. & Rubler, S. (1975) Haemodynamic effects in a new inotropic agent (dobutamine) in chronic cardiac failure. *British Heart Journal*, **37**, 629–634.

Berry, L. J. & Rippe, D. F. (1973) Effect of endotoxin on induced liver enzymes. *Journal of Infectious Disease*, 128, Suppl., S118–S121.

Bland, J. H. L., Laver, M. B. & Lowenstein, E. (1973) Vasodilator effect of commercial 5 per cent plasma protein fraction solutions. *Journal of the American Medical Association*, 224, 1721–1724.

Bowman, H. W. (1953) Clinical evaluation of dextran as a plasma volume expander. *Journal of the American Medical Association*, 153, 24–26.

Brickman, R. D., Murray, G. F., Thompson, W. L. & Ballinger, W. F. (1966) The antigenicity of hydroxyethyl starch in humans. Studies in seven normal volunteers. *Journal of the American Medical Association*, 198, 1277–1279.

Brigham, K. L., Woolverton, W. C., Blake, L. H. & Staub, N. C. (1974) Increased sheep-lung vascular permeability caused by Pseudomonas bacteremia. *Journal of Clinical Investigation*, 54, 792–804.

Brisman, R., Parks, L. C. & Haller, J. A. (1968) Anaphlactoid reactions associated with the clinical use of dextran-70. *Journal of the American Medical Association*, 204, 824–825.

Chaudry, I. H., Sayeed, M. M. & Baue, A. E. (1974a) Effect of hemorrhagic shock on tissue adenine nucleotides in conscious rats. *Canadian Journal of Physiology and Pharmacology*, 52, 131–137.

Chaudry, I. H., Sayeed, M. M. & Baue, A. E. (1974b) Effect of adenosine triphosphate-magnesium chloride administration in shock. *Surgery*, 75, 220–227.

Chaudry, I. H., Sayeed, M. M. & Baue, A. E. (1975) Evidence for enhanced uptake of adenosine triphosphate by muscle of animals in shock. *Surgery*, 77, 833–840.

Chaudry, I. H., Sayeed, M. M. & Baue, A. E. (1976a) Differences in the altered energy metabolism of hemorrhagic shock and hypoxemia. *Canadian Journal of Physiology and Pharmacology*, 54, 750–756.

Chaudry, I. H., Sayeed, M. M. & Baue, A. E. (1976b) Alterations in high-energy phosphates in hemorrhagic shock as related to tissue and organ function. *Surgery*, 79, 666–668.

Chaudry, I. H., Zweig, S., Sayeed, M. M. & Baue, A. E. (1976c) Failure of nicotinamide in the treatment of hemorrhagic shock. *Journal of Surgical Research*, 21, 27–32.

Chiba, S. (1975) Effects of dopamine on the sinus rate and contraction of the canine isolated atrium preparation. *Proceedings of the Western Pharmacology Society*, 18, 23–26.

Clermont, H. G., Williams, J. S. & Adams, J. T. (1974) Steroid effect on the release of the lysosomal enzyme acid phosphatase in shock. *Annals of Surgery*, 179, 917–921.

Courtice, F. C., Adams, E. P., Shannon, A. D. & Bishop, D. M. (1974) Acid hydrolases in the rabbit in haemorrhagic shock. *Quarterly Journal of Experimental Physiology and Cognate Medical Sciences*, 59, 31–42.

Craig, W. M., Gray, H. K. & Lundy, J. S. (1951) Present status of plasma volume expanders in the treatment of shock. *Archives of Surgery*, 63, 742–749.

Crexells, C., Bourassa, M. G. & Biron, P. (1973a) Effects of dopamine on myocardial metabolism in patients with ischemic heart disease. *Cardiovascular Research*, 7, 438–445.

Crexells, C., Chatterjee, K., Forrester, J. S., Dikshit, K. & Swan, H. J. C. (1973b) Optimal level of filling pressure in the left side of the heart in acute myocardial infarction. *New England Journal of Medicine*, 289, 1263–1266.

Crumly, J., Jr, Hinshaw, W. B. & Goldberg, L. I. (1976) Dopamine-like renal and mesenteric vasodilation caused by apomorphine, 6-propylnorapomorphine and 2-amino-6, 7-dihydroxy-1,2,3,4-tetrahydronaphthalene. *Nature*, 259, 584–587.

da Luz, P. L., Shubin, H. & Weil, M. H. (1973) Effectiveness of phentolamine for reversal of circulatory failure (shock). *Critical Care Medicine*, 1, 135–140.

da Luz, P. L., Shubin, H., Weil, M. H., Jacobson, E. & Stein, L. (1975) Pulmonary edema related to changes in colloid osmotic and pulmonary artery wedge pressure in patients after acute myocardial infarction. *Circulation*, 51, 350–357.

Day, M. D. & Blower, P. R. (1975) Cardiovascular dopamine receptor stimulation antagonised by metoclopramide. *Journal of Pharmacy and Pharmacology*, 27, 276–278.

Deysine, M., Lieblich, N. & Aufuses, A. H., Jr (1973) Albumin changes during clinical septic shock. *Surgery, Gynecology and Obstetrics*, 137, 475–478.

Dietzman, R. H., Shatney, C. H. & Lillehei, R. C. (1973) Comparative effects of the salt radical associated with corticosteroids in cardiogenic shock. *Circulation*, 48, IV-108.

Diomi, P., Matheson, A. A., Norman, J. N., Robertson, J. W. & Shearer, J. R. (1969) Effects of dextran 40 on urine flow and composition during pronounced reduction in renal perfusion. *European Surgical Research*, 1, 20–25.

Ehrich, D. A., Biddle, T. L., Kronenberg, M. W. & Yu, P. N. (1977) The hemodynamic response to intra-aortic balloon counterpulsation in patients with cardiogenic shock complicating acute myocardial infarction. *American Heart Journal*, 93, 274–279.

Endoh, M. (1975) Effects of dopamine on sinus rate and ventricular contractile force of the dog heart in vitro and in vivo. *British Journal of Pharmacology*, 55, 475–486.

Erve, P. R., Earnest, W. & Schumer, W. (1975) Antiendotoxic effect of water-soluble analogs of glucocorticoids. *Journal of Surgical Research*, 18, 567–569.

Figueras, J., Stein, L., Diez, V., Weil, M. H. & Shubin, H. (1976) Relationship between pulmonary hemodynamics and arterial pH and carbon dioxide tension in critically ill patients. *Chest*, 70, 466–472.

Figueras, J. & Weil, M. H. (1977) Increases in plasma oncotic pressure during acute cardiogenic pulmonary edema. *Circulation*, 55, 195–199.

Furaukawa, T., Ono, N., Maeda, Y., Nakahara, T. & Yoshihara, K. (1976) A possible mode of cardiovascular actions of dopamine in dogs. *Japanese Journal of Pharmacology*, 26, 481–492.

Furnival, C. M., Linden, R. J. & Snow, H. M. (1971) The inotropic and chronotropic effects of catecholamines on the dog heart. *Journal of Physiology (London)*, 214, 15–28.

Gelin, L. E., Solvell, L. & Zederfeldt, B. (1961) The plasma volume expanding effect of low viscous dextran and macrodex. *Acta chirurgica mavica*, 122, 309–322.

Gelin, L. E. (1962) Personal communication. Cited in Matheson, N. A. (1966) Effect of dextran 40 on urine flow. *Postgraduate Medical Journal*, 42, 457–460.

Gilbert, J. C. & Goldberg, L. I. (1975) Characterisation by cyproheptadine of the dopamine-induced contraction in canine isolated arteries. *Journal of Pharmacology and Experimental Therapeutics*, 193, 435–442.

Goldberg, L. I., Sonneville, P. F. & McNay, J. L. (1968) An investigation of the structural requirements for dopamine-like renal vasodilation: phenylethylamines and apomorphine. *Journal of Pharmacology and Experimental Therapeutics*, 163, 188–197.

Goldberg, L. I. (1972) Cardiovascular and renal actions of dopamine: potential clinical applications. *Pharmacological Reviews*, 24, 1–29.

Goldberg, L. I. (1975) The dopamine vascular receptor. *Biochemical Pharmacology*, 24, 651–653.

Goldberg, L. I. & Toda, N. (1975) Dopamine-induced relaxation of isolated canine renal, mesenteric and femoral arteries contracted with prostaglandin $F_2\alpha$. *Circulation Research*, 36, 37, Suppl. 1, 97–102.

Goldberg, L. I., Hsieh, Y.-Y. & Resnekov, L. (1977) Newer catecholamines for treatment of heart failure and shock: an update on dopamine and a first look at dobutamine. *Progress in Cardiovascular Diseases*, 14, 327–340.

Goldstein, I., Hoffstein, S., Gallin, J. & Weissmann, G. (1973) Mechanisms of lysosomal enzyme release from human leukocytes. microtubule assembly and membrane fusion induced by a component of complement (C5a/chemotaxis cytochalasin B/C AMP: cGMP antagonism). *Proceedings of the National Academy of Sciences of the United States of America*, 70, 2916–2920.

Goldstein, I. M. (1975) Lysosomes and their relation to the cell in shock. In *The Cell in Shock*, ed. Thompson, W. L. New York: Informedia.

Greene, S. I. & Smith, J. W. (1976) Dopamine gangrene. *New England Journal of Medicine*, 294, 114.

Guyton, A. & Lindsey, A. W. (1959) Effect of elevated left atrial pressure and decreased plasma protein concentration on the development of pulmonary edema. *Circulation Research*, 7, 649–657.

Hardaker, W. T., Jr & Wechsler, A. S. (1973) Redistribution of renal intracortical blood flow during dopamine infusion in dogs. *Circulation Research*, 33, 437–444.

Harrison, D. C., Pirages, S., Robinson, S. C. & Wintroub, B. V. (1969) The pulmonary and systemic circulatory response to dopamine infusion. *British Journal of Pharmacology*, 37, 618–626.

Hinds, J. E. & Hawthorne, E. W. (1975) Comparative cardiac dynamic effects of dobutamine and isoproterenol in conscious instrumented dogs. *American Journal of Cardiology*, 36, 894–901.

Hirsch, L. J., Ayabe, T. & Glick, G. (1976) Direct effects of various catecholamines on liver circulation in dogs. *American Journal of Physiology*, 230, 1394–1399.

Holden, W. D., DePalma, R. G., Drucker, W. R. & McKalan, A. (1965) Ultrastructural changes in hemorrhagic shock. Electron Microscopic study of liver, kidney and striated muscle cells in rats. *Annals of Surgery*, 162, 517–534.

Hollenberg, N. K., Adams, D. F., Mendell, P., Abrams, H. L. & Merrill, J. P. (1973) Renal vascular responses to dopamine. Haemodynamics and angiographic observations in normal man. *Clinical Science and Molecular Medicine*, 45, 733–742.

Holloway, E. L., Polumbo, R. A. & Harrison, D. C. (1975) Acute circulatory effects of dopamine in patients with pulmonary hypertension. *British Heart Journal*, 37, 482–485.

Huckauf, H., Ramdohr, B. & Schröder, R. (1976) Dopamine induced hypoxemia in patients with left heart failure. *International Journal of Clinical Pharmacology, Therapy and Toxicology*, 14, 217–224.

Ilhan, M. & Long, J. P. (1975) Inhibition of the sympathetic nervous system by dopamine. *Archives of International Pharmacodynamics*, 216, 4–10.

Ismail-Beigi, F. & Edelman, I. S. (1970) Mechanism of thyroid calorigenesis: role of active sodium transport. *Proceedings of the National Academy of Sciences*, 67, 1071–1078.

Ismail-Beigi, F. & Edelman, I. S. (1971) The mechanisms of calorigenic action of thyroid hormones. Stimulation of Na^+ and K^+-activated adenosinetriphosphate activity. *Journal of General Physiology*, 57, 710–722.

Jewitt, D., Birkhead, J., Mitchell, A. & Dollery, C. (1974) Clinical cardiovascular pharmacology of dobutamine, a selective inotropic catecholamine in patients with severe heart failure. *Lancet*, ii, 363–367.

Kabat, E. A. & Bezer, A. E. (1958) The effect of variation in molecular weight on the antigenicity of dextran in man. *Archives of Biochemistry and Biophysics*, 78, 306–318.

Karliner, J. S. (1975) Usefulness and limitations of dopamine in the therapy of cardiogenic shock. In *Dopamin*, ed. Schröder, R., p. 13. Stuttgart: F. K. Schattauer.

Karlson, K. E., Garzon, A. A., Shaftan, G. W. & Chu, C. (1967) Increased blood loss associated with administration of certain plasma expanders: dextran-75, dextran-40, and hydroxyethyl starch. *Surgery*, 62, 670–678.

Kersting, F., Follath, F., Moulds, R., Mucklow, J., McCloy, R., Sheares, J. & Dollery, C. (1976) A comparison of cardiovascular effects of dobutamine and isoprenaline after open heart surgery. *British Heart Journal*, 38, 622–626.

Krausz, M. D., Perel, A., Eimerl, D. & Cotev, S. (1977) Cardiopulmonary effects of volume loading in patients in septic shock. *Annals of Surgery*, 185, 429–434.

Kveim, M., Cappelen, C., Jr, Froysaker, T. & Hall, K. V. (1976) Intra-aortic balloon pumping in the treatment of cardiogenic shock following open-heart surgery. *Scandinavian Journal of Thoracic and Cardiovascular Surgery*, 10, 231–235.

Lekven, J. & Semb, G. (1974) Effect of dopamine and calcium on lipolysis and myocardial ischemic injury following acute coronary occlusion in the dog. *Circulation Research*, 34, 349–359.

Levine, P. A., McGillavary, M., Klein, M. D., Faxon, D. & Ryan, T. J. (1975) Dopamine dose in cardiogenic shock. *Circulation*, 52, Suppl. 11, 208.

Leob, H. S., Khan, M., Klodyncky, M. L., Sinno, M. Z., Towne, W. D. & Gunnar, R. M. (1975) Haemodynamic effects of dobutamine in man. *Circulatory Shock*, 2, 29–35.

Loeb, H. S., Khan, M., Saudye, A. & Gunnar, R. M. (1976) Acute hemodynamic effects of dobutamine and isoproterenol in patients with low output cardiac failure. *Circulatory Shock*, 3, 55–63.

Lorenz, W., Doenicke, A., Freund, M., Schmal, A., Dormann, P., Praetorius, B. & Shurk-Bulich, M. (1975) Plasma histamine levels in man following infusion of hydroxyethyl starch: a contribution to the question of allergic or anaphylactoid reactions following administration of a new plasma substitute. *Anaesthesist*, 24, 228–230.

Lorenz, W., Doenicke, A., Messmer, K., Relmann, H.-J., Thermann, M., Lahn, W., Berr, J., Schmall, A., Dormann, P., Rogenfus, P. & Hamelmann, H. (1976) Histamine release in human subjects by modified gelatin (haemaccel) and dextran: an explanation for anaphylactoid reactions observed under clinical conditions. *British Journal of Anaesthesia*, 48, 2–14.

MacCannell, K. L., McNay, J. L., Meyer, M. B. & Goldberg, L. I. (1966) The use of dopamine in the treatment of hypotension and shock. *New England Journal of Medicine*, 275, 1389–1398.

Machiedo, G. W., Brown, C. S., Lavigne, J. E. & Rush, B. F., Jr (1976) Beneficial effect of prostaglandin E₁, in experimental hemorrhagic shock. *Surgery, Gynecology and Obstetrics*, 143, 433–436.

Mailloux, L., Swartz, C. D., Capizzi, R., Kim, K. E., Onesti, G., Ramirez, O. & Brest, A. N. (1967) Acute renal failure after administration of low molecular weight dextran. *New England Journal of Medicine*, 277, 1113–1118.

Marino, R. J., Romagnoli, A. & Keats, A. S. (1975) Selective venoconstriction by dopamine in comparison with isoproterenol and phenylephrine. *Anesthesiology*, 43, 570–572.

Maroko, P. R., Libby, P., Covell, J. W., Sobel, B. E., Ross, J., Jr & Braunwald, E. (1972) Precordial ST segment mapping: an atraumatic method for assessing alterations and extent of myocardial ischemic injury: the effects of pharmacologic and hemodynamic interventions. *American Journal of Cardiology*, 29, 223–230.

Maurer, P. H. (1953) Dextran, an antigen in man. *Proceedings of the Society for Experimental Biology and Medicine*, 83, 879–884.

Maurer, P. H. & Berardinelli, B. (1968) Immunologic studies with hydroxyethyl starch (HES) a proposed plasma expander. *Transfusion*, 8, 265–268.

Maycock, W. D. (1952) Analysis of reports on the infusion of dextran solution. *Lancet*, i, 1080–1083.

McCallum, R. E. & Berry, L. E. (1972) Mouse liver fructose-1 disphophatase and glucose-6-phosphatase activities after endotoxin poisoning. *Infection and Immunity*, 6, 883–885.

McDonald, R. H., Jr, Goldberg, L. I., McNay, J. L. & Tuttle, E. D., Jr (1964) Effects of dopamine in man: augmentation of sodium excretion glomerular filtration rate and renal plasma flow. *Journal of Clinical Investigation*, 43, 1116–1124.

McNay, J. L. & Goldberg, L. I. (1966) Comparison of the effects of dopamine, isoproterenol, norepinephrine and bradykinin on canine renal and femoral blood flow after POB. *Journal of Pharmacology and Experimental Therapeutics*, 151, 23–31.

McNeill, I. F., Dixon, J. P. & Moore, F. D. (1963) Effects of hemorrhage and hormones on partition of body water. *Journal of Surgical Research*, 3, 332–343.

Mela, L., Miller, L. D., Bacalzo, L. V., Olofsson, B. S. & White, R. R., IV (1973) Role of Intracellular variations of lysosomal enzyme activity and oxygen tension in mitochondrial impairment in endotoxemia and hemorrhage in the rat. *Annals of Surgery*, 178, 727–735.

Mela, L. M. (1977) Oxygen's role in health and shock. In *The Organ in Shock*, ed. Thompson, W. L. New York: Informedia.

Mentzer, R. M., Jr, Alegre, C. A. & Nolan, S. P. (1976) The effects of dopamine and isoproterenol on the pulmonary circulation. *Journal of Thoracic and Cardiovascular Surgery*, 71, 807–814.

Metcalf, W., Dargan, E. L., Hehre, E. J., Levitsky, S. & Dibuono, T. J. (1962) Clinical physiological characterisation of a new dextran. *Surgery, Gynecology and Obstetrics*, 115, 199–206.

Michelson, E. (1968) Anaphylactoid reactions to dextran. *New England Journal of Medicine*, 278, 552.

Morgan, T. O., Little, J. M. & Evans, W. A. (1966) Renal failure associated with low molecular weight dextran infusion. *British Medical Journal*, ii, 737–739.

Morissette, M., Weil, M. H. & Shubin, H. (1975) Reduction in colloid osmotic pressure associated with fatal progression of cardiopulmonary failure. *Critical Care Medicine*, 3, 115–117.

Mueller, H. S. (1977) The heart and oxygen transport. In *The Organ in Shock*, ed. Thompson, W. L. New York: Informedia.

Murthy, V. V., Gilbert, J.-C., Goldberg, L. I. & Kuo, J. F. (1976) Dopamine-sensitive adenylate cyclase in canine renal artery. *Journal of Pharmacy and Pharmacology*, 28, 567–571.

Nagakawa, B., Goldberg, L., McCartney, J. & Matsumoto, T. (1976) The effect of dopamine on renal microcirculation in hemorrhagic shock in dogs. *Surgery, Gynecology and Obstetrics*, 142, 871–874.

Raflo, G. T., Jones, R. C. W., Jr & Wangensteen, S. L. (1975) Inadequacy of steroids in the treatment of severe hemorrhagic shock. *American Journal of Surgery*, 130, 321–327.

Ramdohr, B., Schuren, K. P., Biamino, G. & Schröder, R. (1973) Der einfluss von dopamin auf hamodynamik und nierenfunktion bei der schweren herzinsuffizienz des menschen. *Klinische Wochenschrift*, 51, 549–556.

Reid, P. R., Pitt, B. & Kelly, D. T. (1973) Effects of dopamine on increasing infarct area in acute myocardial infarction. *Circulation*, 46, 11210.

Replogle, R. L., Kundler, H., Schottenfeld, M. & Spear, S. (1971) Hemodynamic effects of dexamethasone in experimental hemorrhagic shock-negative results. *Annals of Surgery*, 174, 126–130.

Ring, J. & Messmer, K. (1977) Incidence and severity of anaphylactoid reactions to colloid volume substitutes. *Lancet*, i, 446–469.

Rippe, D. F. & Berry, L. J. (1972) Study of inhibition of induction of phosphoenolpyruvate carboxykinase by endotoxin with radial immunodiffusion. *Infection and Immunity*, 6, 766–772.

Robie, N. W., Goetter, W. D. & Goldberg, L. I. (1974a) Systemic and renal hemodynamic effects of dopamine and prostaglandin A alone and in combination. *Blood Vessels*, 11, 86–95.

Robie, N. W., Nutter, D. O. & Moddy, C. (1974b) In vivo analysis of adrenergic receptor activity of dobutamine. *Circulation Research*, 34, 663–671.

Robie, N. W. & Goldberg, L. I. (1975) Comparative systemic and regional hemodynamic effects of dopamine and dobutamine. *American Heart Journal*, 90, 340–345.

Rosenblum, R., Tai, A. R. & Lawson, D. (1972) Dopamine in man: cardiorenal hemodynamics in normotensive patients with heart disease. *Journal of Pharmacology and Experimental Therapeutics*, 183, 256–263.

Ryan, N. T., George, B. C. & Egdahl, R. H. (1974) Chronic tissue insulin resistance following hemorrhagic shock. *Annals of Surgery*, 180, 402–407.

Salvaggio, J., Kayman, H. & Leskowitz, S. (1966) Immunologic responses of atopic and normal individuals to aerosolised dextran. *Journal of Allergy*, 38, 31–40.

Sayeed, M. M. & Baue, A. E. (1973) Na-K transport in rat liver slices in hemorrhagic shock. *American Journal of Physiology*, 224, 1265–1270.

Schöning, B. & Koch, H. (1975) Incidence and severity of anaphylactoid reactions to colloid volume substitutes. *Lancet*, i, 466–469.

Schuler, J. J., Erve, P. R. & Schumer, W. (1976) Glucocorticoid effect on hepatic carbohydrate metabolism in the endotoxin-shocked monkey. *Annals of Surgery*, 345–354.

Schumer, W., Erve, P. R., Kapica, S. K. & Moss, G. S. (1970) Endotoxin effect on respiration of rat liver mitochondria. *Journal of Surgical Research*, 10, 609–612.

Schumer, W., Erve, P. R. & Miller, B. (1975) Biochemical monitoring of the surgical patient. *Surgical Clinics of North America*, 55, 11–20.

Schumer, W. (1976) Steroids in the treatment of clinical septic shock. *Annals of Surgery*, 184, 333–341.

Shannon, A. D., Adams, E. P. & Courtice, F. C. (1974) The lysosomal enzymes acid phosphatase and beta-glucoronidase in muscle following a period of ischemia. *Australian Journal of Experimental Biology and Medical Sciences*, 52, 157–171.

Shimazaki, S., Yoshioka, T., Tanaka, N., Sugimoto, T. & Onji, Y. (1977) Body fluid changes during hypertonic lactated saline solution therapy for burn shock. *Journal of Trauma*, 17, 38–43.

Shires, G. T., Carrico, C. J. & Canizaro, P. C. (1973) *Shock*. Philadelphia: W. B. Saunders Co.

Shoemaker, W. C., Bryan-Brown, C. W., Quigley, L., Stahr, L. & Lewyn, D. H. (1973a) Body fluid shifts in depletion and post-stress states and their correction with adequate nutrition. *Surgery, Gynecology and Obstetrics*, 136, 371–374.

Shoemaker, W. C., Bryan-Brown, C. W. & Elwyn, D. H. (1973b) Therapy of nutritional failure. *Seminars in Drug Treatment*, **3**, 301–313.

Shoemaker, W. C., Elwyn, D. H., Levin, H. & Rosen, A. L. (1974a) Early prediction of death and survival in postoperative patients with circulatory shock by nonparametric analysis of cardiorespiratory variables. *Critical Care Medicine*, **2**, 317–325.

Shoemaker, W. C., Elwyn, D. H., Levin, H. & Rosen, A. L. (1974b) Use of nonparametric analysis of cardiorespiratory variables as early predictors of death and survival in postoperative patients. *Journal of Surgical Research*, **17**, 301–314.

Shoemaker, W. C. (1976a) Effects of transfusion on surviving and nonsurviving postoperative patients. *Surgery, Gynecology and Obstetrics*, **33–40**.

Shoemaker, W. C. (1976b) Comparison of the relative effectiveness of whole blood transfusions and various types of fluid therapy in resuscitation. *Critical Care Medicine*, **4**, 71–78.

Shubin, H., Weil, M. H., Afifi, A. A., Portigal, L. & Chang, P. (1974) Selection of hemodynamic, respiratory and metabolic variables for evaluation of patients in shock. *Critical Care Medicine*, **2**, 326–336.

Silk, M. R. (1966) The effect of dextran and hydroxyethyl starch on renal hemodynamics. *Journal of Trauma*, **6**, 717–723.

Spath, J. A., Jr, Gorczynski, R. J. & Lefer, A. M. (1973) Possible mechanisms of the beneficial action of glucocorticoids in circulatory shock. *Surgery, Gynecology and Obstetrics*, **137**, 597–607.

Strebel, L. & Siegler, P. E. (1968) Experience with clinical testing of dextran solutions. *Archives of Surgery*, **96**, 471–475.

Swan, H. J. C., Ganz, W., Forester, J. S., Marcus, H., Diamond, G. & Ghonette, D. (1970) Catheterisation of the heart in man with use of a flow directed balloon-tipped catheter. *New England Journal of Medicine*, **283**, 447–451.

Swartz, C., Onesti, G., Ramierez, O., Kim, K., Maillous, L. & Brest, A. N. (1967) A tubular resistance theory of dextran-40 acute renal failure (Abstracts). *First Annual Meeting*, American Society of Nephrology, **1**, 64.

Swartz, C., Chinitz, J., Onesti, G., Kim, K., Ramirez, O. & Brest, A. N. (1968) Ethacrynic acid in acute renal failure (Abstracts). *Second Annual Meeting*, American Society of Nephrology, **2**, 66.

Takeuchi, S. (1975) Cardiovascular effects of dopamine after experimental coronary occlusion in the dog. *Japanese Heart Journal*, **16**, 280–292.

Talaat, S. M., Massion, W. H. & Schilling, J. A. (1964) Effects of adenosine triphosphate administration in irreversible hemorrhagic shock. *Surgery*, **55**, 813–819.

Tarrow, A. B. & Pulaski, E. J. (1953) Reactions in man from infusion with dextran. *Anesthesiology*, **14**, 359–365.

Tarrow, A. B. (1955) The plasma volume expanders. *Anesthesiology*, **16**, 598–605.

Thompson, W. L., Britton, J. J. & Walton, R. P. (1962) Persistence of starch derivatives and dextran when infused after hemorrhage. *Journal of Pharmacology and Experimental Therapeutics*, **136**, 126–132.

Thompson, W. L. (1963) Hydroxyethyl starch: a prospective plasma substitute. Dissertation, Medical University of South Carolina, p. 438.

Thompson, W. L. & Walton, R. P. (1964) Elevation of plasma histamine levels in the dog following administration of muscle relaxants, opiates and macromolecular polymers. *Journal of Pharmacology and Experimental Therapeutics*, **143**, 131–136.

Thompson, W. L. & Schwarz, E. (1969) Cardiovascular responsiveness to catecholamines in acute metabolic and respiratory acidosis in dogs. *Federation Proceedings*, **28**, 742.

Thompson, W. L., Fukushima, T., Rutherford, R. B. & Walton, R. P. (1970) Intravascular persistence, tissue storage, and excretion of hydroxyethyl starch. *Surgery, Gynecology and Obstetrics*, **131**, 965–972.

Thompson, W. L. (1975) Rational use of albumin and plasma substitutes. *Johns Hopkins Medical Journal*, **136**, 189–193.

Thompson, W. L., Gurley, H. T., Krug, U., Morris, I. A. & McLouth L. (1975) Dopamine treatment of shock. *Clinical Research*, **23**, 224A.

Thompson, W. L. (1976) Management of shock with infections. In *Use of Dopamine in Shock: I. Septic Shock*, ed. Weil, M. H. Princeton: Excerpta Medica.

Thompson, W. L., Gurley, H. T., Lutz, B. A., Jackson, D. L., Kvols, L. K. & Morris, I. A. (1976) Inefficacy of glucocorticoids in shock (double-blind study). *Clinical Research*, **24**, 258a.

Thompson, W. L. (ed) (1977a) *The Patient in Shock*. New York: Informedia.

Thompson, W. L. (1977b) Dopamine a selective inotropic vasodilator for management of cardiogenic shock. In *Use of Dopamine in Shock: III. Cardiogenic Shock*, ed. Swan, H. C. Princeton: Excerpta Medica (in press).

Thompson, W. L. (1977c) Hydroxyethyl starch. In *Blood Substitutes and Plasma Expanders*, ed. Jamieson, G. A. & Greenwalt, T. J. Proceedings of the American National Red Cross 9th Annual Scientific Symposium, Washington, DC, May 1977. New York: Alan R. Liss, Inc. (in press).

Thompson, W. L., Gurley, H. T., Little, L. R., Morris, I. A. & Drug, U. (1977a) Dopamine: a new inotropic selective visceral vasodilator for hypoperfusion. *Transactions of the Royal Society of Medicine*, (in press).

Thompson, W. L., Bloxham, D. D. & Rudnick, M. S. (1977b) Low molecular weight hydroxyethyl starch—kinetics in dogs. *Federation Proceedings*, **36**, 597.

Thompson, W. L., Gurley, H. T., Little, L. R. & Krug, U. (1977c) Dopamine dose-response relationships in patients with refractory septic or cardiogenic shock. *Proceedings of the Second World Congress on Intensive Care* (in press).

Thompson, W. L., Bloxham, D. D. & Rudnick, M. S. (1977d) Short-persistence hydroxyethyl starch—kinetics in dogs. *Clinical Research*, **25**, 277a.

Thompson, W. L., Bloxham, D. D. & Rudnick, M. S. (1977e) New short-persistence hydroxyethyl starch (HES-S): kinetics and efficacy in dogs and patients. *Proceedings of the Second World Congress on Intensive Care* (in press).

Tinker, J. H., Tarhan, S., White, R. D., Pluth, J. R. & Barnhorst, D. A. (1976) Dobutamine for inotropic support during emergence from cardiopulmonary bypass. *Anesthesiology*, **44**, 281–286.

Toda, N. & Goldberg, L. I. (1975) Effects of dopamine on isolated canine coronary arteries. *Cardiovascular Research*, **9**, 384–389.

Toda, N., Hojo, M., Sakae, K. & Usui, H. (1975) Comparison of the relaxing effect of dopamine with that of adenosine, isoproterenol and acetylcholine in isolated canine coronary arteries. *Blood Vessels*, **12**, 290–301.

Toda, N. (1976) Influence of dopamine and noradrenaline on isolated cerebral arteries of the dog. *British Journal of Pharmacology*, **58**, 121–126.

Trump, B. F. (1975) The role of cellular membrane systems in shock. In *The Cell in Shock*, ed. Thompson, W. L. New York: Informedia.

Turner, F. P., Butler, B. C., Smith, M. E. & Scudder, J. (1949) Dextran-an experimental plasma substitute. *Surgery, Gynecology and Obstetrics*, **88**, 661–675.

Tuttle, R. R. & Mills, J. (1975) Dobutamine: development of a new catecholamine to selectively increase cardiac contractility. *Circulation Research*, **36**, 185–196.

Vargish, T., Turner, C. S., Bond, R. F., Bagwell, C. E. & James, P. M. Jr. (1977) Dose-response relationships in steroid therapy for hemorrhagic shock. *Review of Surgery*, **33**, 363–367.

Vasu, M. A., O'Keefe, D. D., Kapellakis, G. Z., Daggett, W. M. & Powell, W. J. Jr. (1975) Myocardial oxygen consumption and hemodynamic effects of dobutamine, epinephrine, and isoproterenol. *Federation Proceedings*, **34**, 435.

Vatner, S. F., McRitchie, R. J. & Braunwald E. (1974) Effect of dobutamine on left ventricular performance, coronary dynamics and distribution of cardiac output in conscious dogs. *Journal of Clinical Investigation*, **52**, 1265–1273.

Vincenti, F. & Goldberg, L. I. (1977) Combined use of dopamine and prostaglandin A₁ in patients with acute renal failure and hepatorenal syndrome. In press.

Vlachoyannis, J., Weismüller, G. & Schoeppe, W. (1976) Effects of dopamine on kidney function and on the adenyl cyclase phosphodiesterase system in man. *European Journal of Clinical Investigation*, **6**, 131–137.

Walton, R. P., Richardson, J. A. & Thompson, W. L. (1959) Hypotension and histamine release following intravenous injection of plasma substitutes. *Journal of Pharmacology and Experimental Therapeutics*, **127**, 39–45.

Walton, R. P., Hauck, A. L. & Herman, E. H. (1966) Structural specificity of dextran in producing anaphylactoid reactions in rats. *Proceedings of the Society for Experimental Biology and Medicine*, **212**, 272–274.

Weil, M. H. and Afifi, A. A. (1970) Experimental and clinical studies on lactate and pyruvate as indicators of the severity of acute circulatory failure (shock). *Circulation*, **41**, 989–1001.

Whitten, R. H. and Egdahl, R. H. (1976) High-dose glucose-insulin-potassium in treatment of irreversible hemorrhagic shock. *Surgical Forum*, **27**, 60–62.

Wilkinson, A. W. and Storey, I. D. E. (1953) Reactions to dextran. *Lancet*, **2**, 956–958.

Willerson, J. T., Hutton, I., Watson, J. T., Platt, M. R. & Templeton, G. H. (1976) Influence of dobutamine on regional myocardial blood flow and ventricular performance during acute and chronic myocardial ischemia in dogs. *Circulation*, **53**, 828–833.

Williamson, H. R., Refino, C. & LaNoue, K. (1970) Effects of E. coli lipopolysaccharide B treatment of rats on gluconeogenesis, In *Energy Metabolism in Trauma A Ciba Symposium*, eds. Porter, R. & Knight, J., pp. 145–154. London: J & A Churchill.

Wilson, R. F., Sibbald, W. J., Jaanimagi, J. L. (1976) Hemodynamic effects of dopamine in critically ill septic patients. *Journal of Surgical Research*, **20**, 163–172.

Winslow, E. J., Loeb, H. S., Rahimtoola, S. H., Kamath, S. & Gunnar, R. M. (1973) Hemodynamic studies and results of therapy in 50 patients with bacteremic shock. *American Journal of Medicine*, **54**, 421–432.

Wyatt, H. L., da Luz, P. L., Waters, D. D., Swan, H. J. C. & Forrester, J. S. (1977) Contrasting influences of alterations in ventricular preload and afterload upon systemic hemodynamics, function and metabolism of ischemic myocardium. *Circulation*, **55**, 318–324.

Yanchick, V. A. (1966) Urinary excretion of low molecular weight dextran in endotoxin shock. *Parenteral Drug Association Bulletin*, **20**, 173–182.

7. Antiepileptic drugs

Alan Richens

The development of methods for measuring serum concentrations of antiepileptic drugs has been a major advance in the drug treatment of the epilepsies. It has been realised that pharmacokinetic variation is wide, that non-compliance is common, and that a substantial porportion of patients, even those managed in leading neurological centres, have subtherapeutic serum concentrations of the drugs they are receiving. Because adequate control of fits has not been achieved with one drug alone, many patients receive multiple therapy, each drug often being administered in an inadequate dose. This policy has been disastrous for the patient with difficult-to-control epilepsy because the price he has paid in terms of iatrogenic disease has been high and often unjustified for the small degree of control that has been achieved. A number of clinical pharmacologists and psychiatrists have been heard to remark recently that it is regrettable that epilepsy is a neurological disease, for, once the diagnosis is made, most of the problems arising in long-term management are pharmacological, psychiatric or social in nature, three areas which have been sadly neglected in traditional neurological training. It follows that a multidisciplinary approach to the management of the epileptic patient is necessary, and the argument for a special epilepsy clinic in which the neurologist, psychiatrist, social worker, electroencephalographer and clinical pharmacologist pool their resources is a strong one. The latter should be responsible for monitoring serum drug concentrations and for interpreting them in the light of his knowledge of pharmacokinetics. He should be responsible for tailoring the dose of a drug to produce a therapeutic serum level; if this is done properly, most patients' fits will be completely controlled with one drug alone.

PHARMACOKINETICS

Epilepsy is not a single disease entity, but a collection of disorders of brain function in which the common denominator is the fit. However, fits come in many different forms, hence the use of the term 'epilepsies' in this review, and this is probably why no one drug is effective in all types of epilepsy. Nevertheless, a wide range of drugs for a particular type of seizure is always a disadvantage because the clinician's experience is spread thinly rather than concentrated on a small number of drugs, and he is tempted to use them in a variety of permutations and combinations. It is probable that the epilepsies can be completely managed with the following range of drugs: phenytoin (diphenylhydantoin), carbamazepine, phenobarbitone, primidone, sodium valproate, ethosuximide, diazepam and clonazepam. As will be discussed later, however, phenobarbitone and primidone may be replaced by the less toxic carbamazepine in major and focal epilepsies, and sodium valproate may be preferable in petit mal epilepsy. Discussion of the pharmacokinetics of antiepileptic drugs will be confined to

Table 7.1 Summary of pharmacokinetic data on the commonly-used antiepileptic drugs. Modified from Richens (1976).

Drug	Time to peak serum level after single oral dose (h)	Time to peak serum level after single i. m. dose (h)	Apparent Vd (litre/kg)	Elimination half-life in adults (h)	Active metabolites	Major inactive metabolite	% binding to plasma proteins
Phenytoin	4–12 (BP tablets)	Many hours	0.60–0.67	9–140a	None	p-Hydroxyphenytoin (p-HPPH)	89–92
Carbamazepine	6–12	—	0.79–1.4	8.5–19 (chronic therapy) 24–60 (single doses)	10,11-epoxide	10,11-Transdihydro-dihydroxy-carbamazepine	70–80
Phenobarbitone	1–6	1–6	0.50–0.60	53–140 37–73 (children)	None	p-Hydroxypheno-barbitone	46–48
Primidone	0.5–9	—	0.7	3.3–12.5	Phenobarbitone PEMA	p-Hydroxypheno-barbitone	10–15
Sodium valproate	0.5–4	—	0.15–0.42	8–15	None?	Oxidation derivatives	90
Ethosuximide	1–2	—	0.7	60–100 16–68 (children)	None	Hydroxy-derivative	Negligible
Diazepam	1–2	1–3	2.20–2.60	20–42	Desmethyldiazepam Oxazepam	Hydroxy-derivatives	94–98
Clonazepam	1–3	1–3	1.5–4.4	20–60	3-Hydroxy-clonazepam	7-Amino-clonazepam	82

aUsing radioactive tracer doses in volunteers and in patients receiving chronic phenytoin therapy (see text) the abbreviated list given. Table 7.1 summarises the pharmacokinetic data which are most relevant to their clinical use. Suggested therapeutic ranges of serum concentrations are given in Table 7.2 for those drugs for which studies of the relationship between serum concentration and antiepileptic effect have been performed, although in some instances these ranges are tentative only.

Table 7.2 Summary of provisional therapeutic ranges of serum concentrations for the commonly used antiepileptic drugs. The evidence on which those for phenytoin and ethosuximide are based is good, but for the other drugs it is less satisfactory. Some patients with mild epilepsy are likely to be controlled at serum concentrations below these ranges. The values given should be regarded, therefore, as ranges in which optimum control will be achieved in the majority of patients

Drug	Therapeutic range (μmol/litre (μg/ml))
Phenytoin	40– 80 (10–20)
Phenobarbitone (derived from phenobarbitone or primidone)	60–160 (15–40)
Carbamazepine	16– 40 (4–10)
Valproic acid	350–700 (50–100)
Ethosuximide	300–700 (40–100)

Phenytoin

From the pharmacokinetic point of view, this must be the most studied drug in common clinical use. There are several reasons for this: (a) it is a relatively easy drug to measure as its concentration in serum is comparatively high, (b) intersubject variation in serum levels is wide, (c) it has a narrow therapeutic ratio which makes individualisation of dosage important, (d) bioavailability problems and interactions are common, and (e) it exhibits saturation kinetics within the therapeutic range of serum concentrations.

These characteristics make phenytoin a difficult drug to use correctly in practice. The traditional approach has been to increase the dose gradually until either full control of fits has been achieved or signs of intoxication develop, whereupon the dose is cut back slightly. Although this may seem a reasonable approach, in practice it is unsatisfactory and leads to many patients having subtherapeutic serum phenytoin concentrations. Instead of the dose being optimised, it has been usual to add a second or even a third drug in order to achieve control (Shorvon and Reynolds, 1977). Without the feedback provided by monitoring drug concentrations, the physician tends to adhere to standard doses. In a survey performed by Koch-Weser (1975), over 90 per cent of outpatients at the Massachusetts General Hospital were receiving 300 mg daily with the result that only 27 per cent had serum concentrations within the therapeutic range of 40 to 80 μ mol/litre (10–20 μg/ml). It is now clear that tailoring the dose to achieve an optimum serum concentration allows more than 90 per cent of newly presenting outpatients with major epilepsy to be controlled on phenytoin alone (Reynolds, Chadwick and Galbraith, 1976a).

There have been innumerable reports of bioavailability differences between the many marketed preparations of phenytoin. In Sweden, this has been a particular problem (Lund, 1974a). One preparation, Difhydan, contains phenytoin acid in an amorphous form with a highly variable particle size, leading to a very poor bioavailability compared with other preparations with a smaller particle size. The drug is best

F

absorbed from tablets or suspensions of microcrystalline phenytoin. The sodium salt is well absorbed because it dissolves in the gastric juice and reprecipitates as a fine suspension of phenytoin acid at the low pH in the stomach. The most important determinant of phenytoin absorption is therefore particle size, rather than whether the drug is in its acid or salt form. The excipient in a formulation may also influence the bioavailability of the drug by influencing the rate of deaggregation of the particles. When the manufacturers of Dilantin capsules changed the excipient from hydrated calcium sulphate to lactose, the bioavailability of the preparation was substantially increased, resulting in an outbreak of intoxication in Australia (Tyrer et al, 1970).

The parenteral preparation of phenytoin is absorbed only very slowly when injected intramuscularly (Wilensky and Lowden, 1973). The solvent is highly alkaline and when buffered to physiological pH by tissue fluid the drug crystallises out, leading to muscle damage (Serrano and Wilder, 1974). The crystals present a relatively small surface area for absorption so that the serum phenytoin concentration will fall on changing from oral to intramuscular therapy, followed by an overswing perhaps to toxic levels on resumption of oral treatment.

Phenytoin binds to plasma proteins extensively, the most reliable estimates giving values of 90 to 92 per cent bound. There has been some controversy over the importance of intersubject differences in protein binding, one group (Booker and Darcey, 1973) reporting that variation was considerable and that measurement of the free drug gives a much closer correlation with signs of toxicity, while another group (Barth et al, 1976) consider that variation is small provided the plasma albumin concentration is normal. Hypoalbuminaemia will reduce the total amount of drug bound (Porter and Layzer, 1975). In uraemic patients, the total number of binding sites available per molecule of albumin is reduced and therefore phenytoin intoxication can occur at lower total serum concentrations of the drug (Odar-Cederlöff and Borga, 1974).

The possible advantages of measuring free, rather than total, serum concentrations, together with the unpleasantness associated with frequent venepunctures in children, has stimulated interest in measuring salivary phenytoin. There is good evidence that the salivary concentration reflects the level of unbound drug in serum, although there is a considerable scatter of individual values (Reynolds et al, 1976b). It is uncertain whether this variation is real or due to the technical difficulties of separating free and bound drug in serum and the measurement of concentrations only one-tenth of the total serum level. Until this has been resolved, it would be unwise to recommend salivary measurements for routine use because their reliability would be unlikely to meet the requirements of clinical practice—even for total serum concentrations the quality of measurement in many laboratories leaves much to be desired (see Quality Control, below). Mixed saliva appears to give results as good as saliva collected selectively from the parotid duct (Paxton, Whiting and Stephen, 1977) although this may not hold true in a patient who has marked gingival hyperplasia and gingivitis with production of a protein-rich exudate.

One of the major difficulties in using phenytoin effectively is the saturable nature of its metabolism; the dose–serum concentration relationship (Fig. 7.1) obeys Michaelis–Menten kinetics. Within the therapeutic range of serum concentrations the relationship is very steep, such that only a small increment in dose will raise the serum level from subtherapeutic to toxic. This has a number of implications for clinical practice.

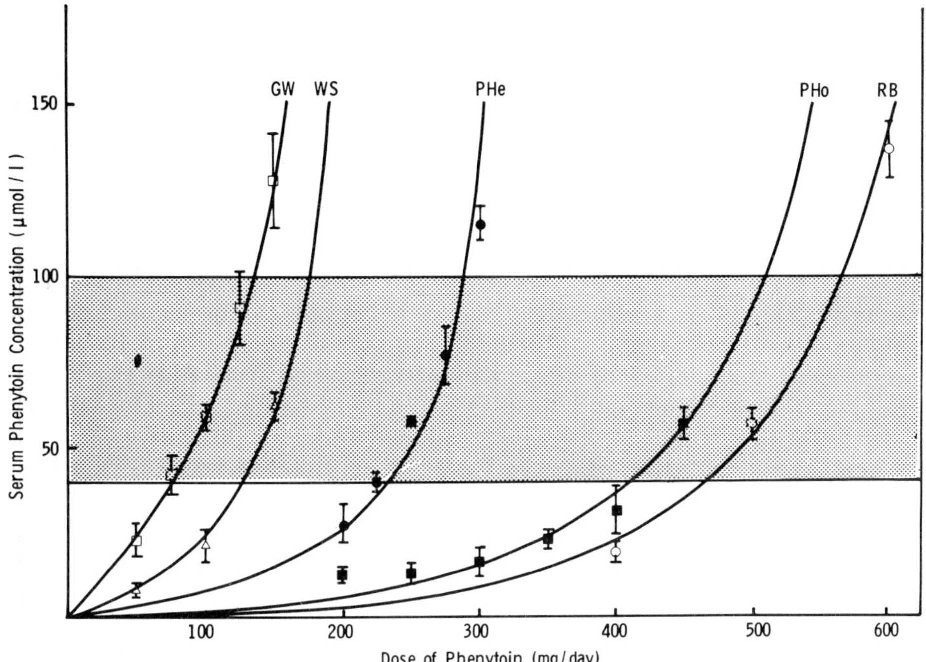

Fig. 7.1   Relationship between phenytoin dose and serum concentration in five epileptic patients. Each point represents the mean ± s.d. of three to eight separate estimations of the serum concentration in steady state. The curves were fitted by computer using the Michaelis–Menten equation. The stippled area indicates the therapeutic range of serum concentrations (a slightly higher upper limit is given than suggested in Table 7.2). (Reproduced from Richens and Dunlop (1975b) by kind permission of the editor)

1. Variations in drug intake due to non-compliance or bioavailability problems will have an exaggerated effect on the serum concentration. The physician may blame the laboratory for inaccurate measurement when fluctuations occur.
2. Increments in dose should be small when the therapeutic range is being approached. Ideally, *Km* and *Vmax* should be derived for each patient so that the optimum dose can be calculated, but in practice this is demanding because it requires at least two widely spaced, reliable measurements of serum phenytoin on different doses of the drug (Ludden et al, 1976), or, preferably, multiple estimations following administration of a single dose (Mawer et al, 1974). Neither approach represents a clinically practical method of individualising drug dosage. An alternative approach is to obtain one reliable measurement of serum phenytoin on a subtherapeutic dose of the drug, and then to predict from a nomogram the dose increment necessary to increase the serum concentration to the therapeutic range (Richens and Dunlop, 1975a). This method is entirely practical in the clinic and, on average, produces satisfactory results, but individual predictions may err on the high or low side because the development of the nomogram required the assumption that variations in *Vmax* rather than *Km* are responsible for intersubject differences, and further work has shown this to be unsound. Nevertheless, it gives better results than clinical judgement alone, although less satisfactory than methods which derive individual Michaelis–Menten parameters (Ludden et al, 1976).

3. Drug interactions resulting in induction or inhibition of phenytoin metabolism will lead to a relatively large change in serum phenytoin concentrations (Richens, 1977a).

4. Monitoring serum concentrations of phenytoin is essential if the drug is to be used correctly. When this is done, a large majority of patients can be controlled on phenytoin alone when previously they would have received multiple therapy (Reynolds et al, 1976a).

It is a disadvantage for a drug to show saturation kinetics, particularly when it has a low therapeutic ratio. It is therefore important that the nature of the metabolism of the commonly used antiepileptic drugs is clarified. Suitable techniques for detecting saturable metabolism are within-patient studies of the relationship between dose and serum concentration and between dose and urinary drug : metabolite ratio, or the use of radiolabelled tracer doses to determine a drug's serum half-life at two or more steady-state concentrations in patients receiving maintenance therapy (Richens, 1975a).

The major metabolite of phenytoin is 5-(p-hydroxyphenyl)-5-phenylhydantoin (p-HPPH). Its renal clearance exceeds the glomerular filtration rate (Bochner et al, 1973) but measurable concentrations, occasionally as high as that of the parent drug (Hoppel et al, 1977) are present in serum, mainly as the glucuronide conjugate. There is evidence in monkeys that p-HPPH causes feedback inhibition of hydroxylation of the parent drug (Glazko et al, 1977), although it was not possible to demonstrate this in three healthy volunteers (Perucca, Makki and Richens, 1977c).

There is now good evidence that the most effective range of serum concentrations for phenytoin is 40 to 80 μmol/litre (10–20 μg/ml) (Lund, 1974b), although patients with mild epilepsy might be expected to show a satisfactory response below this range. In order to achieve a therapeutic serum concentration, careful tailoring of the dose is necessary.

The serum half-life of phenytoin should not, correctly, be calculated from serum concentration data derived from studies in which large single doses of the drug have been administered, because the decay in concentration is not log-linear. Values derived in this way give the impression that the drug is cleared much more rapidly than it is in practice in patients with a therapeutic serum concentration, and hence a partially saturated hydroxylase system. The fluctuation in serum concentration during the course of 24 h is small enough for once daily dosing to give satisfactory control both in children and adults (Cocks et al, 1975).

Carbamazepine (see Penry and Daly, 1975, for review and references)
This compound is being used increasingly because there is good evidence that it is at least as good as phenytoin in tonic-clonic and focal epilepsies, and may even be superior in the latter. Further experience has also shown that it is less toxic on the bone marrow than was originally thought.

Carbamazepine tablets are relatively slowly absorbed from the gastrointestinal tract, and the serum concentration is poorly related to dose, particularly in patients receiving multiple drug therapy. It is metabolised to carbamazepine 10,11-epoxide which, in animal experiments, has antiepileptic activity, although it is only about one-third as potent as the parent compound in this respect. Nevertheless the serum concentration of the epoxide can sometimes be up to 50 per cent of that of the parent compound, and as it is only about 50 per cent bound compared with 75 per cent for the parent drug, it may contribute significantly to the therapeutic effect. This would be especially prominent in children, who metabolise the drug more quickly that adults (Pynnönen et al, 1977), and in those who are receiving concurrent therapy with hepatic microsomal enzyme inducing drugs (phenytoin, phenobarbitone and primidone). Rane, Höjer and Wilson (1976) showed that the average plasma concentration of the epoxide in children on monotherapy was 12 per cent of that of the parent drug, whereas it rose to 24 per cent when more than one drug was prescribed.

In addition to its induction by other compounds, carbamazepine metabolism is auto-inducible, i.e. the drug stimulates its own metabolism (Rawlins et al, 1975). This is reflected by the gradual fall in steady-state serum concentration during the first few weeks following introduction of maintenance therapy, and by the shorter half-lives recorded at the end of chronic therapy. In normal volunteers given single doses, values of 24 to 60 h have been found, but in patients who discontinue chronic therapy the half-life is shortened to 8.5 to 19 h. This phenomenon is likely to reduce the efficacy of the drug as well as to increase the fluctuation in the serum level during a 24 h period. The total dosage and frequency of administration may need to be adjusted to allow for this. Although the relatively short half-life suggests that frequent dosing is necessary, the slow absorption of the drug tends to stabilise the serum concentration so that twice daily dosing is generally acceptable.

Carbamazepine is probably able to induce the metabolism of other compounds, although this appears to have been little studied. Phenytoin levels, however, are lowered by concurrent carbamazepine therapy (Cereghino et al, 1973).

Evidence relating serum carbamazepine concentrations to control of fits is sparse and comes mainly from retrospective studies. The poor correlation shown by some workers may, in part, be explained by the presence of the (unmeasured) active metabolite. At concentrations above 40 μmol/litre (10 μg/ml) adverse effects, particularly dizziness, become common. The salivary concentration closely reflects the level of unbound drug in the serum.

Phenobarbitone and primidone

Phenobarbitone is cleared partly by renal excretion and partly by hepatic metabolism; p-hydroxyphenobarbitone is the major metabolite. Up to 50 per cent of the drug may appear unchanged in the urine but the actual amount is dependent both on the pH and the total volume of the urine (Whyte and Dekaban, 1977). Alkalinisation of the urine, e.g. by concurrent administration of acetazolamide (which is occasionally used in childhood and catamenial epilepsies), is likely to result in a lowering of serum phenobarbitone levels. Variation in the fluid intake or ambient temperature may, by altering urine volume, account for some of the fluctuation observed in serum concentrations in patients who are on a constant dose of the drug and are known to be compliant.

Phenobarbitone is cleared slowly and has a half-life of about four days in the average adult. Once daily dosing before retiring for the night is suitable both in adults and children. There is little evidence that its metabolism is saturable within the therapeutic range of serum concentration in adults, but Wilson and Wilkinson (1973) found evidence for saturation kinetics in a child recovering from an overdose.

The therapeutic range of serum concentrations has been poorly evaluated. Buchthal, Svensmark and Simonsen (1968) described a range of approximately 40 to 105μ mol/

litre (10–25 μg/ml), but in practice many patients are found to have levels greatly in excess of this range without marked adverse effects. The explanation for this may be that tolerance occurs to the central effects of the drug, so that the initial sedative effect on starting chronic therapy may soon be lost (Hutt et al, 1968). It has been questioned whether tolerance occurs to the antiepileptic effect, but if it does occur it would be expected to develop during the gradual rise (over two to four weeks) in serum level to steady state following introduction of therapy, at which time the increase in level would counteract the developing tolerance. Certainly, abruptly stopping phenobarbitone therapy can produce a withdrawal syndrome in which severe fits or status epilepticus can occur. This is a major problem, and even too rapid a reduction in dosage can be a hazardous affair. For this reason phenobarbitone is no longer a drug of first choice in treating the epilepsies.

Phenobarbitone is less extensively bound to plasma proteins than phenytoin and therefore binding interactions are unimportant. Salivary concentrations are a useful guide to the free plasma concentration, although alterations in salivary pH influence the partition of the drug to a greater extent than for phenytoin because the pKa of 7.2 is closer to physiological pH (Mucklow et al, 1977).

Primidone is oxidised in the liver to phenobarbitone and phenylethylmalcnamide (PEMA). The half-life of the parent compound is short, while that of PEMA is intermediate between primidone and phenobarbitone. Although only about 20 to 25 per cent of the dose is converted to phenobarbitone, the latter accumulates so that its concentration in serum is as high as that after administration of phenobarbitone itself. This is likely to account for most of the drug's antiepileptic effect, but the contribution made by unchanged primidone and PEMA has not been adequately assessed in man. In animals, however, both are active (Gallagher, Smith and Mattson, 1970; Baumel, Gallagher and Mattson, 1972).

Although a therapeutic range for primidone has been quoted by many authors, it has no meaning in the absence of evidence that primidone itself has a therapeutic effect in the epileptic patient. Measuring the serum level of derived phenobarbitone gives the most useful information for individualising the dosage.

The oxidation of primidone to phenobarbitone appears to begin slowly on starting chronic therapy; only after several days of therapy is phenobarbitone detectable in serum, perhaps because autoinduction is necessary. The pathway is inducible by concurrent phenytoin administration, resulting in an increase in the serum phenobarbitone : primidone ratio (Reynolds et al, 1975).

Sodium valproate (see Pinder et al, 1977, for review and references)
This is an interesting new compound which differs completely in structure from the established antiepileptic drugs. It is a simple two-chain fatty acid which has been given the alternative names of di-n-propylacetate, 2-n-propylpentanoate and 2-n-propylvalerate. There is evidence that its antiepileptic effects may be mediated by modification of cerebral gamma-aminobutyric acid metabolism. It appears to have a therapeutic effect on all types of epilepsies, and may turn out to be the drug of choice in petit mal and myoclonic epilepsies of childhood when better evaluated.

It is rapidly absorbed and its oral bioavailability is virtually total (Perucca et al, 1977a). Intersubject variation in serum concentrations is wide, as for the other anti-epileptic drugs. It is largely metabolised in the liver by ω-side chain oxidation although a small amount appears in the urine in a conjugated form (Ferrandes and Eymard, 1977). Its serum half-life averages 8 to 9 h in drug-free adult subjects, but no information is so far available in children. Half-lives are shorter in patients receiving concurrent antiepileptic therapy, although the clearance rate is increased to a much greater extent than would be predicted from the half-life. This is probably because other drugs displace valproate from plasma protein binding sites, as evidenced by the larger apparent volume of distribution which was observed in patients receiving polytherapy (Perucca et al, 1977b). The drug normally has a small distribution volume, and as it is about 90 per cent bound to plasma proteins, displacement would be expected to have an appreciable effect on clearance. However, hepatic microsomal enzyme induction is likely to contribute also. It is capable of displacing phenytoin from its binding sites and as a result transient signs of phenytoin intoxication may occur when it is added as a second drug. Serum phenobarbitone concentrations can be increased by valproate, possibly by inhibition of metabolism.

No reports have so far appeared in which the relationship between serum concentration and therapeutic effect has been studied on a prospective basis. From retrospective studies a therapeutic range of 350 to 700 μmol/litre (50–100 μg/ml) has been suggested. However, the drug is relatively non-toxic and it may therefore be safe to exceed this range when control of fits is not achieved at lower levels. It penetrates poorly into saliva, the concentration in this fluid being much lower than would be predicted from its binding characteristics.

The short half-life of valproate suggests that frequent dosing should be necessary. This may not be so, however, because there is evidence that the antiepileptic effect may not fluctuate as much as the serum concentration, and clinical experience suggests that twice daily dosage may be compatible with good control. The possibility of an active metabolite is being investigated.

Ethosuximide (Browne et al, 1975)

The use of this drug is, or should be, confined almost entirely to children and adolescents, for it is effective only in petit mal absences. It is often used inappropriately in the adult, usually because of diagnostic confusion between petit mal and partial (focal) epilepsies (see below). Its pharmacokinetic properties in the child are therefore most relevant to its clinical usage.

Its serum half-life is long enough to give adequate control of absence seizures with once daily dosage, although its gastrointestinal adverse effects may necessitate divided dosage. A daily dose of 20 mg/kg produces a serum concentration of about 430 μmol/litre (60 μg/ml) on average although there is a considerable scatter of individual values, and the younger child may require a rather larger dose. Optimum control of seizures is obtained when concentrations fall between 300 and 700 μmol/litre (40–100 μg/ml) (Browne et al, 1975) although a slightly higher upper limit (850 μmol/litre 120 μg/ml) was suggested in an earlier study (Sherwin and Robb, 1972). Suppression of frequent absences may improve performance on psychometric testing, although mental deterioration has been reported in some studies in which higher doses of the drug were used (Guey et al, 1967).

Clonazepam (see Pinder et al, 1976, for review and references)

Benzodiazepine compounds possess useful antiepileptic activity, particularly in the treatment of status epilepticus. Given chronically, however, they have proved disappointing because tolerance develops (see review by Browne and Penry, 1973). This applies as much to clonazepam as to the other benzodiazepines and therefore its clinical value is likely to be limited. Nevertheless, as an antiepileptic drug it is the most potent of the series, although the question whether its effect is relatively greater than its sedative action has not yet been answered. Clinical experience would suggest that it was not, for sedation is generally dose-limiting and is a major disadvantage, particularly in children. A further drawback to the chronic use of a benzodiazepine compound is that the epileptic patient will be relatively resistant to these drugs should they need to be given in status epilepticus, for which they are drugs of first choice. It is probably wise to reserve the use of oral clonazepam for the myoclonic epilepsies, which are generally difficult to treat with standard drugs, with the exception of sodium valproate. Intravenous clonazepam is effective in status epilepticus, but probably no more effective than diazepam.

Clonazepam is metabolised largely to 7-aminoclonazepam and 7-acetaminoclonazepam which lack antiepileptic effects. In addition, small amounts of 3-hydroxyclonazepam are produced, and this substance appears to be active. A therapeutic range of serum concentrations has not been defined for clonazepam, and as for phenobarbitone, the development of tolerance may make this impossible. Serum concentrations up to 840 nmol/litre (265 ng/ml) have been recorded in patients receiving therapeutic doses, although levels above 200 nmol/litre (60 ng/ml) have usually produced marked sedation.

QUALITY CONTROL OF DRUG MEASUREMENT

For some years, clinical chemists have accepted the need for external quality control of routine laboratory estimations, but in drug measurement the concept is a new one. The unreliability of antiepileptic drug estimations in Europe (Richens, 1977b) and North America (Pippenger et al, 1976) has been highlighted. In the latter study, in which the participating laboratories were unaware that they were under test, the results of phenytoin, phenobarbitone, primidone and ethosuximide estimations in aliquots of pooled sera varied from zero to levels which almost exceeded the solubility of the drugs in serum. The need for external quality control is obvious and urgent. Two schemes in which pooled or spiked serum specimens are sent out at monthly intervals to a large number of laboratories are now available, the St Bartholomew's Hospital Scheme which is organised on an international basis (excluding North America) by the author, and the Epilepsy Foundation of America Scheme covering North America, organised by Dr Charles Pippenger, Columbia University, New York. Although participation in these schemes does not guarantee good quality results, a poor performance by a laboratory has usually stimulated a careful reappraisal of the method used.

THERAPY OF INDIVIDUAL TYPES OF EPILEPSY

Although drug therapy is only one aspect of the management of epilepsy, it remains the only effective method of controlling seizures in the majority of patients. Used correctly, a satisfactory degree of control can usually be achieved. In practice, however, surveys have shown that the results tend to be disappointing (Rodin, 1968). There are many reasons for this, but irrational use of antiepileptic drugs is a common reason for failure. A number of questions need to be considered in the search for an effective drug in the individual patient.

1. *Is it epilepsy?*
Experience in the Special Centres for Epilepsy, which have been set up following the recommendation of the Reid Report (1969), suggests that the incorrect diagnosis of epilepsy is common. It is a diagnosis which should not be made without sound clinical and, if possible, EEG evidence, because its implications both in therapeutic and social terms have far-reaching consequences for the patient.

2. *What type of epilepsy?*
An epileptic fit is only one manifestation of disordered brain function or structure. It follows that the classification of the epilepsies is difficult, and recent attempts have become so cumbersome that they are almost incomprehensible to those who do not specialise in the field. Nevertheless, the accumulation of knowledge and the rationalisation of therapy is dependent upon the development of a logical scheme. In Table 7.3, an outline of the classification proposed by Gastaut (1969) is given; although this has

Table 7.3 Drug treatment of the epilepsies based on an abbreviated version of the International Classification of Epileptic Seizures (Gastaut, 1969)

Type of seizure	Drugs of choice

1. Partial seizures (seizures which produce clinical manifestations referable to a part of one hemisphere)
    (i) With elementary symptomatology (focal motor, sensory and autonomic symptomatology)
    (ii) With complex symptomatology (impaired consciousness and cognitive, affective, psychosensory and psychomotor symptomatology)
    (iii) Becoming secondarily generalised (focal seizure leading to tonic-clonic seizure)
	Carbamazepine
	Phenytoin
	Primidone
	Phenobarbitone

2. Generalised seizures (seizures which do not produce clinical manifestations referable to part of one hemisphere)	
(i) Absences (petit mal and atypical petit mal)	Sodium valproate Ethosuximide
(ii) Bilateral massive epileptic myoclonus (myoclonic jerks)	Clonazepam Sodium valproate
(iii) Infantile spasms	ACTH Clonazepam

(iv) Clonic seizures
    (v) Tonic seizures
    (vi) Tonic-clonic seizures
	Phenytoin
	Carbamazepine
	Primidone
	Phenobarbitone
	Sodium valproate

(vii) Atonic seizures (viii) Akinetic seizures	Sodium valproate Clonazepam
3. Unilateral seizures (tonic clonic or tonic-clonic seizures which are unilateral)	As for 2 (iv)–(vi) above

been accepted internationally, further revision is likely in the near future.

The commonest diagnostic error is confusion between focal fits and petit mal absences. The term 'petit mal' has been used loosely in the past to cover all minor attacks in which a brief alteration of consciousness occurs, and the difference between primary generalised (true petit mal) absences and absences associated with focal epilepsies is still not generally understood. True petit mal absences are uncommon, occur almost entirely in children and adolescents, and are accompanied by 3/s spike and wave abnormality in the EEG. They respond well to succinimide drugs but may be made worse by phenytoin and phenobarbitone. A variety of petit mal variants may occur in childhood, accompanied by slower spike and wave discharges, but from the therapeutic point of view can be considered along with true petit mal absences. Absences occurring in focal epilepsies are common, occur at any age, are not accompanied by regular spike and wave discharges, and do not generally respond to succinimide compounds.

3. *Should it be treated?*

Epilepsy is a liability to recurrent seizures; a single fit does not constitute epilepsy and should not be regarded as an indication for long term therapy. (An exception may be a single febrile convulsion in infancy. Prolonged or recurrent convulsions may lead to Ammon's horn sclerosis, with the subsequent development of temporal lobe epilepsy, and therefore prophylactic treatment during the years of risk may be justifiable — see Lennox-Buchthal, 1973.) If, however, seizures recur without an obvious and remediable precipitating factor, drug treatment will generally be of value, although complex partial seizures appear to be less amenable to therapy than most types of attack. Indeed, in the absence of secondary generalisation, it may not be in the patient's interest for large doses of one or more drugs to be administered in the hope of achieving some degree of reduction in seizure activity.

4. *Which drug?*

Coatsworth (1971) undertook a comprehensive survey of published studies on the efficacy of antiepileptic drugs. Of 110 clinical trials profiled, only three used a control for bias, one with a single-blind and two with a double-blind technique. Not surprisingly, few firm conclusions could be drawn about their effectiveness and indications in the various types of epilepsy. Richens (1975b) was able to include a few more controlled trials in his review, and more recently a number have been published which have added further to our knowledge. Perhaps the most important advance has been in identifying carbamazepine as a highly effective drug, and possibly the drug of choice in complex partial seizures (Penry and Daly, 1975). Sodium valproate appears to be a valuable compound, although its indications require defining more clearly. The current view on the selection of drugs in treating the epilepsies is summarised in Table 7.3.

5. *How should the drug be used?*

Clearly, a knowledge of the clinically relevant pharmacokinetics of a drug is essential for its correct use. Monitoring serum concentrations will then assist in achieving the right dose for the patient. In the author's opinion, monitoring is mandatory when phenytoin is used. The pharmacokinetics of the important antiepileptic drugs has been discussed earlier.

ADVERSE EFFECTS

Most of the commonly used antiepileptic drugs have a low therapeutic ratio, and because they are usually administered for long periods, often in combination, adverse effects are common. These have been the subject of a number of reviews (Richens, 1975; Reynolds, 1975a, 1875b; Pinder et al, 1976, 1977), and therefore no attempt will be made here to give a comprehensive account of them. One development which is of particular importance, however, is the realisation that chronic hepatic microsomal enzyme induction may be responsible for much iatrogenic disease in the epileptic patient. There is good evidence that phenobarbitone, primidone, phenytoin, carbamazepine and pheneturide, and probably all compounds closely related to these drugs, are potent inducers of microsomal enzymes, and as they are all used either alone or in combination in both tonic-clonic and partial epilepsies, the majority of drug-treated epileptic patients are exposed to the consequences of enzyme induction (for reviews, see Richens and Woodford, 1976; Hunter and Chasseaud, 1976).

The generally used indirect indices of microsomal enzyme induction, namely serum antipyrine half-life, serum gamma-glutamyl transpeptidase, and urinary 6-beta-hydroxycortisol or D-glucaric acid, reveal a very marked degree of induction in patients receiving polytherapy. For example, the normal average antipyrine half-life of 12 h may be reduced to a value of 4 h or less. The clearance of other drugs that are normally eliminated by the mixed function oxidase system may also be greatly increased. Naturally, this will lead to a number of interactions between the antiepileptic drugs as well as with other drugs used for general medical purposes (Table 7.4; for references see Richens, 1977a). For drugs whose rate of metabolism is enzyme limited

Table 7.4   Drugs whose metabolism has been shown to be inducible by antiepileptic drug therapy

Phenobarbitone	Quinine
Primidone	Quinidine
Phenytoin	Lignocaine
Carbamazepine	Digitoxin
Sodium valproate	Warfarin and coumarins
Clonazepam and other benzodiazepines	Phenylbutazone
Tricyclic antidepressants	Antipyrine
Phenothiazines	Tolbutamide
Corticosteroids	Metyrapone
Sex hormones (contraceptive pill)	Doxycycline

the serum half-life will decrease, but when liver blood flow is the main determinant of extraction rate the effect of induction may not be noticeable. However, first-pass metabolism may substantially reduce the systemic bioavailability of these latter drugs (e.g. propranolol, lignocaine, paracetamol).

In a few studies, cytochrome P_{450} has been measured in liver needle or wedge biopsy specimens and has been found to be considerably elevated. The clinical techniques for measuring liver size are imprecise, and have generally failed to show an increase. However, hepatic arterial blood blow may increase, as may bile secretion rate. The subnormal serum bilirubin levels that have been demonstrated in epileptic patients may be partly due to this effect, but other contributory factors are an increase in bilirubin uptake by the liver and induction of UDP-glucuronyl transferase, which is responsible for bilirubin conjugation. This effect has been used therapeutically to increase bilirubin clearance in unconjugated hyperbilirubinaemia.

Corticosteroids are normally converted by non-microsomal enzymes to tetrahydroxy-derivatives which are then conjugated with glucuronic acid and excreted as 17-hydroxycorticosteroids. With chronic administration of phenytoin the excretion of 17-hydroxy-compounds diminishes because microsomal 6-beta-hydroxylation is induced causing overall increase in steroid turnover. Patients with an intact pituitary–adrenal axis are able to compensate by increasing their cortisol secretion rate, but if the feedback mechanism is impaired, normal replacement doses of corticosteroids may be inadequate. Also, steroids given for therapeutic purposes, e.g. asthma, may be less effective when enzyme-inducing drugs are given simultaneously. Tests of adrenocortical function, e.g. the dexamethasone suppression test or metyrapone test, may be unreliable because the test drugs are eliminated more rapidly. Sex hormone metabolism is inducible also, although the clinical relevance of this is uncertain. There are reports, however, that breakthrough bleeding is more common in epileptic women receiving the contraceptive pill, and that unwanted pregnancy may occur.

Cholecalciferol (vitamin D_3) is a steroid compound which is normally activated first by 25-hydroxylation in the liver, then by 1-hydroxylation in the kidney. Serum 25-hydroxycholecalciferol levels are often subnormal in drug-treated epileptic patients. Hypocalcaemia occurs frequently and is occasionally accompanied by frank rickets or osteomalacia (see Richens and Woodford, 1976, for reviews). This is probably due to an increased elimination in the bile of biologically inactive dihydroxy-metabolites of vitamin D as a result of enzyme induction. Other mechanisms may, however, contribute to the hypocalcaemia, such as an inhibition of the tissue effects of parathyroid hormone by antiepileptic drugs (Rowe and Harris, 1976). There have been occasional reports of hypocalcaemic fits occurring, which have led to the dose of antiepileptic drugs being increased, only to lead to further aggravation. Although rare, it is important to recognise these iatrogenic fits and to administer vitamin D.

Folic acid deficiency due to antiepileptic drugs has been recognised for 25 years but the mechanism has never been clarified. As the drugs responsible are those with microsomal enzyme inducing properties, it has been suggested that this is the causative mechanism. In support of this hypothesis, it has been shown in the rat that two enzymes concerned with folate metabolism, glutamate formiminotransferase and methylene tetrahydrofolate dehydrogenase, are inducible. An alternative explanation is that folate is necessary as a coenzyme in hydroxylase reactions and the administration of large doses of drugs which require hydroxylation depletes the coenzyme. The resulting folate deficiency might be expected to slow the rate of drug elimination—indeed a fall in serum phenytoin concentrations has been demonstrated when folate is repleted, accounting, perhaps, for the coincidental increase in fit frequency and improvement in mental state which has occasionally been observed (Reynolds, 1973).

REFERENCES

Barth, N., Alvan, G., Borga, O. & Sjöqvist, F. (1976) Twofold interindividual variation in plasma protein binding of phenytoin in patients with epilepsy. *Clinical Pharmacokinetics*, **1**, 444–452.
Baumel, I. P., Gallagher, B. B. & Mattson, R. H. (1972) Phenylethylmalonamide (PEMA). An important metabolite of primidone. *Archives of Neurology (Chicago)*, **27**, 34–41.

Bochner, F., Hooper, W. D., Tyrer, J. H. & Eadie, M. H. (1973) The renal handling of diphenylhydantoin and 5-(p-hydroxyphenyl)-5-phenylhydantoin. *Clinical Pharmacology and Therapeutics*, 14, 791–796.

Booker, H. E. & Darcey, B. (1973) Serum concentrations of free diphenylhydantoin and their relationship to clinical intoxication. *Epilepsia*, 14, 177–184.

Browne, T. R., Dreyfuss, F. E., Dyken, P. R., Goode, D. J., Penry, J. K., Porter, R. J., White, B. J. & White, P. T. (1975) Ethosuximide in the treatment of absence (petit mal) seizures. *Neurology (Minneapolis)*, 25, 515–524.

Browne, T. R. & Penry, J. K. (1973) Benzodiazepines in the treatment of epilepsy. A review. *Epilepsia*, 14, 277–310.

Buchthal, F., Svensmark, O. & Simonsen, H. (1968) Relation of EEG and seizures to phenobarbital in serum. *Archives of Neurology (Chicago)*, 19, 567–572.

Cereghino, J. J., Van Meter, J. C., Brock, J. T., Penry, J. K., Smith, L. D. & White, B. G. (1973) Preliminary observations of serum carbamazepine concentration in epileptic patients. *Neurology (Minneapolis)*, 23, 357–366.

Coatsworth, J. J. (1971) *Studies on the Clinical Efficacy of Marketed Antiepileptic Drugs*, NINDS Monograph No. 12. Washington: US Government Printing Office.

Cocks, D. A., Critchley, E. M. R., Hayward, H. W., Owen, V., Mawer, G. E. & Woodcock, B. G. (1975) Control of epilepsy with a single daily dose of phenytoin sodium. *British Journal of Clinical Pharmacology*, 2, 449–453.

Ferrandes, B. & Eymard, P. (1977) Metabolism of valproate sodium in rabbit, rat, dog and man. *Epilepsia*, 18, 169–182.

Gallagher, B. B., Smith, D. B. & Mattson, R. H. (1970) The relationship of the anticonvulsant properties of primidone to phenobarbital. *Epilepsia*, 11, 293–301.

Gastaut, H. (1969) Clinical and electro-encephalographical classification of epileptic seizures. *Epilepsia*, 10, Suppl., 1–28.

Glazko, A. J., Chang, I., Maschewske, E., Hayes, A. & Dill, W. A. (1977) Role of hydroxylated metabolites of phenytoin in dose-dependency. In *Proceedings of 3rd International Symposium on Microsomes and Drug Oxidation*. Pergamon Press (in press).

Guey, J., Charles, C., Coquery, C. et al (1967) Study of psychological effects of ethosuximide (Zarontin) on 25 children suffering from petit mal epilepsy. *Epilepsia*, 8, 129–141.

Hoppel, C., Garle, M., Rane, A. & Sjöqvist, F. (1977) Plasma concentrations of 5-(4-hydroxyphenyl)-5-phenylhydantoin in phenytoin treated patients. *Clinical Pharmacology and Therapeutics*, 21, 294.

Hunter, J. & Chasseaud, L. F. (1976) Clinical aspects of microsomal enzyme induction. In *Progress in Drug Metabolism*, Vol. 1, pp. 129–192. London: John Wiley.

Hutt, S. J., Jackson, P. M., Belsham, A. & Higgins, G. (1968) Perceptual-motor behaviour in relation to blood phenobarbitone level: a preliminary report. *Developmental Medicine and Child Neurology*, 10, 626–632.

Koch-Weser, J. (1975) The serum level approach to individualisation of drug dosage. *European Journal of Clinical Pharmacology*, 9, 1–8.

Lennox-Buchthal, M. A. (1973) Febrile convulsion. A reappraisal. *Electroencephalography and Clinical Neurophysiology*, Suppl. 32.

Ludden, T. M., Allen, J. P., Valutsky, W. A., Vicuna, A. V., Napp, J. M., Hoffman, S. F., Wallace, J. F., Lacka, D. & McNay, J. L. (1976) Individualisation of phenytoin dosage regimens. *Clinical Pharmacology and Therapeutics*, 21, 287–293.

Lund, L. (1974a) Clinical significance of generic inequivalence of three different pharmaceutical preparations of phenytoin. *European Journal of Clinical Pharmacology*, 7, 119–124.

Lund, L. (1974b) Anticonvulsant effects of diphenylhydantoin relative to plasma levels. A prospective 3-year study in ambulant patients with generalised epileptic seizures. *Archives of Neurology (Chicago)*, 31, 289–294.

Mawer, G. E., Mullen, P. W., Rodgers, M., Robins, A. J. & Lucas, S. B. (1974) Phenytoin dose adjustment in epileptic patients. *British Journal of Clinical Pharmacology*, 1, 163–168.

Mucklow, J. C., Bending, M. R., Kahn, G. C. & Dollery, C. T. (1978) Drug concentrations in human saliva. *Clinical Pharmacology and Therapeutics*. In press.

Odar-Cederlöff, I. & Borga, O. (1974) Kinetics of diphenylhydantoin in uraemic patients: consequences of decreased plasma protein binding. *European Journal of Clinical Pharmacology*, 7, 31–37.

Paxton, J. W., Whiting, B. & Stephen, K. W. (1977) Phenytoin concentrations in mixed, parotid and submandibular saliva and serum measured by radio immuno assay. *British Journal of Clinical Pharmacology*, 4, 185–192.

Penry, J. K. & Daly, D. D. (eds.) (1975) *Complex Partial Seizures and their Treatment. Advances in Neurology*, Vol. 11. New York: Raven Press.

Perucca, E., Gatti, G., Frigo, G. M. & Crema, A. (1978a) Pharmacokinetics of sodium valproate after oral and intravenous administration. *British Journal of Clinical Pharmacology*, 5, 313–318.

Perucca, E., Gatti, G., Frigo, G. M., Crema, A., Calzetti, S. & Visintini, D. (1978b) Disposition of sodium valproate in epileptic patients. *British Journal of Clinical Pharmacology*, 5, 495–500.

Perucca, E., Makki, K. & Richens, A. (1977c) Is phenytoin metabolism subject to feedback inhibition? *Clinical Pharmacology and Therapeutics*. In press.

Pinder, R. M., Brogden, R. N., Speight, T. M. & Avery, G. S. (1976) Clonazepam: a review of its pharmacological properties and therapeutic efficacy in epilepsy. *Drugs*, 12, 321–361.

Pinder, R. M., Brogden, R. N., Speight, T. M. & Avery, G. S. (1977) Sodium valproate: a review of its pharmacological properties and therapeutic efficacy in epilepsy. *Drugs*, 13, 81–123.

Pippenger, C. E., Penry, J. K., White, B. G., Daly, D. D. & Buddington, R. (1976) Interlaboratory variability in determination of plasma antiepileptic drug concentrations. *Archives of Neurology (Chicago)*, 33, 351–355.

Porter, R. J., & Layzer, R. B. (1975) Plasma albumin concentration and diphenylhydantoin binding in man. *Archives of Neurology (Chicago)*, 32, 298–303.

Pynnönen, S., Sillanpaa, M., Frey, H. & Iisalo, E. (1977) Carbamazepine and its 10,11-epoxide in children and adults with epilepsy. *European Journal of Clinical Pharmacology*, 11, 129–133.

Rane, A., Höjer, B. & Wilson, J. T. (1976) Kinetics of carbamazepine and its 10,11-epoxide metabolite in children. *Clinical Pharmacology and Therapeutics*, 19, 276–283.

Rawlins, M. D., Coliste, P., Bertilsson, L. & Palmer, L. (1975) Distribution and elimination kinetics of carbamazepine in man. *European Journal of Clinical Pharmacology*, 8, 91–96.

Reid Report (1969) *People with Epilepsy*. London: HMSO.

Reynolds, E. H. (1973) Anticonvulsants, folic acid, and epilepsy. *Lancet*, i, 1376–1378.

Reynolds, E. H. (1975a) Chronic antiepileptic toxicity: a review. *Epilepsia*, 16, 319–352.

Reynolds, E. H. (1975b) Neurotoxicity of carbamazepine. In *Complex Partial Seizures and their Treatment. Advances in Neurology*, ed. Penry, J. K. & Daly, D. D., Vol. 11, pp. 345–354. New York: Raven Press.

Reynolds, E. H., Fenton, G., Fenwick, P., Johnson, A. & Laundy, M. (1975) Interaction of phenytoin and primidone. *British Medical Journal*, ii, 594–595.

Reynolds, E. H., Chadwick, D. & Galbraith, A. W. (1976a) One drug (phenytoin) in the treatment of epilepsy. *Lancet*, i, 923–926.

Reynolds, F., Ziroyanis, P., Jones, N. & Smith, S. E. (1976b) Salivary phenytoin concentrations in epilepsy and in chronic renal failure. *Lancet*, ii, 384.

Richens, A. (1975a) A study of the pharmacokinetics of phenytoin (diphenylhydantoin) in epileptic patients, and the development of a nomogram for making dose increments. *Epilepsia*, 16, 627–646.

Richens, A. (1975b) *Drug Treatment of Epilepsy*. London: Henry Kimpton.

Richens, A. (1976) Clinical pharmacology and medical treatment. In *A Textbook of Epilepsy*, ed. Laidlaw, J. & Richens, A. Edinburgh: Churchill Livingstone.

Richens, A. (1977a) Interactions with antiepileptic drugs. *Drugs*, 13, 266–275.

Richens, A. (1977b) Evaluation of reliability in determination of antiepileptic drug levels. In *Epilepsy. The Eighth International Symposium*. Ed. Penry, J. K., pp. 115–118. New York: Raven Press.

Richens, A. & Dunlop, A. (1975a) Phenytoin dosage nomogram. *Lancet*, ii, 1305–1306.

Richens, A. & Dunlop, A. (1975b) Serum phenytoin levels in the management of epilepsy. *Lancet*, ii, 247–248.

Richens, A. & Woodford, F. P. (ed.) (1976) *Anticonvulsant Drugs and Enzyme Induction*. Amsterdam: Associated Scientific Publishers.

Rodin, E. A. (1968) *The Prognosis of Patients with Epilepsy*. Thomas, Springfield.

Rowe, D. J. F. & Harris, M. (1976) Effects of anticonvulsant drugs on bone resorption induced by parathyroid extract in vitro. In *Anticonvulsant Drugs and Enzyme Induction*, ed. Richens, A. & Woodford, F. P. Amsterdam: Associated Scientific Publishers.

Serrano, E. E. & Wilder, B. J. (1974) Intramuscular administration of diphenylhydantoin. Histologic follow-up. *Archives of Neurology (Chicago)*, 31, 276–278.

Sherwin, A. L. & Robb, J. P. (1972) Ethosuximide. Relation of plasma levels to clinical control. In *Antiepileptic Drugs*, ed. Woodbury, D. M., Penry, J. K. & Schmidt, R. P., pp. 443–448. New York: Raven Press.

Shorvon, S. D. & Reynolds, E. H. (1977) Unnecessary polypharmacy for epilepsy. *British Medical Journal*, i, 1635–1637.

Tyrer, J. H., Eadie, M. J., Sutherland, J. M. & Hooper, W. D. (1970) Outbreak of anticonvulsant intoxication in an Australian city. *British Medical Journal*, iv, 271–273.

Whyte, M. P. & Dekaban, A. S. (1977) Metabolic fate of phenobarbital. A quantative study of p-hydroxyphenobarbital elimination in man. *Drug metabolism and disposition*, 5, 63–70.

Wilensky, A. J. & Lowden, J. A. (1973) Inadequate serum levels after intramuscular administration of diphenylhydantoin. *Neurology (Minneapolis)*, 23, 318–324.

Wilson, J. T. & Wilkinson, G. R. (1973) Chronic and severe phenobarbital intoxication in a child treated with primidone and diphenylhydantoin. *Journal of Pediatrics*, 83, 484–489.

8. Clinical psychopharmacology

D. G. Grahame-Smith   M. W. Orr

INTRODUCTION

Because of the breadth of the subject this review is highly selective. The reader will find little here in the way of a review of clinical therapeutic trials or advice on the indications for the use of a particular drug since we consider these matters more clinical 'therapeutics' than clinical 'pharmacology'.

Our intention has been to pick out certain topics of interest in the clinical pharmacology of psychotropic drugs, to examine some of their basic and clinical pharmacological effects and the relevance of these to their therapeutic action on the one hand and to the understanding of the abnormalities of brain function present in mental illness and its correction on the other, and lastly to consider the relationship between the pharmacokinetic properties, the pharmacodynamic actions and the therapeutic effects of certain psychotropic drugs with particular reference to the individualisation of dosage schedules and the clinical monitoring of psychotropic drug therapy.

THE INDIVIDUALISATION OF PSYCHOTROPIC DRUG THERAPY: MONITORING TECHNIQUES

The sequence of events which occurs between the administration of a drug and its therapeutic effect is extraordinarily complex. The sequence is diagrammatically depicted in Figure 8.1. This sequence, which is at the core of what follows, ignores one extremely important factor, that of patient compliance with prescribed drug therapy. Blackwell (1973) has looked at this problem and identified certain factors associated with non-compliance. Psychiatric disease he identified as a particular problem because it may erode the capacity to cooperate, and therapy is often prolonged. In a study of patients with schizophrenia Richards (1964) found that those who refused medication expressed unfavourable feelings toward authority. There is little doubt that if the patient has hostility toward the psychiatrist and lack of insight into his illness compliance is likely to be disastrously poor. Multiple medications and frequent dose regimens generally foster poor compliance. The drug treatment should be as simple as possible. The setting in which drugs are prescribed and administered influences compliance. Blackwell (1973) quotes several studies showing that amongst psychiatric patients lack of compliance is worse in out-patients than in in-patients.

What can be done about non-compliance? Firstly keep the treatment as simple as possible and compatible with the patient's everyday habits. The current trend to prescribing tricyclic antidepressants as one dose at night is an example of this. Undoubtedly, chronic neuroleptic therapy in schizophrenia has been aided by the introduction of depot neuroleptics which are given every one to three weeks by injection under supervision. The most important thing is that the physician is aware of the

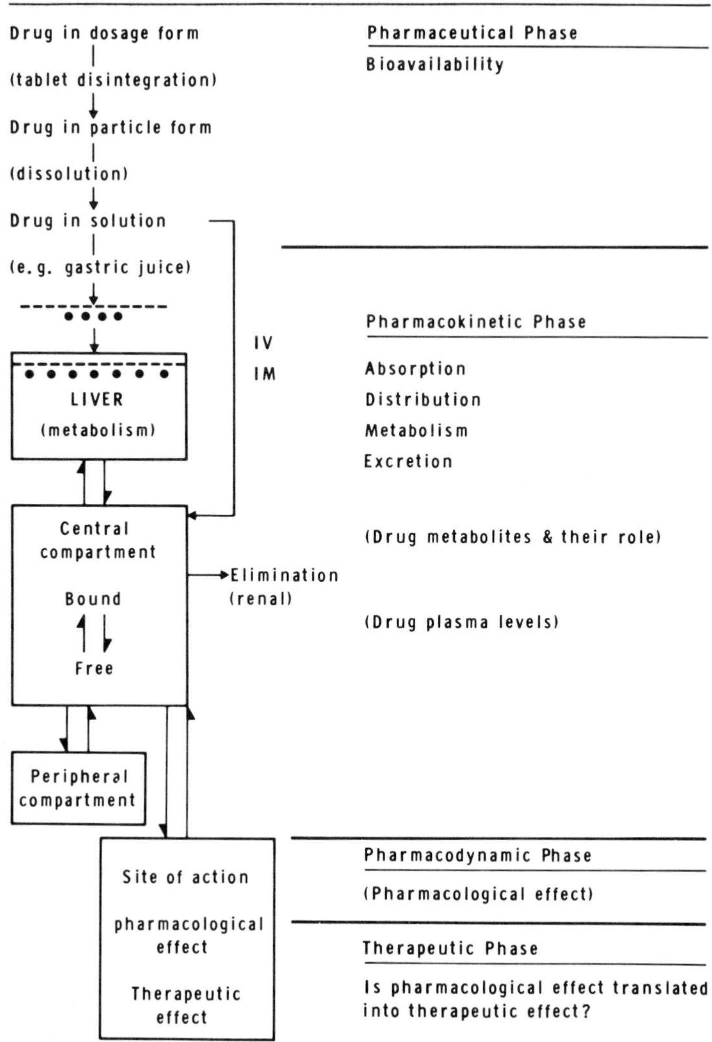

Fig. 8.1 Processes occurring on drug administration

problem of non-compliance as a cause of failure of therapy and is then prepared to go into this as a possibility and to follow this up with appropriate action to overcome it. One cause of non-compliance which is not often appreciated is the adverse effects of drugs.

Many physicians and psychiatrists do not bother to explain to patients the nature of the drug they are receiving. It is no wonder that patients do not cooperate well. Several other ways of improving patient compliance have been discussed by Blackwell (1973). The point of emphasising this matter, is that sophisticated consideration of clinical pharmacology of psychotropic drugs is only relevant if the patient is taking the treatment.

Returning to Figure 8.1, bioavailability though important will not be discussed here. The rest of the sequence can be broken down into three phases (see Grahame-Smith, 1977a):

1. Pharmacokinetic phase

This involves the study and understanding of the absorption, distribution, metabolism and excretion of drugs. This phase is described through the measurement of drug and metabolite concentrations in blood and/or urine over periods of time after dosing. Proper mathematical description of plasma drug concentrations/time curves can tell one a great deal about the disposition of the drug of relevance to its pharmacological effect (Greenblatt and Koch-Weser, 1975). These aspects in regard to psychotropic drugs have been dealt with in some detail by Lader (1976). The pharmacokinetic behaviour of a drug or its metabolites in blood is of major importance in determining its effect because, however many structural and metabolic barriers drug molecules have to pass, the concentration of a drug at its site of action must have the blood concentration as one of its major determinants. The relationship between the blood concentration with time and the pharmacological effect may be a complex one, so complex that it can be difficult to sort out, but logically a relationship must always exist if only we knew how to analyse it properly.

By study of the pharmacokinetic phase inter-individual variability in regard to absorption, distribution, metabolism and excretion of drugs can be defined and the contribution such studies have made to our understanding of the variability of responses to drugs is very considerable.

2. Pharmacodynamic phase

This phase is concerned with understanding of the pharmacological effects of the drug and however ignorant one may be of the mode of action of psychotropic drugs their actions in relationship to their therapeutic effects are still of prime importance and must be interposed between the pharmacokinetic phase and the therapeutic phase. The pharmacodynamic phase is very complex for psychotropic drugs because the parent drug and its metabolites must pass the blood–brain barrier and sometimes neuronal membranes to affect intraneuronal mechanisms. In many cases these multiple barriers through which drugs pass, by passive or active transport mechanisms, obscure the relationship between the plasma level and the therapeutic effect.

Some non-psychotropic drug actions are superficially simple, for example simple pharmacological antagonists such as beta-adrenoreceptor blocking agents and morphine antagonists. Other drugs have much more complex actions involving cascades of biochemical and pharmacological events and such indeed may be the case for many psychotropic agents. In terms of effects with time some drugs are 'on/off', the degree of effect closely following the blood level and in terms of its intoxicant effect alcohol is one of these.

Some drugs, are 'hit and run'. This phenomenon can occur in two ways. First the drug may bind and continue to act (i.e. not immediately reversible) despite a falling blood level (irreversible monoamine oxidase inhibitors); the second mechanism by which this effect may be brought about is when the drug sets in train a sequence of pharmacological effects which take time to run down (one suspects that this might be the case with tricyclic antidepressants and neuroleptics though it is difficult to be sure).

With such drugs the relationship between blood levels and pharmacological effects may be difficult to unravel and subject to great variation in the clinical situation.

3. Therapeutic phase

As a final event the pharmacodynamic effect must be translated into a therapeutic effect and this translation may not always take place. Although it is difficult to be certain, one suspects that many cases of schizophrenia are unresponsive to neuroleptic drug therapy not because the drug is not producing a pharmacological effect but because the disease process is unresponsive to the pharmacological effect of the drug. While our understanding of the neurochemical and neuropharmacological basis of mental illness and the true mode of action of psychotropic drugs is so incomplete it would be foolish to think that just because one achieves a certain pharmacological effect in the brain the mental illness is going to recover. For instance, however much of a positive inotropic effect is feasible with non-toxic doses of digitalis the degree of such an effect might be insufficient to bring about appreciable therapeutic benefit in some cases of severe cardiac failure. It is also debatable as to how much improvement in mortality and morbidity occurs by lowering the blood glucose with oral hypoglycaemics in mild mature-onset diabetes. We merely wish to point out that on occasions one can certainly produce a pharmacological effect without necessarily achieving therapeutic benefit. One cannot help feeling that when depression is truly unresponsive to adequate doses of tricyclic antidepressants and schizophrenia unresponsive to neuroleptics the therapy is probably inappropriate and reflects our lack of understanding of the aetiological process responsible for the condition and/or our ignorance of the mode of action of the drugs.

The investigation and sorting out of the pharmacokinetic, pharmacodynamic, and therapeutic phases and their linkage in psychotropic drug therapy is of importance in two ways. First it has practical benefit in helping to individualise drug therapy for a particular patient. Secondly it leads to a greater understanding of the actions of drugs in the clinical situation and through this, provide clues to disordered brain function underlying the mental illness.

INDIVIDUALISATION OF TRICYCLIC ANTIDEPRESSANT DRUG THERAPY

There is controversy at present about the relationship between the plasma concentrations of tricyclic antidepressants and their therapeutic effects in depression.

Some points are worth emphasising:

1. What holds for one tricyclic antidepressant need not hold for another. There are differences in metabolic pathways, pharmacokinetic properties and pharmacological actions between members of this class of drugs.
2. Diagnostic criteria among studies should be comparable. It is generally agreed that tricyclic antidepressant drug therapy is most effective in classical 'endogenous' depression and less so in 'reactive' depression. Since a relationship between plasma concentration of a drug and its therapeutic effect is only likely to be seen in 'responsive' patients, there is little point, from the purist angle, in studying the relationship in patients who do not respond.
3. Qualitative and quantitative precision of measurement of the drugs and their metabolites in plasma is of crucial importance.

One of the reasons for interest in this problem is the very wide difference in plasma levels of nortriptyline, amitriptyline and imipramine found in patients receiving the same doses of these drugs in steady state (Åsberg, 1974), and this is largely due to genetic differences in metabolic capacity resulting in differences in the rate of the elimination of the drugs from the body (Sjoqvist, 1975). There has been discussion of the role which plasma protein binding might have in accounting for inter-individual differences in response, since only the 'free' fraction of drug in the plasma is likely to be pharmacologically active. Desmethylimipramine, for instance, is about 90 per cent bound to plasma proteins and a 10 per cent decrease in binding would increase the pharmacologically active fraction by 100 per cent. Sjoqvist and his colleagues however (Sjoqvist, 1975) looked at this aspect by comparing the total plasma concentration of desmethylimipramine with the ability of the plasma to inhibit noradrenaline uptake by rat brain slices. There was a very good correlation suggesting that, generally, differences in plasma protein binding are not an important factor.

Nortriptyline

Table 8.1 lists the investigations done with conclusions and comments. It will be seen that in four studies there is evidence that at the least there is a 'therapeutic window' for nortriptyline in which a therapeutic response is likely to occur, i.e. with a 'steady state' plasma level of about 50 to 140 ng/ml. Below 50 ng/ml a therapeutic response is unlikely. Patients with levels >140 ng/ml are less likely to do well but when the dosage is reduced and the plasma level falls to within the therapeutic window they improve again. It has been suggested that at high concentrations nortriptyline might block

Table 8.1   Relationship between nortriptyline plasma concentration and therapeutic effect

Study	Conclusion	Comment
1. Åsberg et al (1971)	Best results obtained with levels 50–140 ng/ml. >140 ng/ml response less. <50 ng/ml response less	Endogenous depressions. Treatment period only two weeks. Other drugs also given
2. Kragh-Sørensen et al (1973)	>170 ng/ml response poor	Endogenous depressions (fairly severe). Four weeks
3. Kragh-Sørensen et al (1976a)	>180 ng/ml poor response. Reduction of level → improvement	Endogenous depression. Four weeks
4. Ziegler et al (1976a)	Best results 50–140 ng/ml >140–260 ng/ml results not so good, particularly at three to six weeks	Depressed patients. Six weeks
5. Lyle et al (1974)	No correlation or upper therapeutic level found	'Depresssed'
6. Burrows et al (1972, 1974)	No correlation	Criticised by Kragh-Sørensen et al (1976b). Mixed groups of depressives. No severe depressives Fluctuations in plasma levels considerable

catecholamine receptors, which could hypothetically account for the fall-off of therapeutic effect at high plasma levels.

Three studies have not shown any correlation between plasma levels and clinical response. These have been criticised on several counts (see Kragh-Sørensen et al, 1976b). Our own impression from reviewing these studies is that in those investigations in which a 'therapeutic window' effect has been found, the conclusion is valid, and it should be possible to replicate the results if the trial methodology and choice of patients is similar. In this field it is essential to compare like studies.

Amitriptyline

The situation in regard to amitriptyline is no less confused. Table 8.2 lists two studies showing some correlation of plasma levels with therapeutic response, in one with both amitriptyline and nortriptyline, its metabolite, and in the other amitriptyline. In a more

Table 8.2 Relationship between amitriptyline plasma concentration and therapeutic effect

Study	Conclusion	Comment
Braithwaite et al (1972)	Linear positive correlation. Amitriptyline 20–278 ng/ml. Nortriptyline 20–228 ng/ml	Measured Amitriptyline and Nortriptyline. 'Depressive' illness undefined
Ziegler et al (1976b)	Response positively correlated with amitriptyline level, not with nortriptyline	Outpatient depressives
Coppen (1977)	No correlations found of plasma levels with therapeutic effect. Good correlation of nortriptyline level with decreased tyramine effect	Multicentre WHO study. Primary depressive illness. Six weeks administration

recent study Coppen (1977) has been unable to confirm some previous results. Certainly no 'therapeutic window' has been found for amitriptyline as for nortriptyline alone. Looking at the evidence on amitriptyline so far it is clear that further carefully designed studies are needed to clear up the matter. From what has been presented up till now it seems that the measurement of plasma amitriptyline (and nortriptyline) levels as a fine guide to amitriptyline therapy is not going to add a great deal.

Imipramine (see Table 8.3)

The early study of Walter (1971) measuring only imipramine fluorometrically suggested a narrow range of levels with a correlation between plasma level and clinical response. Gram et al (1976) and Glassman et al (1977) have gone into the matter in much greater detail. These studies show that on a fixed dose of imipramine plasma levels of imipramine and desipramine vary considerably. However, although a precise correlation between the plasma level of imipramine and/or desipramine and the response may not be possible there is a good indication that there is a therapeutic range of levels below which a response is unlikely and that 33 per cent of patients may not attain that therapeutic range associated with the highest response rate on a fixed dosage schedule of 3.5 mg/kg/day (Glassman et al, 1977). Gram et al (1976) make the point that the

Table 8.3   Relationship between imipramine plasma levels and therapeutic response

Study	Conclusion	Comments
Walter (1971)	Imipramine (only) range 2.5–71 ng/ml. Positive correlation	Endogenous depression. Fluorometric assay
Gram et al (1976)	Responders plasma levels imipramine $\geq$45 ng/ml and desipramine >75 ng/ml. No fall off at high levels	Endogenous depression. Placebo period followed by clinical evaluation on treatment at five to six weeks
Glassman et al (1977)	Positive correlation ($r=0.48$). Pooled imipramine and desipramine plasma levels. Response rate poor with plasma level 150 ng/ml. Response rate improved in range 150–200 ng/ml. Plateaux about 250 ng/ml. No fall off in effect with high plasma levels	Depressed. Unipolar delusional patients—no correlation between plasma level and clinical response. Males with high plasma levels, good response

imipramine/desipramine ratio may be important, that the compounds may have separate effects, and that the ratio is variable from patient to patient and that this is also a source of potential variability in influencing the outcome.

What is to be made of all this?:

1. The studies on nortriptyline showing a therapeutic window (or curvilinear relationship between plasma level and therapeutic response) look reliable. Without access of plasma level determinations the advice given by Åsberg (1976) is useful. A standard dose of nortriptyline of 50 mg three times a day will produce therapeutic plasma levels in about 65 per cent of patients. If in three weeks there is no response, lower the dose to 25 mg three times a day (since it is most probable that the level is too high). Wait one week and if no effect, raise the dose to 75 mg three times a day. If still no response change to another antidepressant agent, she suggests clomipramine.
2. A case can be made for measuring plasma imipramine and desipramine levels in patients treated with imipramine to ensure that they are in the therapeutic range (i.e. combined levels between 150 and 250 ng/ml).
3. The situation in regard to amitriptyline is difficult and more work is needed to clarify the matter.
4. There are now several studies showing excellent correlations between the inhibition of the tyramine pressor response and the plasma level of amitriptyline and nortriptyline yet the actual correlations with the therapeutic response in depression are usually rather weak. This means that the peripheral pharmacodynamic effect does not mirror the central effect through which the therapeutic response is mediated. This points to either pharmacokinetic differences existing between the compartment housing the sympathetic nervous system and the brain compartment *or* pharmacodynamic differences, i.e. is the mechanism of action by which tricyclic antidepressants effectively produce their antidepressant effects really inhibition of monoamine re-uptake? If inhibition of monoamine re-uptake is not the mechanism by which the tricyclic antidepressant drugs effectively produce the therapeutic action

and if their therapeutic action depends upon longer term complex changes in monoamine turnover, metabolism or changes in receptor sensitivity and so on, then simple relationships between plasma levels and therapeutic response are unlikely to be found. We believe that the work that has been done in this field suggests that such a complexity does exist and that further work is needed to verify or refute the hypothesis that inhibition of monoamine re-uptake is the mechanism by which these drugs act to relieve depression. If another mechanism is discovered it would change our thinking about the likely relationship between the pharmacokinetic properties of the drugs and what at present are believed to be their important pharmacodynamic effect.

INDIVIDUALISATION OF NEUROLEPTIC DRUG THERAPY IN SCHIZOPHRENIA

The variability in response to neuroleptic drug therapy in schizophrenia is well known. Is this variability due to the differences in the pharmacokinetic handling of the drug, in its pharmacodynamic effects or in the link between its pharmacodynamic effects and the therapeutic action?

A major difficulty in the identification of pharmacological factors which might account for some of the observed variability in drug response in schizophrenia (as in depression) is that patients do not form uniform groups. It may be thought that in some patients clinical improvement does bear a good relationship to adequate plasma levels and central pharmacodynamic effects. Other patients may remit or remain well without medication, the natural course of the illness being the main determinant. Others may prove resistant to therapy however adequate the plasma levels and pharmacodynamic effects of the drugs at present being used. Again, as with antidepressants this heterogeneity may obscure the factors relating drug prescription to therapeutic response.

Another important complicating factor is that in general, factors which are of prognostic value for the natural course of schizophrenia bear a similar relationship to the outcome of drug treatment, but neither prognostic factors nor environmental factors such as social stresses or family influences explain in a satisfactory way, the wide variation in the clinical course of treated patients. In schizophrenia certain clinical factors have been shown to be associated with a good response to treatment (Leff and Wing, 1971) and certain psychosocial factors are associated with an increased risk of relapse (Vaughn and Leff, 1976). The point here is that the disturbance in brain function (whatever that may be!) in schizophrenia, the drug used to treat it, and the influence of environmental factors on that disturbed brain function, all interact, certainly in the context of long term out-patient therapy.

Most of the work on plasma levels in neuroleptic drugs has been carried out with chlorpromazine and in a series of early studies, Curry, Davis and Janowsky (1970) showed that there were wide variations in the plasma levels of chlorpromazine in patients receiving the same dose, though, within patients, dosage and plasma levels varied in a consistent way. In a later study Sakalis et al (1972) showed however that intra-individual consistency was poor in a group of acutely ill psychotic patients who were monitored during the early phases of treatment. The low correlation between dose and plasma levels has been widely confirmed (Rivera-Calimlim et al, 1976; Wiles et al,

1976); the overall relationship between dosage and plasma levels is, however, not simple and Wiles et al (1976) have suggested that though plasma chlorpromazine levels increase with dosage up to a daily dose of 400 mg, patients receiving larger doses had a lower mean level of chlorpromazine — this confirmed similar findings reported by Mackay, Healey and Baker (1974) with chlorpromazine and Martensson and Roos (1974) with thioridazine.

The variability in the relationship between plasma levels and dosage is accompanied by a variability in the relationship between plasma levels of chlorpromazine and clinical effects. Most workers report a plasma level range of 0 to 110 ng/ml in patients receiving conventional doses of chlorpromazine by mouth; there does not appear to be a 'therapeutic range' of levels for patients receiving chlorpromazine. A number of studies (Curry et al, 1970; Mackay et al, 1974; Rivera-Calimlim et al, 1973, 1976; Wiles et al, 1976; Kolakowska et al, 1976) have shown that clinical improvement in both acute and chronic schizophrenic patients treated with chlorpromazine was associated with a wide range of plasma levels; furthermore there were no significant differences in the plasma levels of patients who responded and patients who did not respond.

However, results have not been uniformly negative. Sakalis et al (1972) showed that clinical changes in the first fortnight of treatment in acute patients were related to plasma chlorpromazine levels, though the correlation was not maintained throughout treatment. Rivera-Calimlim et al (1976) showed a relationship between plasma chlorpromazine levels and clinical improvement for certain symptoms of schizophrenia and suggested that a plasma level range of 50 to 300 ng/ml was associated with improvement in thought disorder and paranoid ideation, but not with some negative symptoms of schizophrenia such as withdrawal, retardation, blunting of affect and somatic concern. This suggests that it might be possible to show a relationship between plasma levels of a neuroleptic drug and certain aspects of a patient's symptomatology, which would have been masked by a lack of correlation between plasma levels and global clinical response.

Plasma levels of chlorpromazine have also been shown to correlate positively with plasma levels of prolactin, which may be an indication of the dopamine blocking action of chlorpromazine in the hypothalamus (Kolakowska et al, 1975; Wiles et al, 1976). In addition, extrapyramidal side effects have been shown to be associated with higher levels of plasma chlorpromazine and prolactin in acutely ill schizophrenic patients (Wiles et al, 1976) though this relationship did not hold in chronic patients (Kolakowska et al, 1976).

The search for active metabolites has suggested that metabolic pathways might be important in determining the outcome of treatment with neuroleptic drugs. Sakalis et al (1974) and Mackay et al (1974) have reported higher levels of a pharmacologically active metabolite of chlorpromazine, 7-hydroxychlorpromazine, in patients who had improved clinically, and Wiles et al (1976) found that acutely ill patients who failed to respond to treatment had a greater proportion of chlorpromazine sulphoxide, a pharmacologically inactive metabolite, in plasma samples taken just before a dose. Chlorpromazine has a multiplicity of metabolites and these studies have been concerned with only a few; it will therefore be difficult to show a positive relationship between only a fraction of what could be the total amount of pharmacologically active drug and metabolites and any clinical changes.

Relationships between plasma levels and clinical changes after a single dose of the drug may not necessarily be observed after multiple doses or during long-term treatment, either as a result of the persistence and accumulation of the drug in the body, the development of tolerance or changes in other factors influencing the disease process. Tolerance is a particularly interesting phenomenon and clinical observation has suggested that long-term administration of neuroleptic drugs leads to the development of tolerance to some of the side effects. Tolerance could be due to pharmacokinetic factors or to changes in the sensitivity of those areas of the brain affected by the drug. The relationship observed between plasma chlorpromazine levels, extrapyramidal side effects and prolactin levels in acute patients does not hold for chronic patients and no relationship could be shown between plasma levels of chlorpromazine and plasma levels of prolactin or extrapyramidal side effects in chronic patients who had been receiving chlorpromazine for a prolonged period. (Kolakowska et al, 1976) Both prolactin levels and extrapyramidal side effects are related to the dopamine blocking effects of neuroleptics in the brain and the finding that, in chronic patients, these indices of dopamine blockade were lower than in acute patients in spite of similar plasma levels would suggest that there could be acquired tolerance to some of the dopamine blocking effects of neuroleptic drugs without any apparent interference in their capacity to maintain their therapeutic activity. One wonders whether these aspects of tolerance might be related to the *increased* sensitivity of animals to the behavioural effects of central 5-HT and dopamine action after long-term neuroleptic drug administration (Heal et al, 1976), perhaps indicating increased receptor sensitivity subsequent to receptor block.

In animals the effects of neuroleptic drugs on dopamine turnover in the brain are also different during acute and chronic treatment; Wiesel et al (1975) showed that, while a single dose of chlorpromazine led to increases in levels of homovanillic acid (HVA) in the rat striatum which correlated with plasma and brain levels of the drug, HVA levels after repeated dosage correlated only with brain levels and not with plasma levels. There is evidence that the effects of repeated administration of neuroleptics vary between one area of the brain and another and this could explain why tolerance to extrapyramidal side effects can occur without any lessening in therapeutic effects. Sayers et al (1975) have shown that repeated administration of chlorpromazine produces smaller rises in HVA in the caudate nucleus than a single dose given acutely, while others (Bowers and Rozitis, 1974) have shown no difference between the effects of acute and chronic chlorpromazine treatment on HVA levels in the limbic system and in the hypothalamus. In man, Goodwin, Post and Sack (1975) showed an increase in HVA in cerebrospinal fluid in patients shortly after the start of phenothiazine treatment, but not in patients who had been on phenothiazines for more than five weeks.

These studies confirm the clinical impression that there is a dissociation between the therapeutic effects of neuroleptic drugs and their capacity to produce extrapyramidal side effects; they also suggest important implications for the prescription of anticholinergic drugs in the management of drug-induced extrapyramidal side effects in patients on chronic treatment. There is some evidence that some anticholinergic drugs lead to a reduction in plasma levels of chlorpromazine (Rivera-Calimlim et al, 1976), perhaps by interfering with absorptive mechanisms, but this finding has not been confirmed by others (Wiles et al, 1976); it has also been shown (Singh and Smith, 1976) that anticholinergic drugs prescribed during acute treatment occasionally lead to a therapeutic reversal with an exacerbation of symptoms. It is also well known that withdrawal of anti-Parkinsonian drugs carries very little risk of a recurrence of Parkinsonian symptoms (Orlov et al, 1971) and that the routine long-term prescription of these drugs can increase the intensity and duration of dyskinetic symptoms in tardive dyskinesia and sometimes lower the threshold for the manifestation of tardive dyskinesia (Klawans and Rubovits, 1974).

A large number of factors are known to affect the relationship between plasma levels of a drug and clinical changes and these have been reviewed elsewhere (Curry, 1974). With chlorpromazine, such factors as the presence of intestinal contents and the pharmaceutical formulation of the drug were shown to affect the concentration of chlorpromazine in plasma (Curry et al, 1970). As chlorpromazine is 95 to 98 per cent bound to plasma proteins and as this binding is reversible and has been shown to vary in the interval between doses, variations in binding theoretically could also lead to fluctuations in plasma level concentrations and non-linear relationship between levels and clinical effect.

Similar non-linear relationships between plasma levels and therapeutic effects have been shown with thioridazine (Martensson and Roos, 1974). Forsman et al (1974) have recently developed a gas-chromatographic method for determining plasma levels of haloperidol and have shown a one- to ten-fold variation in serum levels in patients on the same dose and, as with other neuroleptics it has been difficult to identify a therapeutic range which might serve as a guide to treatment.

There have been no reports so far relating plasma levels of the long acting depot neuroleptic preparations to therapeutic effects. This is because it has proved difficult to develop an assay sensitive enough to measure the very low plasma levels obtained with these drugs. It is possible that inter-individual variability in plasma levels may be less of a problem with these drugs than with other neuroleptics as they are administered parenterally. A sensitive radioimmunoassay for fluphenazine is now available (Wiles and Franklin, 1977) and preliminary results on a small group of patients receiving usual maintenance doses of fluphenazine decanoate (Modecate) suggests that patients on different dose regimens show a narrow range of plasma levels (1–3 ng/ml) with very little change within patients between one injection cycle and the next (Wiles et al, in preparation).

The absence of a linear relationship between plasma levels of chlorpromazine and other neuroleptic drugs and therapeutic responses has led to a series of studies relating the concentration of phenothiazines in red blood cells to therapeutic responses. Garver et al (1976) showed that acute extrapyramidal side effects of butaperazine, a piperazine phenothiazine, were more clearly related to quantities of the drug bound to red cells than to plasma levels. In a more recent study (Garver et al, 1977), butaperazine bound to red cells was also found to correlate more closely with therapeutic effects of the drug than plasma levels. The rationale for measuring red cell bound drug was based upon the possibility that the factors which affected the accumulation of a drug in a red blood cell might be similar to those affecting the passage of a drug into the brain and its localisation at relevant receptor sites in the central nervous system.

PHARMACODYNAMIC APPROACHES

1. Neuroendocrine approach

Rotrosen, Angrist and Gershon (1976) have produced some tantalising data on growth hormone responses to apomorphine and L-dopa in schizophrenics. Unusually high growth hormone responses to apomorphine were seen in schizophrenics who failed subsequently to respond to neuroleptic drug therapy. Conversely lower growth hormone responses to apomorphine occurred in schizophrenics subsequently responding. In this study due care was taken that to avoid interference by prior neuroleptic drug therapy. If these findings can be confirmed such responses might be a guide to therapeutic management and also reveal something of the sensitivity of the monoamine systems mediating neuroendocrine responses which might mirror the sensitivity of the monoamine systems underlying the behavioural abnormality.

It is plain that neuroendocrine abnormalities are going to play an increasing role in the understanding of drug effects and the abnormalities of brain function in psychiatric disease. The effect—at least acutely—of phenothiazines and butyrophenones on serum prolactin levels is striking, even though these changes so far do not mirror the therapeutic response. In the field of depression, the work of Carroll, Curtis and Mendels (1976) clearly shows that in endogenous depression as opposed to reactive depression, the control of ACTH release is abnormal such that these workers have suggested that in depression there is a disinhibition of hypothalamo-pituitary-adrenal function probably reflecting an abnormal limbic system drive on the release of corticotrophin releasing factor.

2. Cellular biochemical pharmacology

This aspect of the pharmacodynamic approach to drug therapy involves the study of the effects which drugs have on the cellular components of the blood which might reflect changes which occur in the target organ—in this case the brain. This approach has been used in the study of the effects of digoxin where changes in the Rb^{86} uptake by the patient's red blood cells caused by the digoxin which he takes correlates with certain aspects of the therapeutic effect of the drug on the heart (see Grahame-Smith, 1977a).

In applying this approach to the study of neuroleptic drug therapy the work of Mills and Roberts (1967) was a starting point. They showed that chlorpromazine in concentrations which approximate to those that are now known to exist in patients receiving the drug, inhibited the aggregation of human blood platelets produced by 5-hydroxytryptamine (5-HT) in vitro. This was confirmed and extended to include some of the metabolites of chlorpromazine by Boullin et al (1975a). Interestingly the potency of chlorpromazine and its metabolites to inhibit platelet aggregation was very similar to their potency in inhibiting the dopamine sensitive adenylate cyclase in the rat caudate nucleus in vitro. Changes in 5-HT induced aggregation in the plasma of patients receiving chlorpromazine were however found to be completely opposite. In a pilot study on nine schizophrenic patients receiving chlorpromazine, platelet aggregation responses to 5-HT were shown to be considerably enhanced (Boullin et al, 1975b).

The relevance of changes in platelet aggregation as a pharmacological index of phenothiazine activity rests on the hypothesis that such changes reflect a drug effect on the platelet membrane which might mirror changes in the brain which are manifest clinically as antipsychotic activity. The relationship between changes in 5-HT induced platelet aggregation and clinical changes have been examined in a group of acutely ill psychotic patients and a group of chronic schizophrenic patients receiving chlorpromazine (Orr et al, in preparation) and a group of chronic schizophrenic patients receiving fluphenazine (Orr and Boullin, 1976).

In acutely ill patients receiving chlorpromazine for the first time, enhanced aggregation responses were closely related to clinical improvement. In a group of 34 chronic schizophrenic patients receiving chlorpromazine, enhanced aggregation responses were seen in 25 patients. Enhancement was no longer present when chlorpromazine was substituted with placebo and the disappearance and reappearance of enhanced responses was closely related to changes in clinical symptoms in a small group of patients who relapsed clinically during the placebo period. Preliminary work in 20 patients receiving fluphenazine showed that enhanced responses were present in only half (Orr and Boullin, 1976). Patients showing enhanced responses had better controlled psychiatric symptoms and fewer extrapyramidal side effects than those who showed no change.

The pharmacological basis for this response of the platelet is not yet fully understood but there may be a relation to the behavioural effects of acute and chronic chlorpromazine administration to rats. After a single dose of chlorpromazine, the hyperactivity syndrome observed in rats produced by increasing brain 5-HT function and dopamine function is inhibited but when chlorpromazine is administered for six days, the hyperactivity syndromes produced by increasing 5-HT and dopamine function in the brain are enhanced (Heal et al, 1976). It is possible that the mechanisms whereby enhancement of both aggregation and of the hyperactivity syndrome occur could be due to receptor supersensitivity following on receptor blockade in the platelet and brain respectively (see Table 8.4).

Table 8.4   Effects of chlorpromazine (CPZ) on platelet aggregation (man) and 5-HT and dopamine-induced hyperactivity syndromes (rat)

	5-HT induced platelet aggregation (man)	5-HT and dopamine-induced hyperactivity syndromes (rat)
Acute CPZ	CPZ added to platelet rich plasma 5-HT induced platelet aggregation inhibited	One dose CPZ Hyperactivity syndromes inhibited
Chronic CPZ	Chronic CPZ therapy 5-HT-induced platelet aggregation enhanced	Chronic daily CPZ. CPZ administration (stop CPZ for 24 h) Hyperactivity syndromes enhanced

DEPOT NEUROLEPTICS

The long-acting depot neuroleptic drugs are now firmly established as the maintenance treatment of choice in schizophrenia (Hirsch et al, 1973). Intramuscular administration ensures that patients receive the drug and bypasses problems of absorption from the gut and first-pass metabolism in the liver (Adamson et al, 1973). Of the two preparations in common use, fluphenazine decanoate (Modecate) and flupenthixol decanoate (Depixol), the latter is reputed to carry a lesser risk of causing depression, which was reported in some patients receiving fluphenazine (de Alarcon and Carney, 1969). Penfluridol, a diphenylbutylpiperidine derivative related to pimozide (Orap) and fluspirilene (Redeptin) differs from other long-acting neuroleptics in being administered by mouth and clinical studies (Gallant et al, 1974) indicate that it provides safe and adequate control of symptoms in schizophrenic patients. Until recently, it has not been possible to examine the pharmacokinetics of these compounds as 'therapeutic' plasma levels are very low and proved difficult to measure; a radioimmunoassay has now been developed which allows the detection of very low levels of fluphenazine in plasma (Wiles and Franklin, 1977) and preliminary results indicate that the range of 'therapeutic' levels is a relatively narrow one and the patients on different but effective dose regimens shared the same range of levels, suggesting that clinicians were prescribing the drug in a way which produced steady plasma levels within a narrow range (Wiles et al, in preparation). The precise relationship between dosage, plasma levels and therapeutic and unwanted effects has still to be explored. On clinical grounds, anti-psychotic effects and extrapyramidal side effects appear to be dose dependent, but effective dose regimes show a wide scatter (Johnson, 1975). A comprehensive review of the practical matters involved in the use of depot neuroleptics in schizophrenia has been provided by Johnson (1977).

Propranolol in schizophrenia

Atsmon, Blum and Fischl (1972) noted that when large doses of propranolol were given to reduce tachycardia and the blood pressure in a patient with acute porphyria, the psychotic features associated with the syndrome disappeared. Steiner et al (1972) went on to show that symptoms in schizophrenic patients remitted when propranolol was given in increasing dosage every 2 to 3 h. In a pilot study Yorkston et al (1974) reported marked improvement in an impressive proportion of schizophrenic patients treated with propranolol. The same group (Yorkston et al, 1976) have confirmed and extended their findings in a larger group of schizophrenic patients. They found that while the drug was effective in controlling schizophrenic symptoms it was less effective in treating relapses. The dose of propranolol used ranged from 160 to 3000 mg daily and the average maintenance dose was 500 mg/day. Acute toxic effects were a problem early on in these studies but improved monitoring of patients decreased the incidence of acute toxic effects and so far no chronic toxic effects have been observed. Apart from potentially improving the therapy of schizophrenia these trials also raise questions about the mode of action of propranolol and secondarily implications concerning the abnormalities in the brain underlying the schizophrenic illness.

Green and Grahame-Smith (1976b) found that in rats ($\pm$)-propranolol (40 mg/kg, i.p.) inhibited the hyperactivity syndrome resultant upon increasing the functional activity of brain 5-HT but did not inhibit the hyperactivity produced by increasing the functional activity of dopamine. This action of ($\pm$)-propranolol racemate was found to be due to($-$)-propranolol (i.e. the beta-blocking isomer) (Weinstock and Schechter, 1975).

Green and Grahame-Smith (in preparation) have now studied a series of beta-adrenergic blocking agents for their activity in blocking 5-HT induced hyperactivity syndromes in the rat. The results are shown in Table 8.5. It can be seen that several beta-adrenergic blocking agents block 5-HT induced hyperactivity. None of them affects dopamine-induced hyperactivity and in more recent experiments it has been shown that beta-adrenergic blocking agents have no effect on another model for the functional activity of dopamine in brain, i.e. the rat with a unilateral nigrostriatal lesion in which rotational behaviour occurs with dopamine agonist treatment. It is uncertain yet as to whether the features which distinguish those beta-blocking agents which do

Table 8.5   The relative effects of beta-adrenergic blocking agents on the hyperactivity syndrome produced by L-tryptophan and tranylcypromine in rats

Beta-blocker	mg/kg (dose)	Block of 5-HT response	Entry to brain
Sotalol	40	+ +	
			+ +
	20	+ +	
Timolol	40	+ +	
			+ +
	20	+	
Pindolol	40	+ +	+ +
Alprenolol	40	+ +	
			+ +
	20	+	
Acebutolol	40	+ +	
			+ +
	20	+ +	
Metoprolol	40	+	+ +
Oxprenolol	40	+	+ +
Labetalol	40	−	−
Atenolol	40	−	−
Practolol	40	−	−

inhibit 5-HT induced hyperactivity from those which do not is due to the ease with which the former enter the brain or whether there is some intrinsic specificity of action in regard to this effect. Middlemiss, Blakebrough and Leather (1977) have recently shown that (−)-propranolol inhibits the specific binding of 5-HT to brain membranes, perhaps indicating that propranolol can block the binding of 5-HT to brain receptor sites.

If the conclusions are correct that propranolol inhibits central 5-HT neurotransmission or its behavioural effects in some way and if future studies confirm its efficacy in the treatment of schizophrenia there are several implications. The dopamine receptor blocking action of neuroleptics, as their mechanism of action as antipsychotic drugs, is one of the corner-stones of the so-called 'dopamine hypothesis' of the causation of schizophrenia. If propranolol inhibits the central effects of 5-HT but not dopamine, and if it is effective through this mechanism in schizophrenia, then this points indirectly to an involvement of 5-HT as well as dopamine in this condition. If indeed 5-HT mechanisms are involved at a higher organisational level than dopaminergic mechanisms then the action of current neuroleptics could still be explained by their action on dopaminergic mechanisms since the central functional activity of 5-HT, at least as far as the hyperactivity syndrome is concerned, is crucially dependent upon intact dopaminergic mechanisms for its behavioural expression (Green and Grahame-Smith, 1974a).

THE IMPLICATIONS OF NEUROPHARMACOLOGY IN CONSIDERATION OF CEREBRAL MECHANISMS OF MOOD AND BEHAVIOUR

It is exceedingly difficult at the present time to see how the intimate biochemical and pharmacological functioning of the human brain in vivo can be directly investigated. A good deal of the hypotheses which implicate one neurotransmitter or another in the

abnormal functioning of the brain underlying manic-depressive disease and schizophrenia are based on the knowledge of the pharmacological actions of drugs which,
largely serendipitously, have been found to have a beneficial effect in these conditions.

Drugs are exogenous molecules which interact with endogenous molecules and set in
train a sequence of events by which a biological process is manipulated. When this
molecular interaction is put to therapeutic ends a disordered physiological process is
either returned to normal or altered in such a way that the symptoms or manifestations
of the disease are ameliorated.

Two points follow from this which are relevant to the biology of normal and abnormal
mental function and which, although self evident, are none the less worth stating:

1. Whatever the rationale for the use of the drug in mental illness, if the drug can be
   shown by clinical trial to produce benefit, then at some level a potentially definable
   biological process is involved. This does not help very much because it is tantamount
   to saying that you must have a brain to be mad.
2. It is reasonable to suppose that an understanding of the actions of the drug whether
   from studies in man, animals, intact organs, cells, particles or at the molecular level,
   might give some insight into the pathological processes involved in the mental illness.
   There are two corollaries to this which have been used by those interested in this
   field. First when drugs worsen or change the quality of mental illness the study of the
   actions of such drugs may give insight into the underlying processes (eg studies on
   amino acid administration in schizophrenia; see Grahame-Smith, 1973). Second, if
   certain drugs produce in normal people states of mind, altered behaviour or mental
   symptoms which mimic certain aspects of spontaneous mental illness the study of the
   actions of such drugs might lead to the understanding of the biology of the mental
   illness or symptoms which are mimicked (e.g. hallucinogens, amphetamine; see
   Grahame-Smith, 1973).

It is this kind of reasoning which has caused so much attention to be focused upon the
role of the brain monoamines noradrenaline, dopamine and 5-hydroxytryptamine in
the brain mechanisms underlying schizophrenia (Grahame-Smith, 1973; Snyder et al,
1974), manic depressive disease (Schildkraut, 1969; Shopsin et al, 1974; Van Praag,
1974), and the mental syndromes produced by reserpine and psychotomimetic drugs.
Table 8.6 (a, b) shows some general current hypotheses concerning the pharmacological actions of some of the drugs used in the treatment of mental illness or which
produce mental syndromes, together with the over-simplified but quite widely held
belief linking their pharmacological actions to the aetiology of mental illness. The table
does an injustice to the arguments and open-mindedness of the workers propounding
the hypotheses but it is these shorthand conclusions that get taken up into the general
body of knowledge and need examination.

There is a big snag in this whole approach which might be explained by an artificial
analogy. Suppose we knew as little about the pathophysiology of heart failure as we do
of brain function in mental illness. Suppose too that by serendipity a powerful diuretic
was discovered and used empirically and with benefit in this uncharted syndrome of
'heart failure'. If the mode of action of this drug was then investigated the investigations
would reveal that its action was on the kidney and the conclusion would be drawn that
the syndrome of 'heart failure' was due to a primary disturbance in renal tubular sodium
excretion and indeed this might be considered a normal response to the altered

Table 8.6(a)   Some current shorthand hypotheses concerning the role of monoaminergic function in the causation of mental illness based upon the mode of action of psychotropic drugs

Drug	Illness	Possible mechanism of action	Shorthand 'aetiological' conclusions
Phenothiazines Butyrophenones Thioxanthenes	Schizophrenia Mania	Dopamine receptor blockade (see Snyder, 1974)	Overactivity of dopaminergic systems
Tricyclic anti-depressants	Depression	Inhibition of presynaptic monoamine re-uptake → increased monoaminergic function (see Iversen, 1973)	Decreased monoaminergic function
Monoamine oxidase inhibitors	Depression	Decreased metabolism of monoamines → increased monoaminergic function (see Iversen, 1973)	Decreased monoaminergic function
Lithium	'Prophylaxis' of manic	Increased functional activity of 5-HT (see Green and Grahame-Smith,1975)	Disturbance in 5-HT function
ECT	Depression	Increased sensitivity to behavioural actions of 5-HT and dopamine (Grahame-Smith and Green, 1977)	Decreased 5-HT or dopamine function or 'sensitivity'

Table 8.6(b)   Drugs 'mimicking' certain aspects of mental illness, their mode of action and conclusions on aetiology

Drug	Clinical effects	Action	Conclusions
Reserpine	Depression	Depletion of brain monoamines (see Iversen, 1973)	Depression 'due to' decreased monoaminergic function
LSD	'Psychotic' symptoms	5-HT agonist/antagonist (see Grahame-Smith, 1973)	Aspects of schizophrenia due to 5-HT dysfunction
Amphetamine	Syndrome-like paranoid schizophrenia	Dopamine release (see Snyder et al, 1974)	Aspects of schizophrenia due to dopaminergic overactivity

haemodynamic state produced by the heart failure but although a renal abnormality is involved, excessive and undivided attention upon it would distract from the primary cause of heart failure.

Consider schizophrenia in this light. There is a very impressive correlation between the ability of phenothiazines and other neuroleptics to block the actions of dopamine in the brain and their antipsychotic potency. In addition the similarity between amphetamine psychosis and paranoid schizophrenia coupled with the actions of amphetamine to release brain dopamine also fits into this picture. This has led to the proposition of a 'dopamine hypothesis' for the causation of schizophrenia (see Snyder et al, 1974). It is difficult to be sure exactly what is meant by 'the dopamine hypothesis of schizophrenia' except that it implies that somehow or other a disturbance of dopaminergic neuronal function is involved. This may be so but it would be naive at this stage to consider it a primary disturbance. The neuroleptics could equally well be acting at a secondary level (Grahame-Smith, 1973). Curare would prevent physical violence ensuing from a schizophrenic paranoid delusion but it would be foolish to invoke therefore a 'peripheral cholinergic hypothesis' as the cause of paranoid schizophrenia. There is nothing in the indirect evidence culled from drug studies implicating dopaminergic mechanisms in schizophrenia which convincingly shows that an abnormality in dopaminergic function is a *primary* aetiological factor. Indeed, just as the kidney in heart failure is responding in a normal physiological manner to the change in the haemodynamic state produced by heart failure it might be that the dopaminergic systems in the brain are over-functioning as a normal response to some other more fundamental disturbance. The neuroleptics then would dampen down this overactivity without affecting the primary disturbance. This is rather destructive reasoning, particularly when there are few ideas as to what the primary disturbance might be. One can speculate upon two other possibilities. First, one can imagine a disturbance of subcortical systems lying at an even more 'primitive' level than the monoaminergic systems but requiring monoaminergic systems for its linkage to cortical functions. Second, a subtle neurohumoral mechanism acting within the brain, altering in a diffuse way the function of monoaminergic systems or the reactivity of neuronal systems to their action.

These are not entirely idle speculations for there are now precedences upon which they may be based. In regard to the first speculation it has been shown that in rats the syndrome of a distinctive form of hyperactivity produced by increasing brain 5-HT levels or by central 5-HT agonists depends for its expression upon brain dopaminergic function. If one interferes with dopaminergic function pharmacologically either by decreasing brain dopamine levels or by pharmacologically blocking the action of brain dopamine then the pharmacological stimulation of 5-HT receptors no longer brings about abnormal hyperactive behaviour (see Green and Grahame-Smith, 1974a; Heal et al, 1976). The precedence is therefore set for dopaminergic function in some way playing a linking or permissive role in the expression of behavioural syndromes produced by the abnormal function of non-dopaminergic pathways.

The second speculation is more hazy, but is based upon the effects which small polypeptides, such as thyrotrophin releasing hormone (TRH) (Green and Grahame-Smith, 1974b), melanocyte stimulating hormone release inhibitory factor (MIF) (Plotnikoff et al, 1972), and inhibitors of brain protein synthesis such as cycloheximide, and perhaps ECT, have on the behaviour of rats and mice. These effects involve changes in the hyperactivity syndromes produced by raising brain 5-HT levels or by the administration of 5-HT agonists, the hyperactivity syndrome produced by raising brain dopamine levels with L-dopa and a monoamine oxidase inhibitor, pentylenetetrazol produced convulsions, pentobarbitone induced sleeping time, and the turning behaviour produced by dopaminergic influences in rats with unilateral nigrostriatal lesions. TRH potentiates the hyperactivity syndromes without having much effect on monoamine synthesis and turnover and shortened pentobarbitone induced sleeping time. Cycloheximide on the other hand does the opposite (Green et al, 1976). The actions of TRH on these behavioural syndromes is not mediated by its action on the pituitary to release TSH since its behavioural actions occur in hypophysectomised rats. These phenomena suggest that polypeptides like TRH and MIF may in some way modulate the activity of monoaminergic systems or the response of other neuronal systems to their actions. Inhibitors of protein synthesis like cycloheximide could be acting either by preventing the synthesis of some neuromodulating polypeptides or by preventing either the release of monoamines or the mediation of their action. The changes in brain function brought about by electroconvulsive shock in animals which is discussed a little later is also suggestive of a rather diffuse change in the function of monoaminergic systems or the reactivity of neuronal systems to their action. However unclear the picture may be at the moment there is sufficient evidence to consider systems internal to the brain, possibly mediated by polypeptides, which modulate neuronal activity in monoaminergic systems or systems influenced by them. If this turns out to be the case then an abnormality in such a neurohumoral control mechanism could result in overactivity or underactivity of neuronal systems such as those subserved by the monoamines. The cyclic nature of manic depressive disease, the latency of action of tricyclic antidepressants, the waxing and waning nature of several psychiatric syndromes, the usual requirement of a course of ECT, are phenomena, the time course of which might be explained by gradual biochemical and pharmacological changes requiring more primary changes in protein/polypeptide synthesis.

One can apply the same types of argument to the actions of tricyclic antidepressants, monoamine oxidase inhibitors and the known effect of reserpine to produce monamine depletion in the brain and then to the 'serotonin' or 'noradrenaline' hypotheses of manic depressive disease. Here again the primacy of involvement of monoaminergic systems in the aetiology of such conditions are based upon rather shaky evidence. The evidence culled from the action of antidepressive drugs could be equally applied to a monoaminergic function at a secondary level mediating some other primary disturbance. Such abnormalities in CSF, monoamine metabolites in depression as have been demonstrated, particularly the low levels of 5-HIAA and its decreased rise on the administration of probenecid (see Van Praag, 1974, 1977) need not necessarily imply a primary abnormality in monoaminergic function. However, Van Praag's work (1977) showing that 5-HTP can alleviate the depressive syndrome, this effect being potentiated by clomipramine, a relatively selective inhibitor of 5-HT re-uptake, and a negative correlation between 5-HT turnover in the CNS and the therapeutic effect of clomipramine, does go some way towards implicating an abnormality in 5-HT function of a primary rather than a secondary nature. There are criticisms of a biochemical nature which can be levelled at the significance of monoamine metabolism (such as 5-HIAA) in the CSF (Green and Grahame-Smith, 1975; Bulat, 1977). Be that as it may, the work of Van Praag (1977) and of Åsberg, Träskman and Thorén (1976) does suggest that whatever the reason, there might be alterations in CSF 5-HIAA in depression. Van Praag and his colleagues showed that within a group of patients with endogenous depression the rise in 5-HIAA in response to probenecid was decreased in about 40 per cent of patients. Åsberg and her colleagues have shown a bimodal distribution of 5-HIAA in the CSF in depressed patients, one group having very low CSF 5-HIAA levels and the other group more normal levels. In the group with low CSF 5-HIAA levels, Åsberg and her colleagues showed that the lower the level the worse the depression, and indeed that the incidence of suicide of a violent form was increased in those with the lowest 5-HIAA levels. These findings are extremely important since they do suggest that there is a group of endogenous depressives with abnormal 5-HT function or metabolism. It remains to be seen whether this is a primary or secondary phenomenon.

G

So much of current psychopharmacological research and therapeutic practice is based upon monoaminergic mechanisms that it is well to ask the question 'What do these mechanisms do?' Moore (1971) has summed it up succinctly in a general way, 'Highly integrated neural functions such as those involving thought processes, which are generally considered to take place in cortical structures, may be modified by primitive, chronically active subcortical neuronal systems (e.g. limbic and retricular activating systems). Accordingly a dysfunction of these delicately balanced primitive systems may result in derangement of mental processes and behaviour.'

Because we know so little of the functional neuroanatomy of human thought processes, mood and behaviour, it is necessary to play the game of association between the effects of drugs in man, the known actions of drugs, the functional neuroanatomy of animal behaviour, and the effects of drugs with known actions on animal behaviour and to try by this game, by intuitive reasoning and with a fair share of serendipity to come out with some sensible answers. Crucial to all these considerations is the mode of action of the relevant drugs. Green and Grahame-Smith (1976a) have summarised their findings on the mode of action of drugs affecting the processes regulating the functional activity of brain 5-HT. Lithium, phenytoin, reserpine, phenothiazines, tricyclic anti-depressants, dopamine depletors, inhibitors of brain protein synthesis and elec-troconvulsive shock can all be shown to affect the hyperactivity syndrome in rats produced by raising brain 5-HT levels through the administration of tryptophan and a monoamine oxidase inhibitor or by the administration of 5-HT agonists. It is possible to dissect out whether the drugs affect the synthesis, compartmentation, release, re-uptake and immediate postsynaptic action or the function of other neuronal pathways mediating or permitting the immediate postsynaptic action of 5-HT to be expressed as a behavioural response.

One of the interesting and more recent findings in neuropharmacological work is that the chronic effects of drugs appear different to and involve unsuspected phar-macological actions on monoamine metabolism and function when compared with the acute effects of those drugs. For instance acute chlorpromazine administration to animals undoubtedly blocks the action of dopamine in the brain and will inhibit the hyperactivity syndromes produced by increasing brain 5-HT or dopamine function. Chronic chlorpromazine treatment however leads to a situation in which, when the chlorpromazine is stopped, the hyperactivity syndrome produced by increasing brain 5-HT or dopamine function is enhanced, suggesting that 5-HT or dopamine receptor supersensitivity has been induced by chronic pharmacological inhibition. There is an interesting contrast between the effects of chronic chlorpromazine and chronic haloperidol administration. Chronic chlorpromazine administration enhances both 5-HT and dopamine-induced behavioural responses whilst chronic haloperidol enhances only dopamine-induced behavioural responses. This suggests that acutely chlorpromazine blocks both 5-HT and dopamine and haloperidol only dopamine.

Another example of the chronic effect of treatment on the brain involves recent findings on electroconvulsive shock in rats. *Repeated* electroconvulsive shock (ECS) in rats enhances the behavioural responses to increased brain 5-HT, dopamine (DA), and probably noradrenaline (NA) agonist activity (Modigh, 1975; Evans et al, 1976). This enhancement of monoamine action has been found in several model systems (see Grahame-Smith and Green, 1977):

1. The hyperactivity syndrome in rats produced by raising brain 5-HT or by 5-HT agonists.
2. The hyperactivity syndrome in rats produced by raising brain DA or by DA agonists.
3. The rotational behaviour produced by either amphetamine (ipsilateral turning) or apomorphine (contralateral turning) in rats with a unilateral nigrostriatal lesions.
4. The hyperactivity produced by apomorphine and clonidine (?noradrenaline agonist activity) in mice (Modigh, 1975).
5. The increased secretion of growth hormone produced by apomorphine (Modigh, 1977).

Note that in all of these experiments the behavioural responses are tested 24 h after the last shock.

The time course of the effects of ECS are interesting. For the enhancement of monoamine function to occur a shock a day for at least six days are needed, (routinely we give a shock a day for 10 days). Recently though, Costain et al (in preparation) have found that monoamine responses are enhanced by a 'clinical' regimen of ECS (i.e. one shock daily on Monday, Wednesday and Friday on three consecutive weeks). After a shock a day for 10 days the enhanced behavioural responses to 5-HT agonist activity are still present three days after cessation of shock and last for a total of six to seven days. Subconvulsive ECS (90 V for 1 s) given otherwise comparably to convulsive ECS (150 V, 50 cycles/s, sinusoidal for 1 s), does not produce enhanced responses to monoamine agonist activity. Green (1977) has shown that flurothyl (Indoklon), a convulsive gas which has been used as an alternative to ECT in the treatment of depression, produces changes in brain monoamine mediated behavioural responses similar to those produced by ECS.

Overall there are rather minor biochemical changes in the synthesis, turnover and re-uptake of the monoamines, which certainly do not explain the marked changes in monoamine induced behavioural responses. Largely by exclusion it seems that ECS is producing some change postsynaptically and the questions which arise are:

1. Does ECS produce increased postsynaptic receptor sensitivity to the brain monoamines?
2. Does ECS alter the activity of neuronal systems modulating the through-put resultant upon the stimulation of postsynaptic monoamine receptors?
3. Does ECS release neuromodulatory substances within the brain such that the reactivity of neuronal systems stimulated by primary monoamine stimuli is increased?

Grahame-Smith and Green (1977) have discussed the relevance of this work on ECS to the clinical effect of ECT and the neuropharmacology of depression. The action of ECS to enhance brain monoamine function fits in generally with the known pharmacological actions of tricyclic antidepressants and monoamine oxidase inhibitors, and considering all the evidence so far it would be a cruel joke on nature's part if the increase in the functional activity of brain monoamines produced by repeated ECS did not have something to do with its therapeutic effect in depression. It is of some importance to find out how ECS produces these effects because it may be possible to substitute drug therapy for ECT and to produce similar biological changes with less hazard and perhaps fewer side effects.

The effects of repeated administration of neuroleptics, lithium and now ECS force one to consider the role that 'adaptative' changes in brain function play in both the therapeutic and adverse effects of these therapies. For instance tardive dyskinesia induced by chronic neuroleptic therapy might be dependent upon dopamine receptor sensitivity induced by chronic dopamine receptor blockade. It is difficult to know whether the latency of onset of the action of lithium in mania and of tricyclic antidepressants in depression is due to the time taken to reach a pharmacokinetic steady-state or due to delayed effects which these drugs might have. This is particularly important in considering the links between the pharmacokinetic, pharmacodynamic and therapeutic phases of psychotropic drug therapy. If a drug actually produces its therapeutic effect by its early acute pharmacological action (A), (i.e. A → therapeutic effect) then hopefully this set of conditions is fairly easy to analyse. But if the acute pharmacological action (A) leads to chronic 'adaptative' pharmacological actions (C) which are responsible for the therapeutic effect (i.e. A → C → therapeutic effect), then this situation becomes much more difficult to analyse.

There are some topics of importance which we have omitted in this review both for reasons of space and because they have been dealt with elsewhere. We should particularly like to refer the reader to reviews on

1. The recent work on opiate receptors and internal opiates (Kosterlitz, 1976; Klee, 1977; Snyder, 1977).
2. The current status of lithium therapy (Fieve, 1977).
3. Drug interactions in psychopharmacology (Grahame-Smith, 1977b; Lader, 1977; Marley, 1977).

REFERENCES

Adamson, L., Curry, S. H., Bridges, P. K., Firestone, A. F., Lavin, N. I., Lewis, D. M., Watson, R. D., Xavier, C. M. & Anderson, J. A. (1973) Fluphenazine decanoate trial in chronic in-patient schizophrenics failing to absorb oral chlorpromazine. *Diseases of the Nervous System*, **34**, 181–191.

Åsberg, M. (1974) Individualisation of treatment with tricyclic compounds. *Medical Clinics of North America*, **58**, 1083–1092.

Åsberg, M. (1976) Treatment of depression with tricyclic drugs: pharmacokinetic and pharmacodynamic aspects. *Pharmakopsychiatrie Neuro-Psychopharmakologie*, **9**, 18–26.

Åsberg, M., Cronholm, B., Sjoqvist, F. & Tuck, D. (1971) Relationship between plasma level and therapeutic effect of nortriptyline. *British Medical Journal*, **iii**, 331–334.

Åsberg, M., Träskman, L. & Thorén, P. (1976) 5-HIAA in the cerebrospinal fluid. A biochemical suicide predictor? *Archives of General Psychiatry*, **33**, 1193–1197.

Atsmon, A., Blum, I. & Fischl, J. (1972) Treatment of an acute attack of porphyria variegata with propranolol. *South African Medical Journal*, **46**, 311–314.

Blackwell, B. (1973) Drug therapy: patient compliance. *New England Journal of Medicine*, **289**, 249–252.

Boullin, D. J., Grahame-Smith, D. G., Grimes, R. P. J. & Woods, H. F. (1975a) Inhibition of 5-hydroxytryptamine-induced human blood platelet aggregation by chlorpromazine and its metabolites. *British Journal of Pharmacology*, **53**, 121–125.

Boullin, D. J., Woods, H. F., Grimes, R. P. J., Grahame-Smith, D. G., Wiles, D., Gelder, M. G. & Kolakowska, T. (1975b) Increased platelet aggregation responses to 5-hydroxytryptamine in patients taking chlorpromazine. *British Journal of Clinical Pharmacology*, **2**, 29–35.

Bowers, M. G. Jr & Rozitis, A. (1974) Regional differences in homovanillic concentrations after acute and chronic administration of antipsychotic drugs. *Journal of Pharmacy and Pharmacology*, **26**, 743–745.

Braithwaite, R. A., Goulding, R., Theano, G., Bailey, J. & Coppen, A. (1972) Plasma concentration of amitriptyline and clinical response. *Lancet*, **i**, 1297–1300.

Bulat, M. (1977) On the cerebral origin of 5-hydroxyindoleacetic acid in the lumbar cerebrospinal fluid. *Brain Research*, **122**, 388–391.

Burrows, G. D., Davies, B. & Scoggins, B. A. (1972) Plasma concentrations of nortriptyline levels in endogenous depression. *Lancet*, **ii**, 619–623.

Burrows, G. D., Scoggins, B. A., Turecek, L. R. & Davies, B. (1974) Plasma nortriptyline and clinical response. *Clinical Pharmacology and Therapeutics*, **16**, 639–644.

Carroll, B. J., Curtis, G. C. & Mendels, J. (1976) Neuroendocrine regulation in depression I and II. *Archives of General Psychiatry*, **33**, 1039–1044, 1051–1058.

Coppen, A. (1977) Personal communication.

Curry, S. H. (1974) *Drug Disposition and Pharmacokinetics*. Oxford: Blackwell.

Curry, S. H., Davis, J. M. & Janowsky, D. S. (1970) Factors affecting chlorpromazine plasma levels in psychiatric patients. *Archives of General Psychiatry*, **22**, 209–215.

De Alarcon, R. & Carney, M. W. P. (1969) Severe depressive mood changes following slow-release intramuscular fluphenazine injection. *British Medical Journal*, **iii**, 564–567.

Evans, J. P. M., Grahame-Smith, D. G., Green, A. R. & Tordoff, A. F. C. (1976) Electroconvulsive shock increases the behavioural responses of rats to brain 5-hydroxytryptamine accumulation and central nervous system stimulant drugs. *British Journal of Pharmacology*, **56**, 193–199.

Fieve, R. R. (1977) The clinical use of lithium in affective disorders. *Drugs*, **13**, 458–466.

Forsman, A., Mårtensson, E., Nyberg, G. & Öhman, R. (1974) A gas-chromatographic method for determining haloperidol. *Naunyn-Schmiedebergs Archives of Pharmacology*, **286**, 113–124.

Gallant, D. M., Mielke, D. H., Sprites, M. A., Swanson, W. C. & Bost, R. (1974) Penfluridol: an efficacious long-acting oral antipsychotic compound. *American Journal of Psychiatry*, **131**, 699–702.

Garver, D. L., Davis, J. M., Dekirmenjian, H., Jones, F. D., Casper, R. & Haraszti, J. (1976) Pharmacokinetics of red blood cell phenothiazine and clinical effects: acute dystonic reactions. *Archives of General Psychiatry*, **33**, 862–866.

Garver, D. L., Dekirmenjian, H., Davis, J. M., Casper, R. & Eriksen, S. (1977) Neuroleptic drug levels and therapeutic response: preliminary observations with red-cell bound butaperazine. *American Journal of Psychiatry*, **134**, 304–307.

Glassman, A. H., Perel, J. M., Shostak, M., Kantor, S. J. & Fleiss, J. L. (1977) Clinical implications of imipramine plasma levels for depressive illness. *Archives of General Psychiatry*, **34**, 197–204.

Goodwin, F. K., Post, R. M. & Sack, R. L. (1975) Clinical evidence for neurochemical adaptation to psychotropic drugs. In *Neurobiological Mechanisms of Adaptation and Behaviour*, ed. Mandell, A. J. New York: Raven Press.

Grahame-Smith, D. G. (1973) Pharmacological aspects of schizophrenia. *Biochemical Society Special Publications*, **1**, 197–207.

Grahame-Smith, D. G. (1977a) Monitoring drug therapy: the use of cellular biochemical and pharmacological techniques. *Netherlands Journal of Medicine*, **20**, 36–45.

Grahame-Smith, D. G. (1977b) General aspects of drug interactions in psychopharmacology. In *Drug Interactions*, ed. Grahame-Smith, D.G., p. 147. London: Macmillan.

Grahame-Smith, D. G. & Green, A. R. (1977) The effect of electroconvulsive shock on brain monoamine function in the rat. In *Depression*. Symposium Medica Hoechst (to be published).

Gram, L., Reisby, N., Ibsen, I., Nagy, A., Dencker, S. J., Petersen, G. O. & Christiansen, J. (1976) Plasma levels and the antidepressant effect of imipramine. *Clinical Pharmacology and Therapeutics*, **19**, 318–324.

Green, A. R. (1977) Repeated exposure of rats to the convulsant agent fluorothyl enhances 5-hydroxytryptamine and dopamine mediated behavioural responses. *British Journal of Pharmacology* (to be published).

Green, A. R. & Grahame-Smith, D. G. (1974a) The role of dopamine in the hyperactivity syndrome produced by increased 5-hydroxytryptamine synthesis in rats. *Neuropharmacology*, **13**, 949–959.

Green, A. R. & Grahame-Smith, D. G. (1974b) TRH potentiates behavioural changes following increased brain 5-hydroxytryptamine accumulation in rats. *Nature*, **251**, 524–526.

Green, A. R. & Grahame-Smith, D. G. (1975) 5-Hydroxytryptamine and other indoles in the central nervous system. In *Handbook of Psychopharmacology*, ed. Iversen, S. D., Iversen, L. L. & Snyder, S. H., Vol. 3, pp. 169–245. New York: Plenum Press.

Green, A. R. & Grahame-Smith, D. G. (1976a) The effect of drugs on the processes regulating the functional activity of brain 5-hydroxytryptamine. *Nature*, **260**, 487–491.

Green, A. R. & Grahame-Smith, D. G. (1976b) (−)-Propranolol inhibits the behavioural responses of rats to increased 5-HT in the central nervous system. *Nature*, **262**, 594–596.

Green, A. R., Heal, D. J., Grahame-Smith, D. G. & Kelly, P. H. (1976) The contrasting actions of TRH and cycloheximide in altering the effects of centrally acting drugs: evidence for the non-involvement of dopamine sensitive adenylate cyclase. *Neuropharmacology*, **15**, 591–599.

Greenblatt, D. J. & Koch-Weser, J. (1975) Clinical pharmacokinetics. *New England Journal of Medicine*, **293**, 702–705.

Heal, D. J., Green, A. R., Boullin, D. J. & Grahame-Smith, D. G. (1976) Single and repeated administration of neuroleptic drugs to rats: effects on striatal dopamine-sensitive adenylate cyclase and locomotor activity produced by tranylcypromine and L-tryptophan or L-dopa. *Psychopharmacology*, **49**, 287–300.

Hirsch, S. R., Gaind, R., Rohde, P. D., Stevens, B. C. & Wing, J. K. (1973) Outpatient maintenance of chronic schizophrenic patients with long-acting fluphenazine. *British Medical Journal*, i, 633–637.

Iversen, L. L. (1973) Monoamines in the mammalian central nervous system and the action of antidepressant drugs. *Biochemical Society Special Publications*, 1, 81–96.

Johnson, D. A. W. (1975) Observations on the dose regime of fluphenazine decanoate in maintenance therapy of schizophrenia. *British Journal of Psychiatry*, 126, 457–461.

Johnson, D. A. W. (1977) Practical considerations in the use of depot neuroleptics for the treatment of schizophrenia. *British Journal of Hospital Medicine*, 17, 546–560.

Klawans, H. L. & Rubovits, R. (1974) Effect of cholinergic and anticholinergic agents on tardive dyskinesia. *Journal of Neurology, Neurosurgery and Psychiatry*, 37, 941–947.

Klee, W. A. (1977) Endogenous opiate peptides. In *Peptides in Neurobiology*, ed. Gaint, H., pp. 375–396. New York: Plenum Press.

Kolakowska, T., Wiles, D. H., McNeilly, A. S. & Gelder, M. G. (1975) Correlation between plasma levels of prolactin and chlorpromazine in psychiatric patients. *Psychological Medicine*, 5, 214–216.

Kolakowska, T., Wiles, D. H., Gelder, M. G. & McNeilly, A. S. (1976) Clinical significance of plasma chlorpromazine levels, II. Plasma levels of the drug, some of its metabolites and prolactin in patients receiving long-term phenothiazine treatment. *Psychopharmacology Bulletin*, 49, 101–107.

Kosterlitz, H. W. (ed.) (1976) *Opiates and Endogenous Opioid Peptides*. Amsterdam: North-Holland.

Kragh-Sørensen, P., Åsberg, M. & Eggert-Hansen, C. (1973) Plasma nortriptyline levels in endogenous depression. *Lancet*, i, 113–115.

Kragh-Sørensen, P., Hansen, Chr. E., Baastrup, P. Chr. & Hvidberg, E. F. (1976a) Self-inhibiting action of nortriptylines antidepressive effect at high plasma levels. *Psychopharmacologia (Berlin)*, 45, 305–312.

Kragh-Sørensen, P., Eggert-Hansen, Chr., Baastrup, P. Chr. & Hvidberg, E. F. (1976b) Relationship between antidepressant effect and plasma level of nortriptyline: clinical studies. *Pharmakopsychiatrie Neuro-psycho-pharmacologie (Stuttgart)*, 9, 27–32.

Lader, M. (1976) Clinical Psychopharmacology. In *Recent Advances in Psychiatry*, ed. Granville-Grossman, K., pp. 1–30. Edinburgh: Churchill Livingstone.

Lader, M. (1977) Drug interactions and the major tranquillisers. In *Drug Interactions*, ed. Grahame-Smith, D. G., p. 159. London: Macmillan.

Leff, J. P. & Wing, J. K. (1971) Trial of maintenance therapy in schizophrenia. *British Medical Journal*, iii, 599–604.

Lyle, W. H., Brooks, P. W., Early, D. F., Leggett, W. P., Silverman, G., Braithwaite, R. A., Cuthill, J. M., Goulding, R., Pearson, I. B. & Snaith, R. P. (1974) Plasma concentration of nortriptyline as a guide to treatment. *Postgraduate Medical Journal*, 50, 282–287.

Mackay, A. V. P., Healey, A. F. & Baker, J. (1974) The relationship of plasma chlorpromazine to its 7-hydroxy and sulphoxide metabolites in a large population of schizophrenics. *British Journal of Clinical Pharmacology*, 1, 425–430.

Marley, E. (1977) Monoamine oxidase inhibitors and drug interactions. In *Drug Interactions*, ed. Grahame-Smith, D. G., p. 171. London: Macmillan.

Martensson, E. & Roos, B. E. (1974) Serum levels of thioridazine in psychiatric patients and healthy volunteers. *European Journal of Clinical Pharmacology*, 6, 181–186.

Middlemiss, D. N., Blakeborough, L. & Leather, S. R. (1977) Direct evidence for an interaction of beta-adrenergic blockers with the 5-HT receptor. *Nature*, 267, 289–290.

Mills, D. C. B. & Roberts, G. C. K. (1967) Membrane active drugs and the aggregation of human blood platelets. *Nature*, 213, 35–38.

Modigh, K. (1975) Electroconvulsive shock and post-synaptic catecholamine effects: increased psychomotor stimulant action of apomorphine and clonidine in reserpine pretreated mice by repeated ECS. *Journal of Neural Transmission*, 36, 19–32.

Modigh, K. (1977) Personal communication.

Moore, K. E. (1971) In *Introduction to Psychopharmacology*, ed. Rech, R. H. & Moore, K. E., p. 117. New York: Raven Press.

Orlov, P., Kasparian, G., Dimaxio, A. & Cole, J. O. (1971) Withdrawal of anti-Parkinson drugs. *Archives of General Psychiatry*, 25, 410–412.

Orr, M. W. & Boullin, D. J. (1976) The relationship between changes in 5-HT induced platelet aggregation and clinical state in patients treated with fluphenazine. *British Journal of Clinical Pharmacology*, 3, 925–928.

Plotnikoff, N. P., Prange, A. J., Breese, G. R., Anderson, M. S. & Wilson, I. C. (1972) TRH: enhancement of DOPA activity by a hypothalamic hormone. *Science*, 178, 417–418.

Richards, A. D. (1964) Attitude and drug acceptance. *British Journal of Psychiatry*, 110, 46–52.

Rivera-Calimlim, L., Castanida, L. & Lasagna, L. (1973) Effects of mode of management on plasma chlorpromazine in psychiatric patients. *Clinical Pharmacology and Therapeutics*, 14, 978–986.

Rivera-Calimlim, L., Nasrallah, H., Strauss, J. & Lasagna, L. (1976) Clinical response and plasma levels: effect of dose, dosage schedules and drug interactions on plasma chlorpromazine levels. *American Journal of Psychiatry*, **133**, 646–652.

Rotrosen, J., Angrist, B. M. & Gershon, S. (1976) Dopamine receptor alteration in schizophrenia: neuroendocrine evidence. *Psychopharmacology*, **51**, 1–7.

Sakalis, G., Curry, S. H., Mould, G. P. & Lader, M. H. (1972) Physiologic and clinical effects of chlorpromazine and their relationship to plasma level. *Clinical Pharmacology and Therapeutics*, **13**, 931–946.

Sakalis, G., Chan, T. L., Gershon, S. & Park, S. (1974) The possible role of metabolites in therapeutic response to chlorpromazine treatment. *Psychopharmacologia (Berlin)*, **32**, 279–284.

Sayers, A. C., Burki, H. R., Ruch, W. & Asper, H. (1975) Neuroleptic induced hypersensitivity of striatal dopamine receptors in the rat as a model of tardive dyskinesia. Effects of clozapine, haloperidol, loxapine and chlorpromazine. *Psychopharmacologia (Berlin)*, **41**, 97–104.

Schildkraut, J. J. (1969) Rationale of some approaches used in the biochemical studies of the affective disorders: the pharmacological bridge. In *Psychochemical Research in Man*, ed. Mandell, A. J. & Mandell, M. P. New York: Academic Press.

Shopsin, B., Wilk, S., Sathananthan, G., Gershon, S. & Davis, K. (1974) Catecholamines and affective disorders raised. A critical assessment. *Journal of Nervous and Mental Disease*, **158**, 369–383.

Singh, M. M. & Smith, J. M. (1973) Reversal of some therapeutic effects of an antipsychotic agent by an anti-Parkinsonian drug. *Journal of Nervous and Mental Disease*, **157**, 50–58.

Sjoqvist, F. (1975) Assessment of antidepressants; pharmacokinetic aspects. In *Advanced Medicine Topics and Therapeutics*, ed. Breckenridge, A. M. London: Pitman Medical.

Snyder, S. H. (1977) Opiate receptors and internal opiates. *Scientific American*, **236**, 44–50.

Snyder, S. H., Banerjee, S. P., Yamamura, H. I. & Greenburg, D. (1974) Drugs, neurotransmitters and schizophrenia. *Science*, **184**, 1243–1253.

Steiner, M., Blum, I., Wijsenbeek, H. & Atsmon, A. (1972) Results of the treatment of psychoses with propranolol. The implications on the biochemical mechanisms of psychotic disorders. *Kupat-Holim Yearbook*, **2**, 201–209.

Van Praag, H. M. (1974) Towards a biochemical typology of depression? *Pharmakopsychiatria*, **7**, 281–292.

Van Praag, H. M. (1977) The significance of biochemical parameters in the diagnosis, treatment and prevention of depressive disorders. *Biological Psychiatry*, **12**, 101–131.

Vaughn, C. E. & Leff, J. P. (1976) The influence of family and social factors on the course of psychiatric illness: a comparison of schizophrenic and depressed neurotic patients. *British Journal of Psychiatry*, **129**, 125–137.

Walter, C. J. S. (1971) Clinical significance of plasma imipramine levels. *Proceedings of the Royal Society of Medicine*, **64**, 282–285.

Weinstock, M. & Schecter, Y. (1975) Antagonism by propranolol of the ganglion stimulant action of 5-hydroxytryptamine. *European Journal of Pharmacology*, **32**, 293–301.

Wiesel, F.-A., Alfredson, G., Likwornik, V. & Sedvall, G. (1975) A relation between drug concentrations in brain and striatal homovanillic acid levels in chlorpromazine treated rats. *Life Sciences*, **16**, 1145–1156.

Wiles, D. H. & Franklin, M. (1978) Radioimmunoassay for fluphenazine in human plasma. *British Journal of Clinical Pharmacology*, **5**, 265–268.

Wiles, D. H., Kolakowska, T., McNeilly, A. S., Mandelbrote, B. M. & Gelder, M. G. (1976) Clinical significance of plasma chlorpromazine levels. I. Plasma levels of the drug, some of its metabolites and prolactin during acute treatment. *Psychological Medicine*, **6**, 407–415.

Yorkston, N. J., Zaki, S. A., Malik, M. K. V., Morrison, R. C. & Havard, C. W. H. (1974) Propranolol in the control of schizophrenic symptoms. *British Medical Journal*, **iv**, 633–635.

Yorkston, N. J., Zaki, S. A., Themen, J. F. A. & Havard, C. W. H. (1976) Propranolol to control schizophrenic symptoms: 55 patients. In *Neuropsychiatric Effects of Adrenergic Beta-receptor Blocking Agent*, ed. Carlsson, C., Engel, J. & Hansson, L. Müchen–Berlin–Wien: Urban & Schwanzenberg.

Ziegler, V. E., Clayton, P. J., Taylor, J. R., Co, B. T. & Biggs, J. T. (1976a) Nortriptyline plasma levels and therapeutic response. *Clinical Pharmacology and Therapeutics*, **20**, 458–463.

Ziegler, V. E., Co, B. T., Taylor, J. R., Clayton, P. J. & Biggs, J. T. (1976b) Amitriptyline plasma levels and therapeutic response. *Clinical Pharmacology and Therapeutics*, **19**, 795–801.

9. Drug toxicity

L. F. Prescott

L. F. Prescott

INTRODUCTION

The use of drugs has increased enormously in recent years, and although great therapeutic progress has been made with their aid, toxicity is an ever-increasing problem. Unlike their predecessors, modern drugs are potent biologically active agents which demand much more knowledge of their properties by prescribers. There is no such thing as an effective and completely safe drug, and the risks of toxicity must always be balanced against the anticipated benefits of treatment. Adverse drug reactions are an important cause of illness and death, a burden on the health services and a source of economic loss. The mechanisms of drug toxicity are often poorly understood and the ultimate objective must be to elucidate the basis of cell damage at the molecular level.

EPIDEMIOLOGY

The true incidence and significance of adverse drug reactions is unknown. Not only must prescription drugs be taken into account, but also the great consumption of non-prescription remedies and the illicit use of drugs of abuse. Many hospital surveys of drug reactions have been carried out but the reported incidence depends on the extent of drug usage, the type of patient, and the criteria used for definition of an adverse reaction. The latter vary widely and investigators cannot agree over the diagnosis of a drug reaction (Koch-Weser, Sellers and Zacest, 1977). In addition, many adverse reactions are subjective in nature, occurring also with placebo, and attention has been drawn to the lack of adequately controlled studies (Karch and Lasagna, 1975).

Incidence of adverse drug reactions

In an analysis of the combined results of 11 prospective surveys in medical wards totalling 8562 patients, 17.5 per cent developed adverse reactions to drugs while in hospital. About 5 per cent were admitted because of drug toxicity, and of these 30 per cent developed further reactions in hospital (Gardner and Cluff, 1970). In a recent extensive study of 7423 medical admissions over a period of 3½ years, 1318 drug reactions were observed in 928 patients (17.9 per cent) (Caranasos et al, 1976), and similar results have been obtained in many other studies. Little is known of the incidence of drug reactions in general practice, but these accounted for 2.5 per cent of consultations in one survey (Mulroy, 1973). Of the many factors predisposing to drug toxicity, the over-prescribing of drugs and polypharmacy are the most important and the easiest to remedy. Patients with asthma, eczema or a history of previous drug reactions are more susceptible, and reactions are more likely to occur in women than in men.

Mortality and cost of adverse drug reactions

Estimates of the overall mortality caused by drugs in hospital patients have varied from 0 to 2.3 per cent and the incidence of 0.22 per cent in 7423 medical in-patients reported by Caranasos et al (1976) is probably representative. In this study, most patients who died were admitted because of drug toxicity. Although many deaths occurred in seriously ill patients, two died from gastrointestinal haemorrhage after taking aspirin on the instructions of doctors. In one report 25 per cent of all deaths on medical wards were attributed to drugs (Ogilvie and Ruedy, 1967) while in another, drugs were considered an important contributory factor in the deaths of 20 of 100 hospital patients examined at autopsy. Cessation of drug therapy was implicated in only four cases (Wade, 1975).

The length of hospital stay is increased by drug toxicity and one-seventh of all days spent in hospital in the USA are devoted to the care of drug toxicity at an annual cost of $3000 million (Melmon, 1971). In Belfast, 4.5 per cent of the total cost of hospital care in a survey of 1268 patients was attributed to adverse drug reactions, not to mention the associated loss of earnings (Hurwitz, 1969).

Drug regulation and the reporting of adverse reactions

The official drug regulatory agencies in many countries include a voluntary reporting system for adverse drug reactions. These may be useful for defining 'toxicity profiles' for individual drugs but no conclusions can be drawn regarding the incidence of reactions. The great majority of adverse reactions go unreported, and the number of patients at risk at any time is unknown. Emphasis is placed on new drugs, reporting is greatly influenced by publicity and new or unusual forms of toxicity are unlikely to be recognised. Thus, the system failed to pick up the oculocutaneous syndrome caused by practolol despite one million patient-years of use. In 1976 only 1013 reports were received by the New Zealand Committee on Adverse Drug Reactions. Yet two hospital monitoring groups observed 342 reactions and a further 904 were found in only two months in a general practice survey. In the latter group 43 drug reactions were major and 13 life threatening (McQueen, 1976). Because of the serious underreporting of drug toxicity to the Committee on Safety of Medicines, a system of intensive monitoring of selected drugs has been proposed (Dollery and Rawlins, 1977).

Much information is gained from pre-clinical and early clinical studies of new drugs but the true potential for toxicity can only be established after the drug has been in general use for many years. Animal toxicity studies may be misleading because of species differences in susceptibility, metabolism and pharmacokinetics. Teratogenicity and carcinogenicity studies are particularly difficult to extrapolate to man. The intensive monitoring of hospital patients by groups such as the Boston Collaborative Drug Surveillance Program has yielded valuable information on interactions, the incidence of reactions with specified drugs and drugs most often associated with particular reactions (Porter and Jick, 1977).

RECOGNITION OF DRUG TOXICITY

Major problems arise through the failure of clinicians to recognise drug toxicity. Patients suffer reactions needlessly, much time and money is wasted on unnecessary and sometimes dangerous investigation and additional drugs are often prescribed to counteract the unwanted effects of those already given. Doctors are unwilling to accept that their treatment actually causes the patient harm, especially if the drug in question is highly valued for its therapeutic effects. Recognition is easier if a drug produces an immediate dramatic effect ('light switch' phenomenon) such as collapse from hypotension after the first dose of prazosin. But subtle or delayed effects may pass unnoticed for many years. It took the medical profession almost 40 years to recognise the gastrointestinal haemorrhage and ulceration produced by therapeutic doses of as familiar and widely used a drug as aspirin, and 75 years to appreciate its disastrous effects on mother and child when taken regularly during pregnancy (Collins and Turner, 1975; Turner and Collins, 1975). With increasing use and variety of drugs, detection of long-term effects is becoming more and more difficult. Teratogenesis, mutagenesis and carcinogenesis are particularly difficult to recognise since the effects are delayed for many months or years after exposure. Toxicity may not be apparent until the second generation, as in the development of vaginal adenocarcinoma in young women whose mothers had been prescribed stilboestrol during pregnancy (Herbst, Ulfelder and Poskanzer, 1971). Again, psychoactive drugs prescribed during pregnancy may produce long-lasting disturbance of cerebral function in the offspring without obvious structural abnormalities (Lewis et al, 1977).

The recognition of drug toxicity is complicated enormously by the fact that it so often mimics naturally occurring disease. Thus the use of phenylbutazone has been associated with such 'natural' conditions as skin eruptions, fever, arthropathy, lymphadenopathy, parotid enlargement ('phenylbutazone mumps'), haematological changes resembling infectious mononucleosis, gastrointestinal irritation, haemorrhage and ulceration, impaired haemostasis, iron deficiency and megaloblastic anaemias, thrombocytopenia, agranulocytosis, aplastic anaemia, leukaemoid reactions, acute leukaemias, bronchospasm, fluid retention, oedema, increased blood pressure, cardiac failure, pericarditis, pleural effusion, oliguria, nephrotic syndrome, renal papillary necrosis, acute renal failure, hepatitis, goitre, hypothyroidism and delayed wound healing, not to mention numerous drug interactions (Prescott, 1975a). Many new 'diseases' have subsequently been shown to be caused by drugs. The outbreak of subacute myelo-optic neuropathy (SMON) in Japan was probably related to the uncontrolled use of clioquinol (Meade, 1975), chronic active hepatitis is often caused by drugs such as oxyphenisatin and nitrofurantoin (Strömberg and Wengle, 1976) and 'dialysis dementia'—a previously inexplicable and usually fatal condition—seems to be caused by the inappropriate use of benzodiazepines and other CNS depressants in patients with renal failure (Taclob and Needle, 1976). Drugs may produce such unusual and bizarre effects (e.g. plastic peritonitis induced by practolol) that the relationship with drug therapy is not appreciated. Difficulty also arises when drug effects are complicated by underlying disease and the inevitable polypharmacy. Toxicity caused by analgesics, laxatives and alkalis bought without prescription is often unrecognised because many doctors and most patients do not think of these remedies as drugs. One patient with aspirin-induced gastrointestinal bleeding spent more than two months in hospital and experienced three sigmoidoscopies, four barium enemas, three barium meals and a laparotomy before the correct diagnosis was made (Vickers and Stanley, 1963).

CLASSIFICATION OF ADVERSE REACTIONS AND DRUG TOXICITY

The mechanisms of drug toxicity encountered in clinical practice often differ from those involved in other areas of toxicology and it is important to distinguish between minor reversible reactions, unwanted effects related to pharmacological actions and 'true' toxic reactions. The potential for toxicity of a drug depends on its physicochemical and biological properties, route of administration, the dose and duration of treatment and interaction with host factors, particularly disease, adaption (tolerance) and the ability to repair cell damage.

Exaggerated therapeutic effect

This is very common and is due to increased susceptibility or excessive dosage. A faimilar example is excessive lowering of blood pressure in the elderly causing syncope, strokes, myocardial infarction, and death as a result of inappropriate and over-enthusiastic antihypertensive drug therapy.

Secondary pharmacological actions

Many drugs have several pharmacological actions at normal doses, and although these may be beneficial they are often undesirable. Thus drowsiness with an antihistamine could be beneficial in a sleepless patient with urticaria at home but disastrous in a thirsty long-distance lorry driver. Many of the acute clinical problems of drug overdosage and poisoning result from a combination of exaggerated therapeutic effects and secondary pharmacological actions.

Allergic and hypersensitivity reactions

Many drug reactions have an immunological basis, and these may range in severity from minor evanescent skin reactions to rapidly fatal anaphylaxis. The immunological basis of drug toxicity is described in more detail below.

Idiosyncrasy

Bizarre, unexpected and inexplicable immediate reactions are sometimes referred to as 'idiosyncracy'. The mechanisms are unknown.

Organ-specific toxicity

This form of toxicity is usually predictable from animal studies and is a function of dosage and duration of treatment. For example, as a group, the non-steroid acidic anti-inflammatory drugs cause gastrointestinal ulceration and renal papillary necrosis, benzodiazepines cause CNS depression and digitalis preparations are cardiotoxic. Drugs may also produce local toxicity at the site of application such as conjunctivitis with eye drops, muscle necrosis and fibrosis after intramuscular injections and gastrointestinal ulceration with slow release or enteric coated potassium chloride.

Changes in drug effects due to disease

The response to drugs may be profoundly altered by disease either through enhanced sensitivity of receptors or because of pharmacokinetic abnormalities (Prescott, 1975b). Many examples are known and adverse reactions are most likely to occur in seriously ill patients. Patients with hypothyroidism, respiratory failure and advanced liver disease, are particularly sensitive to CNS depressants (Branch et al, 1976), patients with burns, uraemia, peripheral nerve injury and muscle wasting may respond to usual doses of succinyl choline with the release of large amounts of K^+ causing ventricular arrhythmias (Tolomie, Joyce and Mitchell, 1967). The explanation for increased drug toxicity in certain diseases is often obscure. For example, it is difficult to understand why salicylate hepatotoxicity should be confined to young patients with rheumatoid arthritis and collagen diseases (Prescott, 1977). Sometimes drugs produce the opposite effect to that expected. Saralasin may increase blood pressure in some hypertensive patients and isoprenaline and theophylline may aggravate bronchospasm in some patients with cystic fibrosis (Shapiro et al, 1976).

Disease may alter drug distribution. The volume of distribution is decreased in cardiac and peripheral circulatory failure with increased drug concentrations in the central, well-perfused tissues (Benowitz and Meister, 1976). In addition, the binding of acidic drugs to plasma proteins is reduced in patients with hypoalbuminaemia and renal failure (Reidenberg, 1976). In severe cardiac failure there is also reduced hepatic and renal blood flow, and in such circumstances the elimination of drugs with high hepatic extraction ratios (e.g. lignocaine) may be grossly impaired (Prescott, Adjepon-Yamoah and Talbot, 1976a).

Many pathological factors influence the activity of drug metabolising enzymes, and toxicity may be enhanced or diminished, depending on whether it is mediated by the parent drug or metabolites (Mitchell et al, 1975; Drayer, 1976). There may be gross impairment of drug metabolism in chronic advanced liver disease (Adjepon-Yamoah, Nimmo and Prescott, 1974) but marked prolongation of the plasma half-life of one drug is not necessarily associated with correspondingly delayed elimination of other drugs. The underlying pathology, hepatic blood flow and extraction ratio must all be taken into account. Thus the plasma half-life of lignocaine is prolonged to a much greater extent than that of paracetamol or antipyrine in patients with chronic liver disease (Forrest et al, 1977). Drug metabolism is impaired with acute hepatic damage resulting from paracetamol overdosage but enhanced following recovery from barbiturate poisoning (Forrest et al, 1974). Biliary tract obstruction interferes with the elimination of drugs with extensive biliary secretion such as rifampicin.

Dietary deficiencies, malnutrition, starvation and consumption of ethanol and other compounds may alter intracellular reduced glutathione (GSH) concentrations and thus predispose to toxicity and neoplasia caused by alkylating drug metabolites which are normally inactivated by conjugation with GSH (McLean and Day, 1975; Buttar, Chow and Downie, 1977).

Drug effects may be enhanced in advanced renal disease because of increased receptor sensitivity, changes in drug distribution, decreased plasma protein binding, changes in drug metabolism, abnormalities of acid-base and electrolyte balance and decreased clearance of drugs and active metabolites (Reidenberg, 1976; Fabre and Balant, 1976). Many drugs are eliminated primarily by renal excretion and will cumulate progressively as the creatinine clearance falls below 20 to 30 ml/min unless the dosage interval is increased. Polar drug metabolites which normally have little or no biological activity, cumulate to a remarkable degree in advanced renal failure and may cause serious toxicity. Thus clofibrate can produce severe myopathy (Pierides et al, 1975) and benzodiazepines and tricyclic antidepressants can cause fatal dialysis dementia (Taclob and Needle, 1976). The nephrotoxicity of drugs may be enhanced by dehydration since this increases the corticomedullary and luminal-interstitial concentration gradients while changes in urine pH can have profound effects on the solubility, renal clearance and intrarenal distribution of weak organic acids and bases.

Thus the systemic and renal toxicity of high-dose methotrexate therapy is reduced by making the urine alkaline and increasing its aqueous solubility. This simultaneously increases its renal clearance and reduces the risk of its intrarenal precipitation (Stoller et al, 1975). The nephrotoxicity of organic acids may also be modified by compounds which compete for active tubular transport. Probenicid, for example, reduces the renal tubular necrosis induced by cephaloridine, aspirin and oxyphenbutazone (Arnold, Collins and Starmer, 1976).

Interference with natural defence mechanisms and host resistance

Cytotoxic drugs, immunosuppressive agents, anti-inflammatory drugs and corticosteroids modify the normal physiological responses to injury and infection. Susceptibility to infection is increased, physical signs may be suppressed and patients may succumb to fulminating sepsis (Weitzman and Aisenberg, 1977). Infection is a common cause of death in patients given cytotoxic and immunosuppressive agents, and organisms which are not normally highly pathogenic may be responsible. Relief of pain in arthritic weight-bearing joints by anti-inflammatory drugs may permit excessive loads and abnormal movements resulting in joint destruction.

Interference with nutrient absorption, protein synthesis and growth

Drugs may interfere with absorption of nutrients and vitamins (Clark, 1976). Chronic therapy with colcnicine, p-aminosalicylate, phenformin, neomycin and mefenamic acid may cause malabsorption syndromes while oral contraceptives, anticonvulsants, and salicylazosulphapyridine may rarely cause folate deficiency. In high dosage, corticosteroids have a catabolic action and the resultant impairment of collagen synthesis causes dermal atrophy and osteoporosis. These drugs also impair growth in children. Some drugs produce toxic effects by interfering with the action of vitamins. Thus the peripheral neuropathy induced by isoniazid is reversed by pyridoxine, and co-trimoxazole occasionally causes megaloblastic anaemia in the malnourished by inhibiting the conversion of folate to essential tetrahydrofolic acid.

Inhibition of cell division

Cytotoxic drugs, alkylating agents and antimetabolites produce a characteristic spectrum of toxicity by inhibiting normal cell division. Rapidly dividing cells are affected most with resultant myelodepression and gastroenteritis. These drugs are usually potent teratogens.

Teratogenesis

The welfare of the developing fetus is threatened by the maternal use of drugs. Despite the awful lesson of thalidomide (Spiers, 1961), drugs are still prescribed for over 97 per cent of mothers-to-be in Edinburgh and 65 per cent take non-prescription drugs (Nelson and Forfar, 1971). The fetus is most susceptible to teratogens during the critical period of organogenesis in the first trimester of pregnancy, and the incidence of phocomelia was almost 100 per cent when thalidomide was taken between the 34th and 45th day after the last menstrual period. Teratogens are thought to act by interfering with normal cell division during development. Such commonly used drugs as aspirin, benzodiazepines, warfarin and phenytoin seem to be teratogenic in man (Nelson and Forfar, 1971; Hanson et al, 1976; Holzgreve, Carey and Hall, 1976; Safra and Oakley, 1975).

Carcinogenesis

The carcinogenic potential of most drugs remains unknown and drug-induced neoplasia is particularly difficult to detect because of the long induction period and exposure of most of the population to multiple drugs. Animal studies are difficult to assess because of species differences and the multifactorial aetiology of neoplasia. The use of some commonly used drugs is associated with malignant disease in man. About 10 per cent of patients with analgesic nephropathy in Sweden develop transitional cell tumours of the renal pelvis (Johansson et al, 1974) and controversy is raging over the apparent five-fold increase in the risk of endometrial carcinoma in women prescribed oestrogens for postmenopausal symptoms (Smith et al, 1975). The carcinogenicity of immunosuppressive and alkylating agents is well known, but they are being used increasingly (and often with doubtful benefit) for the treatment of non-malignant conditions. The use of azathioprine, melphalan, and cyclophosphamide has been associated with leukaemias, sarcomas and tumours of the skin and bladder (Wall and Clausen, 1975; Sieber, 1975; *Lancet*, 1977). The incidence of malignant tumours in renal transplant patients receiving immunosuppressive therapy is about 100 times that of the general population, and some patients develop multiple tumours (Mendelsohn, 1976).

Genetically determined toxicity

Many examples are known of genetically determined drug toxicity caused by abnormal or atypical receptors and enzymes (Vesell, 1975). Examples include drug-induced haemolysis, prolonged paralysis with succinyl choline and genetically controlled differences in drug metabolising enzyme activity. The peripheral neuropathy associated with isoniazid therapy occurs predominately in slow acetylators and is apparently caused by the parent drug while hepatotoxicity is caused by acetylhydrazine metabolites and is observed most often in fast acetylators (Mitchell et al, 1976a). Similarly, the systemic lupus erythematosus syndrome caused by hydralazine and procainamide has been related to the acetylator phenotype (Davies, Beedle and Rawlins, 1975). Other examples of genetically determined toxicity dependent on drug metabolism include porphyria, methaemoglobinaemia and haemolysis induced by phenacetin and salicylazosulphapyridine and slow hydroxylation of phenytoin. Genetic factors are involved in some immunological reactions to drugs.

Drug withdrawal

These reactions are different in that they occur in the absence of drug. Functional adaption, or tolerance, occurs at the cellular level with chronic exposure to some drugs, particularly those acting on the CNS (e.g. narcotic analgesics, most hypnotics, amphetamines, and ethanol). Increasing doses are required to maintain the initial response and abrupt withdrawal of the drug results in a 'rebound' effect with manifestations opposite to those produced by the drug. Withdrawal from CNS depressants such as barbiturates and ethanol taken in large doses is characterised by restlessness, agitation, insomnia, tachycardia, fever, hyperventilation, tremor, confusion, delirium, hallucinations and convulsions. The rebound wakefulness and increased rapid-eye-movement (REM) sleep following sudden withdrawal of hypnotics is a major factor in perpetuation of the widespread dependence on these drugs. Contrary to popular belief, disturbed sleep follows the withdrawal of nitrazepam (Adam et al, 1976) and abrupt cessation of diazepam may cause convulsions (Rifkin, Quitkin and Klein, 1976). The severity of withdrawal reactions depends, amongst other factors, on the rate at which drug and active metabolite concentrations fall after the last dose. Thus drugs with long biological half-lives such as phenobarbitone, methadone and benzodiazepines have a lower withdrawal and dependence potential than those with a shorter duration of action such as amylobarbitone, pethidine and ethanol.

Abrupt withdrawal of other drugs may also cause problems. Acute adrenal insufficiency may follow withdrawal of corticosteroids, severe hypertension may occur when clonidine is discontinued, and sudden withdrawal of propranolol in patients with ischaemic heart disease may exacerbate angina and precipitate fatal myocardial infarction (Miller et al, 1975). A most unusual withdrawal effect has been reported in which massive hepatic necrosis occurred in Australia-antigen (HB$_S$ Ag) positive patients following cessation of therapy for malignant disease with cytotoxic drugs. This was attributed to sudden restoration of immunocompetence in the presence of the virus (Galbraith et al, 1975).

Drug dependence

Drug abuse in the young is a serious problem and a most pernicious form of toxicity. Drug dependence also occurs in older age groups as a result of the inappropriate repeat prescription of hypnotics, tranquillisers and narcotics such as dipipanone, d-propoxyphene and dihydrocodeine.

Social effects of drugs

Psychoactive drugs are widely prescribed and have important effects on alertness, judgement, memory, coordination and psychomotor skills. Important decisions are undoubtedly taken under the influence of these drugs, and they also contribute to the toll of death and injury on the roads. Hypnotics, sedatives, tranquillisers, antidepressants, antihistamines, anticonvulsants, narcotic analgesics (including pentazocine, d-propoxyphene and codeine derivatives), clonidine and alpha-methyldopa may cause drowsiness, impair judgement and prolong reaction times. These effects may persist for many hours or even days after the last dose and are greatly increased by consumption of alcohol (Molander and Duvhök, 1976). Some 3 to 5 per cent of drivers in the UK are taking psychoactive drugs at any given time (not to mention alcohol) (Silverstone, 1974), and doctors rarely mention the dangers of these drugs when they prescribe them. In Oslo, more than 20 per cent of drivers admitted to hospital after road accidents were found to have diazepam in their blood (Haffner, Bø and Lunde, 1974) and a Glasgow train driver passed through three sets of red signal lights and crashed his passenger train into another under the influence of diazepam (*The Times*, 1975). Particular problems arise with drugs with long biological half-lives (e.g. benzodiazepines) because drug and active metabolite concentrations increase gradually over many days with repeated doses and the progressive impairment of performance may not be appreciated.

Drug interaction

Drug interactions have a pharmacodynamic or pharmacokinetic basis. Many are avoidable, and polypharmacy is an important contributory factor. The subject has been extensively reviewed (Morselli, Cohen and Garattini, 1974) and relatively few of the thousands of potential interactions are of major clinical importance (Prescott, 1973). These include mutual potentiation by CNS depressants, and interactions involving oral anticoagulants, cytotoxic agents, antacids, anticonvulsants, anti-inflammatory drugs (especially phenylbutazone) and inhibition or induction of microsomal enzymes.

Errors of drug formulation
Faulty drug manufacture is rare but has resulted in serious toxicity. A recent outbreak of digitalis poisoning was traced to tablets containing 0.2 mg of the more potent digitoxin and 0.05 mg of digoxin instead of the proper content of 0.25 mg of digoxin (Leby and Van Enter, 1970).

Toxicity caused by additives or vehicle
Additives, solvents or contaminants may cause toxicity rather than the drug itself. A notorious example was the use of ethylene glycol as solvent in a sulphonamide elixir resulting in many deaths in the USA (Geiling and Cannon, 1937).

BIOCHEMICAL MECHANISMS OF TOXICITY

Drugs produce biological effects by interfering with some aspect of cell structure or function. The mechanisms involved include non-specific membrane effects, interaction with physiological receptors, enzyme inhibition, covalent binding (often after metabolic activation) and stimulation of immunological responses. Only the toxic effects of drugs unrelated to therapeutic actions will be discussed here.

Enzyme inhibition
This is an important mechanism of drug toxicity. Inhibition may be relatively specific as with methotrexate, in which case the action is selective, or there may be interference with many enzymes causing multiple and widespread effects. Substrate analogues often inhibit enzymes competitively and reversibly, but in some cases inhibition is irreversible (e.g. monoamine oxidase inhibitors). Drugs may also reduce enzyme activity by reacting or competing with cofactors, such as the inhibition of pyridoxal phosphate-dependent enzymes by isoniazid. Some enzymes contain metals and are susceptible to inactivation by chelating agents. Unexpected death has followed the use of nitroprusside, but this should not be surprising because it undergoes a rapid non-enzymatic reaction with haemoglobin to release cyanide (Smith and Kruszyna, 1974). Cyanide inactivates cytochrome oxidase by combining avidly with its ferric iron and the resultant inhibition of cell respiration causes widespread metabolic effects. Other examples of generalised metabolic effects include phenformin-induced lactic acidosis, and inactivation of vital enzymes by heavy metals which bind strongly to SH groups. Salicylates cause uncoupling of oxidative phosphorylation with inhibition of many of the enzymes of intermediary metabolism dependent on ATP for their energy (Smith and Smith, 1966).

Metabolic activation and covalent binding
Most drugs undergo metabolic transformation to some extent, and metabolites are an important cause of toxicity (Gillette, 1974; Mitchell et al, 1975; Oesch, 1976). Highly reactive metabolites can be formed by the action of cytochrome P-450-dependent

microsomal oxidases, and the liver is a major target organ. Other organs may be damaged by metabolites formed locally or released into the circulation from the liver. The urinary tract is vulnerable because most drugs and metabolites are concentrated in renal tissue and remain in contact with bladder epithelium for long periods. Bladder epithelium in patients with vesical tumours may contain large amounts of beta-glucuronidase, and this may facilitate local hydrolysis of conjugates releasing active carcinogenic metabolites (Boyland, Wallace and Wallace, 1957).

Hepatotoxins and carcinogens such as the senecio pyrrolizidine alkaloids, aflatoxins, dimethylnitrosamine, carbon tetrachloride and bromobenzene produce their effects through the formation of highly reactive alkylating metabolites within the liver cell. Similar mechanisms have recently been established for such commonly used drugs as paracetamol, frusemide, isoniazid and possibly halothane (Mitchell et al, 1974, 1976a, 1976b; Sipes and Brown, 1976). The toxic metabolites generated by microsomal oxidation include free radicals, epoxides and N-hydroxy compounds which bind covalently to vital cell constituents causing necrosis. The extent of liver damage is directly related to the degree of covalent binding and susceptibility to the hepatotoxicity of many of these agents can be greatly influenced by treatments which alter microsomal enzyme activity. Induction with 3-methylcholanthrene or phenobarbitone generally increases toxicity while inhibition with piperonyl butoxide or SKF525A usually protects (Mitchell et al, 1973, 1975). Similarly, reduction in microsomal enzyme activity produced by feeding a low-protein diet decreases the hepatic metabolism of carbon tetrachloride and dimethylnitrosamine and greatly reduces their hepatotoxicity (Mitchell et al, 1973). In the case of dimethylnitrosamine, decreased hepatic metabolism increases the exposure of the kidneys to the compound and protein-deficient animals die later from renal tumours rather than early from hepatic necrosis. Other enzymes are usually involved in the inactivation of toxic intermediate metabolites and the overall effects of enzyme induction and inhibition are complex and unpredictable (Gillette, 1974).

Paracetamol hepatotoxicity
Acute centrilobular hepatic necrosis following paracetamol overdosage is an increasing problem and a common cause of fulminant hepatic failure in the UK. It is caused by the formation of a minor arylating metabolite which binds covalently to hepatocytes (Mitchell et al, 1974, 1975). With therapeutic doses this toxic metabolite is inactivated by preferential conjugation with reduced glutathione (GSH) and excreted in the urine as cysteine and mercapturic acid conjugates of paracetamol. With toxic doses, GSH is depleted and the metabolite is free to bind covalently with vital cell constituents (Mitchell et al, 1974, 1975). As expected, patients who have previously taken microsomal inducing agents such as barbiturates or ethanol are more vulnerable (Wright and Prescott, 1973). There is a threshold dose for paracetamol hepatotoxicity, and covalent binding does not occur until hepatic GSH stores have been reduced to about 30 per cent of normal. Prior depletion with diethyl maleate or a yeast diet greatly increases paracetamol hepatotoxicity (Mitchell et al, 1974; McLean and Day, 1975). Administration of GSH itself is not very effective in preventing hepatic necrosis, but good results have been obtained in animals with precursors and other SH donors such as L-cysteine, L-methionine, cysteamine and dithiocarb (Mitchell et al, 1974; McLean and Day, 1975; Strubelt, Siegers and Schütt, 1974). Cysteamine is very effective in preventing

severe liver damage after paracetamol poisoning provided it is given within 10 h of overdosage in adequate dosage (Prescott et al, 1976b). Similar results have been obtained with L-cysteine and N-acetylcysteine, but L-methionine is less effective and does not always prevent severe liver damage.

The mechanisms of protection by these agents are unknown. Although cysteine and cysteamine replete hepatic GSH levels in animals (Strubelt et al, 1974) this is unlikely to account for protection in man since they do not increase the urinary excretion of the cysteine and mercapturic acid conjugates of paracetamol after overdosage. The severity of liver damage is directly related to the urinary excretion of the cysteine conjugate and inversely related to paracetamol sulphate excretion (Howie, Adriaenssens and Prescott, 1977). Cysteamine inhibits cytochrome P-450 reductase and probably acts by inhibiting the oxidation of paracetamol to the arylating metabolite.

SH donors such as cysteamine, L-cysteine and dithiocarb also protect against ionising radiation and the toxicity of alkylating agents, carbon tetrachloride, bromobenzene and heavy metals. They may act by the common mechanism of trapping reactive metabolites and radicals which might otherwise attack vulnerable SH groups of essential proteins and enzymes. Many compounds including hepatotoxins, carcinogens (including polycyclic hydrocarbons and diethyl stilboestrol) and ethacrynic acid are conjugated with GSH and excreted as mercapturic acid conjugates (Chasseaud, 1973) and GSH probably plays a vital biological role in protecting essential thiol and other groups from attack by reactive metabolites and other alkylating agents (Mitchell et al, 1974, 1975).

Phenacetin

Phenacetin, a precursor of paracetamol, also causes acute hepatic necrosis in animals, and has long been suspected as a cause of renal papillary necrosis. Again, the severity of liver damage is related to covalent binding of phenacetin and depletion of hepatic GSH, and is increased by pretreatment with 3-methylcholanthrene and decreased by piperonyl butoxide. Phenacetin also binds covalently to renal tissue and depletes renal glutathione. These effects of phenacetin are unlikely to be due to its prior conversion to paracetamol and the toxic metabolite is probably N-hydroxyphenacetin. The excretion of the latter as labile N-O-glucuronide or sulphate conjugates may be related to the occurrence of renal pelvic tumours in analgesic abusers (Mitchell et al, 1975).

Isoniazid and frusemide hepatotoxicity

Isoniazid and frusemide also cause acute hepatic necrosis through the formation of reactive alkylating metabolites. Isoniazid hepatotoxicity occurs predominately in fast acetylators, and is caused by acetylhydrazine produced by the hydrolysis of acetyl isoniazid to isonicotinic acid. Acetylhydrazine is converted by hepatic cytochrome P-450-dependent oxidases to N-hydroxyacetylhydrazine which dehydrates to acetyldiazine. The latter or a further derivative is a potent alkylating agent which binds covalently to hepatocytes. Again, covalent binding and hepatic necrosis is increased by phenobarbitone and decreased when the hydrolysis of acetylisoniazid to acetylhydrazine is inhibited by bis-p-nitrophenylphosphate. A similar sequence of metabolic activation was demonstrated for iproniazid, another hepatotoxin (Mitchell et al, 1976a).

In high doses, frusemide causes massive hepatic necrosis in animals through covalent binding via the furan ring. The reactive metabolite is probably an epoxide, and hepatotoxicity is reduced by inhibition of microsomal oxidases. The lack of toxicity of frusemide at low doses with a dose-threshold effect is due to extensive plasma protein binding with saturation at high plasma concentrations (Mitchell et al, 1976b). Structural analogues of frusemide and other furans are hepatotoxic, and some also cause renal and pulmonary damage (Mitchell et al, 1975). Nitrofurantoin is well known to cause pulmonary toxicity with chronic use, and it has also been implicated in the aetiology of chronic active hepatitis (Strömberg and Wengle, 1976). It is conceivable that these lesions are caused by metabolic activation of nitrofurantoin.

Cephaloridine and cephalothin

The nephrotoxicity of cephaloridine is potentiated by frusemide, and it contains a thiophene ring which resembles a furan ring with the oxygen replaced by sulphur. Many thiophene-containing compounds cause hepatic and renal tubular necrosis, and cephaloridine-induced tubular necrosis is prevented by inhibition of microsomal oxidases with piperonyl butoxide or cobaltous chloride. Unlike other furan and thiophene compounds, frusemide and cephaloridine do not deplete renal GSH stores (Mitchell et al, 1975). With the exception of cephalothin, other cephalosporins in clinical use do not contain a thiophene ring and do not seem to cause renal damage. However, like cephaloridine, cephalothin may cause acute renal failure (Burton et al, 1974).

Halothane, fluroxene and methoxyflurane

Halothane occasionally causes acute hepatic necrosis, especially after repeated exposure (Walton et al, 1976). As with other halogenated hydrocarbons, this form of toxicity may be caused by reactive alkylating metabolites since halothane binds covalently and produces acute hepatic necrosis in animals pretreated with a microsomal enzyme inducing agent (Sipes and Brown, 1976). Fluroxene is another anaesthetic gas which causes liver damage. Its hepatotoxicity in animals is greatly potentiated by phenobarbitone pretreatment (Mitchell et al, 1975) and fatal massive hepatic necrosis has been recorded after its use in a patient taking phenobarbitone and phenytoin (Reynolds, Brown and Vandam, 1972). Similarly, the nephrotoxicity of methoxyflurane depends upon microsomal drug metabolising enzyme activity (Bell, Hitt and Mazze, 1975).

Carcinogenesis

Chemical carcinogens are thought to act by binding covalently to DNA, and any drug which forms active alkylating metabolites is a potential carcinogen. Of the examples mentioned above, isoniazid and oestrogens are carcinogenic in animals and use of the latter has been associated with endometrial carcinoma and hepatoma in women (Smith et al, 1975; Davis et al, 1975). Chemically reactive drugs such as cytotoxic alkylating agents probably cause neoplasia by direct binding with DNA, but many other carcinogens must first be converted to alkylating metabolites (Miller and Miller, 1966). The polycyclic hydrocarbons are converted by microsomal enzymes to carcinogenic 'K' region epoxides, which in common with many other chemically reactive epoxides are conjugated with GSH and excreted in the urine as mercapturic acids (Chasseaud, 1973; Oesch, 1976). Once again, GSH assumes a vital protective role. Aromatic amines undergo N-hydroxylation, and the carcinogenic metabolites may be N-O-sulphate esters (Mitchell et al, 1975). Carcinogenicity is usually associated with mutagenicity.

Immunological drug reactions

Most drug reactions are considered by clinicians to be immunological in nature and to be caused by 'allergy' or 'hypersensitivity'. Drugs may stimulate the formation of antibodies directly ('complete antigens') but more often this only occurs after metabolic activation and conjugation with proteins to form haptenes (Remmer and Schüppel, 1972).

Drug toxicity can be produced by several different types of immunological reaction. Anaphylactic and immediate reactions are mediated by IgE antibodies produced by previous exposure to the drug in sensitive individuals. Immunoglobulin IgE becomes attached to the surface of cells including mast cells and basophils. Subsequent administration of the drug causes the rapid release of kinins and vasoactive compounds resulting in oedema, erythema, pruritus, bronchoconstriction, hypotension and collapse. Drugs and their metabolites can also stimulate the formation of IgM or IgG antibodies. Again, this response can occur directly, or as a result of the combination of drug or metabolites with plasma or cell-membrane proteins. The subsequent antigen–antibody reaction involves fixation of complement and results in lysis of the cell, e.g. haemolysis, thrombocytopenia or agglutination of leucocytes. In some cases of haematotoxicity (e.g. amidopyrine agranulocytosis) agglutinins may be active only in the presence of the drug.

Another type of immunological drug reaction involves the combination of circulating antigen and antibody with the formation of immune complexes. These complexes activate complement and are deposited in small vessels giving rise to inflammation and necrosis as a result of release of kinins, lysosymes and proteases. The primary lesion is a vasculitis and the clinical manifestations include skin rashes, fever, arthropathy and glomerulitis. These vasculonecrotic reactions usually develop after the drug has been taken for 7 to 14 days and are generalised with multisystem involvement.

Drugs may also stimulate the development of autoantibodies directed against specific cells or cell nuclei. The mechanisms involved are unknown. Examples include haemolytic anaemia with methyldopa and mefenamic acid, and the systemic lupus erythematosus syndrome caused by procainamide and hydralazine. Autoantibodies, as shown by positive antiglobulin (Coombs) and antinuclear factor tests may appear within a few weeks of starting therapy with these drugs, but overt clinical manifestations do not usually appear for many months. The oculocutaneous syndrome caused by beta-adrenergic blocking drugs may have a similar basis. A further type of reaction is delayed hypersensitivity to drugs applied to the skin. This response is thought to be mediated by T (thymus-derived) lymphocytes at the site of contact (Whittingham and Mackay, 1976).

A variety of immunological tests have been employed in attempts to prove an immunological basis for adverse drug reactions (Greaves, 1973). With a few exceptions they are unreliable and results are often difficult to interpret. Provocation tests can be highly dangerous, even with very small doses of drug, and cross-reaction may occur not only with related drugs, but also with food additives and colouring agents. Although the yellow dye tartrazine cross-reacts with anti-inflammatory drugs causing asthma and urticaria (Stenius and Lemola, 1976), it is still, unbelievably, being used to colour formulations of antibiotics and bronchodilators taken by asthmatics.

REFERENCES

Adam, K., Adamson, L., Brezinova, V., Hunter, W. M. & Oswald, I. (1976) Nitrazepam: lastingly effective but trouble on withdrawal. *British Medical Journal*, **i**, 1558–1560.

Adjepon-Yamoah, K. K., Nimmo, J. & Prescott, L. F. (1974) Gross impairment of hepatic drug metabolism in a patient with chronic liver disease. *British Medical Journal*, iv, 387–388.

Arnold, L., Collins, C. & Starmer, G. A. (1976) Studies on the modification of renal lesions due to aspirin and oxyphenbutazone in the rat and the effects on the kidney of 2 : 4-dinitrophenol. *Pathology*, 8, 179–184.

Bell, L. E., Hitt, B. A. & Mazze, R. I. (1975) The influence of age on the distribution, metabolism and excretion of methoxyflurane in Fischer 344 rats: a possible relationship to nephrotoxicity. *Journal of Pharmacology and Experimental Therapeutics*, 195, 34–40.

Benowitz, N. L. & Meister, W. (1976) Pharmacokinetics in patients with cardiac failure. *Clinical Pharmacokinetics*, 1, 389–405.

Boyland, E., Wallace, D. M. & Wallace, D. C. (1957) Enzyme activity in relation to cancer. Inhibition of urinary beta-glucuronide of patients with cancer of the bladder by oral administration of 1 : 4-saccharolactone and related compounds. *British Journal of Cancer*, 11, 578–589.

Branch, R. A., Morgan, M. H., James, J. & Read, A. E. (1976) Intravenous administration of diazepam in patients with chronic liver disease. *Gut*, 17, 975–983.

Burton, J. R., Lichtenstein, N. S., Colvin, R. B. & Hyslop, N. E., Jr (1974) Acute renal failure during cephalothin therapy. *Journal of the American Medical Association*, 229, 679–682.

Buttar, H. S., Chow, A. Y. K. & Downie, R. H. (1977) Glutathione alterations in rat liver after acute and subacute oral administration of paracetamol. *Clinical and Experimental Pharmacology and Physiology*, 4, 1–6.

Caranasos, G. J., May, F. E., Stewart, R. B. & Cluff, L. E. (1976) Drug-associated deaths of medical inpatients. *Archives of Internal Medicine*, 136, 872–875.

Chausseaud, L. F. (1973) The nature and distribution of enzymes catalysing the conjugation of glutathione with foreign compounds. *Drug Metabolism Reviews*, 2, 195–220.

Clark, F. (1976) Drugs and vitamin deficiency. *Adverse Drug Reaction Bulletin*, 57, 196–199.

Collins, E. & Turner, G. (1975) Maternal effects of regular salicylate ingestion in pregnancy. *Lancet*, ii, 335–338.

Davies, D. M., Beedie, M. A. & Rawlins, M. D. (1975) Antinuclear antibodies during procainamide therapy and drug acetylation. *British Medical Journal*, iii, 682–684.

Davis, M., Portmann, B., Searle, M., Wright, R. & Williams, R. (1975) Histological evidence of carcinoma in a hepatic tumour associated with oral contraceptives. *British Medical Journal*, iv, 496–498.

Dollery, C. T. & Rawlins, M. D. (1977) Monitoring adverse reactions to drugs. *British Medical Journal*, i, 96–97.

Drayer, D. E. (1976) Pharmacologically active drug metabolites: therapeutic and toxic activities, plasma and urine data in man, accumulation in renal failure. *Clinical Pharmacokinetics*, 1, 426–443.

Fabre, J. & Balant, L. (1976) Renal failure, drug pharmacokinetics and drug action. *Clinical Pharmacokinetics*, 1, 99–120.

Forrest, J. A. H., Finlayson, N. D. C., Adjepon-Yamoah, K. K. & Prescott, L. F. (1977) Antipyrine, paracetamol and lignocaine elimination in chronic liver disease. *British Medical Journal*, i, 1384–1387.

Forrest, J. A. H., Roscoe, P., Stevenson, I. H. & Prescott, L. F. (1974) Abnormal drug metabolism following barbiturate and paracetamol overdosage. *British Medical Journal*, iv, 499–502.

Galbraith, R. M., Eddleston, A. L. W. F., Williams, R., Zuckerman, A. J. & Bagshawe, K. D. (1975) Fulminant hepatic failure in leukaemia and choriocarinoma related to withdrawal of cytotoxic drug therapy. *Lancet*, ii, 528–530.

Gardner, P. & Cluff, L. E. (1970) The epidemiology of adverse drug reactions. A review and perspective. *Johns Hopkins Medical Journal*, 126, 77–87.

Geiling, E. M. K. & Cannon, P. R. (1937) Pathologic effects of elixir of sulfanilamide (ethylene glycol) poisoning. *Journal of the American Medical Association*, 111, 919–926.

Gillette, J. R. (1974) A perspective on the role of chemically reactive metabolites of foreign compounds in toxicity I and II. *Biochemical Pharmacology*, 23, 2785–2793, 2927–2938.

Greaves, M. W. (1973) Detecting the culprit in adverse drug reactions. *Adverse Drug Reaction Bulletin*, No. 39, 124–127.

Haffner, J. F. W., Bø, O. & Lunde, P. K. M. (1974) Alcohol and drug consumption as causal factors in road traffic accidents in Norway. *Journal of Traffic Medicine*, 2, 52–56.

Hanson, J. W., Myrianthopoulos, N. C., Sedgwick, A. & Smith, D. W. (1976) Risks to offspring of women treated with hydantoin anticonvulsants with emphasis of fetal hydantoin syndrome. *Journal of Pediatrics*, 89, 662–668.

Herbst, A. L., Ulfelder, H. & Poskanzer, D. C. (1971) Adenocarcinoma of the vagina: association of maternal stilbestrol therapy with tumour appearance in young women. *New England Journal of Medicine*, 284, 878–881.

Holzgreve, W., Carey, J. C. & Hall, B. D. (1976) Warfarin-induced fetal abnormalities. *Lancet*, ii, 914–915.

Howie, D., Adriaenssens, P. I. & Prescott, L. F. (1977) Paracetamol metabolism following overdosage: application of high performance liquid chromatography. *Journal of Pharmacy and Pharmacology*, 29, 235–237.

Hurwitz, N. (1969) Admissions to hospital due to drugs. *British Medical Journal*, i, 539–540.

Johansson, S., Angervall, L., Bengtsson, U. & Wahlqvist, L. (1974) Uroepithelial tumours of the renal pelvis associated with the abuse of phenacetin containing analgesics. *Cancer (Philadelphia)*, **33**, 743–753.

Karch, F. E. & Lasagna, L. (1975) Adverse drug reactions—critical review. *Journal of the American Medical Association*, **234**, 1236–1241.

Koch-Weser, J., Sellers, E. M. & Zacest, R. (1977) The ambiguity of adverse drug reactions. *European Journal of Clinical Pharmacology*, **11**, 75–78.

Lancet (1977) Therapy-linked leukaemia. i, 519–520.

Leby, A. H. & Van Enter, C. M. J. (1970) Large-scale digitoxin intoxication. *British Medical Journal*, iii, 737–740.

Lewis, P. D., Patel, A. J., Bendek, G. & Balazs, R. (1977) Do drugs acting on the nervous system affect cell proliferation in the developing brain? *Lancet*, i, 399–401.

McLean, A. E. M. & Day, P. A. (1974) The effect of diet on the toxicity of paracetamol and the safety of paracetamol–methionine mixtures. *Biochemical Pharmacology*, **24**, 37–42.

McQueen, E. G. (1976) New Zealand Committee on Adverse Drug Reactions. 11th Annual Report 1976. *New Zealand Medical Journal*, **84**, 450.

Meade, T. W. (1975) Subacute myelo-optic neuropathy and clioquinol. An epidemiological case-history for diagnosis. *British Journal of Preventive and Social Medicine*, **29**, 157–169.

Melmon, K. L. (1971) Preventable drug reactions—causes and cures. *New England Journal of Medicine*, **284**, 1361–1367.

Mendelsohn, G. (1976) Multiple tumors in a renal transplant recipient. *Johns Hopkins Medical Journal*, **139**, 253–256.

Miller, E. C. & Miller, J. A. (1966) Mechanisms of chemical carcinogenesis: nature of proximate carcinogens and interactions with macromolecules. *Pharmacology Reviews*, **18**, 805–838.

Miller, R. R., Olson, H. G., Amsterdam, E. A. & Mason, D. T. (1975) Propranolol-withdrawal rebound phenomenon. Exacerbation of coronary events after abrupt cessation of antianginal therapy. *New England Journal of Medicine*, **293**, 416–418.

Mitchell, J. R., Jollow, D. J., Gillette, J. R. & Brodie, B. B. (1973) Drug metabolism as a cause of drug toxicity. *Drug Metabolism and Disposition*, **1**, 418–423.

Mitchell, J. R., Thorgeirsson, S. S., Potter, W. Z., Jollow, D. J. & Keiser, H. (1974) Acetaminophen-induced hepatic injury: protective role of glutathione in man and rationale for therapy. *Clinical Pharmacology and Therapeutics*, **16**, 676–684.

Mitchell, J. R., Potter, W. Z., Hinson, J. A., Snodgrass, W. R., Timbrell, J. A. & Gillette, J. R. (1975) Toxic drug reactions. In *Concepts in Biochemical Pharmacology: Handbook of Experimental Pharmacology*, XXVIII/3, ed. Gillette, J. R. & Mitchell, J. R., pp. 383–419. Berlin: Springer-Verlag.

Mitchell, J. R., Zimmerman, H. J., Ishak, K. G., Thorgeirsson, U. P., Timbrell, J. A., Snodgrass, W. R. & Nelson, S. D. (1976a) Isoniazid liver injury: clinical spectrum, pathology and probable pathogenesis. *Annals of Internal Medicine*, **84**, 181–192.

Mitchell, J. R., Nelson, W. L., Potter, W. Z., Sasame, H. A. & Jollow, D. J. (1976b) Metabolic activation of furosemide to a chemically reactive hepatotoxic metabolite. *Journal of Pharmacology and Experimental Therapeutics*, **199**, 41–52.

Molander, L. & Duvhök, C. (1976) Acute effects of oxazepam, diazepam and methylperone, alone and in combination with alcohol on sedation, coordination and mood. *Acta pharmacologica et toxicologica*, **38**, 145–160.

Morselli, P. L., Cohen, S. N. & Garattini, S. (eds.) (1974) *Drug Interactions*. New York: Raven Press.

Mulroy, R. (1973) Iatrogenic disease in general practice: its incidence and effects. *British Medical Journal*, ii, 407–410.

Nelson, M. M. & Forfar, J. O. (1971) Associations between drugs administered in pregnancy and congenital abnormalities of the fetus. *British Medical Journal*, i, 523–527.

Oesch, F. (1976) Metabolic transformation of clinically used drugs to epoxides: new perspectives in drug–drug interactions. *Biochemical Pharmacology*, **25**, 1935–1937.

Ogilvie, R. I. & Ruedy, J. (1967) Adverse reactions during hospitalisation. *Canadian Medical Association Journal*, **97**, 1445–1450.

Pierides, A. M., Alvarez-Ude, F., Kerr, D. N. S. & Skillen, A. W. (1975) Clofibrate-induced muscle damage in patients with chronic renal failure. *Lancet*, ii, 1279–1281.

Porter, J. & Jick, H. (1977) Drug-induced anaphylaxis, convulsions, deafness and extrapyramidal symptoms. *Lancet*, i, 587–588.

Prescott, L. F. (1973) Clinically important drug interactions. *Drugs*, 5, 161–186.

Prescott, L. F. (1975a) Anti-inflammatory analgesics and drugs used in rheumatoid arthritis and gout. In *Meyler's Side Effects of Drugs*, ed. Dukes, M. N. G., Vol. VIII, pp. 207–240. Amsterdam: Excerpta Medica.

Prescott, L. F. (1975b) Pathological and physiological factors affecting drug absorption, distribution, elimination and response in man. In *Concepts in Biochemical Pharmacology: Handbook of Experimental Pharmacology*, XXVIII/3, ed. Gillette, J. R. & Mitchell, J. R., pp. 234–257. Berlin: Springer-Verlag.

Prescott, L. F. (1977) Antipyretic analgesics. In *Side Effects of Drugs*, Annual I. ed. Dukes, M. N. G., pp. 64–85. Amsterdam: Excerpta Medica.

Prescott, L. F., Adjepon-Yamoah, K. K. & Talbot, R. G. (1976a) Impaired metabolism of lignocaine in patients with myocardial infarction and cardiac failure. *British Medical Journal*, i, 939–941.

Prescott, L. F., Park, J., Sutherland, G. R., Smith, I. J. & Proudfoot, A. T. (1976b) Cysteamine, methionine, and penicillamine in the treatment of paracetamol poisoning. *Lancet*, ii, 109–113.

Reidenberg, M. M. (1976) The binding of drugs to plasma proteins from patients with poor renal function. *Clinical Pharmacokinetics*, 1, 121–125.

Remmer, H. & Schüppel, R. (1972) The formation of antigenic determinants. In *Hypersensitivity to Drugs*, ed. Samter, M. & Parker, C. W., Vol. 1, pp. 67–89. Oxford: Pergamon Press.

Reynolds, E. S., Brown, B. R., Jr & Vandam, L. D. (1972) Massive hepatic necrosis after fluroxene anesthesia—a case of drug interaction. *New England Journal of Medicine*, 286, 530–531.

Rifkin, A., Quitkin, F. & Klein, D. F. (1976) Withdrawal reaction to diazepam. *Journal of the American Medical Association*, 236, 2172–2173.

Safra, M. J. & Oakley, G. P. (1975) Association between cleft lip with or without cleft palate and prenatal exposure to diazepam. *Lancet*, ii, 478–480.

Shapiro, G. G., Bamman, J., Kanarek, P. & Bierman, C. W. (1976) Paradoxical effect of adrenergic and methylxanthine drugs in cystic fibrosis. *Pediatrics*, 58, 740–743.

Sieber, S. M. (1975) Commentary: Cancer chemotherapy agents and carcinogenesis. *Cancer Chemotherapy Reports*, 59, 915–918.

Silverstone, T. (1974) Drugs and driving. *British Journal of Clinical Pharmacology*, 1, 451–454.

Sipes, I. G. & Brown, B. R. (1976) An animal model of hepatotoxicity associated with halothane anesthesia. *Anesthesiology*, 45, 622–628.

Smith, R. P. & Kruszyna, H. (1974) Nitroprusside produces cyanide poisoning via a reaction with hemoglobin. *Journal of Pharmacology and Experimental Therapeutics*, 191, 557–563.

Smith, M. J. H. & Smith, P. K. (1966) *The Salicylates. A Critical Bibliographic Review*, pp. 49–105. London: Interscience Publishers.

Smith, D. C., Prentice, R., Thompson, D. J. & Herrmann, W. L. (1975) Association of exogenous estrogen and endometrial carcinoma. *New England Journal of Medicine*, 293, 1164–1167.

Spiers, A. L. (1962) Thalidomide and congenital abnormalities. *Lancet*, i, 303–305.

Stenius, B. S. M. & Lemola, M. (1976) Hypersensitivity to acetylsalicylic acid (ASA) and tartrazine in patients with asthma. *Clinical Allergy*, 6, 119–129.

Stoller, R. G., Jacobs, S. A., Drake, J. C., Lutz, R. J. & Chabner, B. A. (1975) Pharmacokinetics of high-dose methotrexate (NSC-740). *Cancer Chemotherapy Reports*, 6, 19–24.

Strömberg, A. & Wengle, B. (1976) Chronic active hepatitis induced by nitrofurantoin. *British Medical Journal*, ii, 174–175.

Strubelt, O., Siegers, C. P. & Schütt, A. (1974) The curative effects of cysteamine, cysteine, and dithiocarb in experimental paracetamol poisoning. *Archiv für Toxicology (Berlin)*, 33, 55–64.

Taclob, L. & Needle, M. (1976) Drug-induced encephalopathy in patients on maintenance haemodialysis. *Lancet*, ii, 704–705.

The Times (1975) Drug warning in report on train collision. 13th March, p. 5.

Tolomie, J. D., Joyce, T. H. & Mitchell, G. D. (1967) Succinylcholine danger in the burned patient. *Anesthesiology*, 28, 467–470.

Turner, G. & Collins, E. (1975) Fetal effects of regular salicylate ingestion in pregnancy. *Lancet*, ii, 338–339.

Vesell, E. S. (1975) Pharmacogenetics. *Biochemical Pharmacology*, 24, 445–450.

Vickers, N. F. & Stanley, M. M. (1963) Aspirin gastritis: gastroduodenoscopic observations. *Gastroenterology*, 44, 419–423.

Wade, O. L. (1975) The incidence of adverse reactions to drugs. *Journal of Clinical Pathology*, 28, Suppl. 9, 7–13.

Wall, R. L. & Clausen, K. P. (1975) Carcinoma of the urinary bladder in patients receiving cyclophosphamide. *New England Journal of Medicine*, 293, 271–273.

Walton, B., Simpson, B. R., Strunin, L., Doniach, D., Perrin, J. & Appleyard, A. J. (1976) Unexplained hepatitis following halothane. *British Medical Journal*, i, 1171–1176.

Weitzman, S. & Aisenberg, A. C. (1977) Fulminant sepsis after the successful treatment of Hodgkin's disease. *American Journal of Medicine*, 62, 47–50.

Whittingham, S. & Mackay, I. R. (1976) Adverse reactions to drugs: relationship to immunopathic disease. *Medical Journal of Australia*, i, 486–492.

Wright, N. & Prescott, L. F. (1973) Potentiation by previous drug therapy of hepatotoxicity following paracetamol overdosage. *Scottish Medical Journal*, 18, 56–58.

Index

Acebutolol
  effect on hyperactivity syndrome, 177
  properties, 111
  selectivity, 49
Acecainide
  in arrhythmias, 105
  structure, 105
N–Acetylprocainamide *see* Acecainide
Adrenaline
  in hypertension, 61–3
  in shock, 129–30
Adrenergic receptor blocking drugs in hypertension, 72–6
  alpha, 72
  beta, 72–6
Ajmaline in arrhythmias, 115
Albumin, human serum, in shock, 127
Allergy, drug reaction, 192, 201
Alpha–adrenergic blocking drugs in hypertension, 72
Alprenolol
  after acute myocardial infarction, 112
  effect on hyperactivity syndrome, 177
  in hypertension, 75
  properties, 110–11
Amiloride in hypertension, 81
Amitriptyline, 168, 169
  plasma concentration and therapeutic effect, 168
Amphetamine, 'mimicking' mental illness, 179
Angiotensin II, 63–4
Antazoline in arrhythmias, 114
Antiarrhythmic drugs, 93–122
  see also specific drugs
Antiepileptic drugs, 147–62
  individual types, therapy, 156–8
  pharmacokinetics, 147–9
  quality control of drug measurement, 156
  see also specific drugs
Antihypertensive drugs
  individualisation, 82
  pharmacology, 65–81
  see also specific drugs and systems
Aprindine in arrhythmias, 108–9
  adverse effects, 109
  structure, 108
Arachidonic acid metabolism, simplified scheme, 17
Arrhythmias, drugs, 93–122
  see also specific drugs
Aspirin and aspirin–like drugs
  in Bartter's syndrome, 27
    relation to PGs, 27

Aspirin–*continued*
  in cancer, 21
    relation to PGs, 21
  causing gastric bleeding, 23
    relation to PGs, 23–4
  effect on thrombosis, 19
Asthma
  treatment with beta–adrenoceptor agonists, 37–41, 44, 46
  see also Beta–adrenoceptor agonists
Atenolol
  effect on hyperactivity syndrome, 177
  in hypertension, 75
  properties, 111
  selectivity, 48, 49
Autonomic
  ganglia, drugs blocking in hypertension, 68
  nervous system, role in blood pressure regulation, 55–8

Barbiturates, withdrawal symptoms, 195
Bartter's syndrome, prostaglandin levels, and aspirin–like drugs, 27
Behaviour and mood, cerebral mechanisms, neuropharmacology, 177–84
Beta–adrenoceptors, 31–54
  agonists, and antagonists, terminology, 31–2
    properties, 42
    selectivity, 37–42
      determination, 40–1
      mechanisms, 39–40
    in treatment of asthma, 37–41
      cardiotoxicity, 38
      determination of selectivity, 39–40
      evaluation, 39
      mechanisms of selectivity, 40–1
  antagonists, cardiac conditions, 42–7
    conditions treated, 43, 44–7
    selectivity, 42–50
      assessing, 43–45
      individual drugs, 47–50
      significance of selectivity, 46–50
  in arrhythmias, 110–14
  cardioselectivity, 111
  effect on hyperactivity syndrome, 176–7, 180
  in hypertension, 72–6
  intrinsic sympathomimetic activity, 111–12
  membrane stabilising action, 112
  partial agonist activity, 112
  pharmacokinetics, 110–11

Beta–adrenoceptors, *continued*
  prophylaxis of sudden death, 112–3
  selectivity
    individual tissues, 36–7
    mechanism, 32
      tissue selectivity and sub–types, 32–3, 37
        and physicochemical factors, 33–6
      subdivision hypothesis, 36–7
  toxicity, 113
  withdrawal phenomenon, 113
Bethanidine in hypertension, 70–1
Blood
  pressure, regulation, physiology, 55–8
    see also Hypertension
  transfusion in shock, 124
  volume in shock, 124
Bone
  metastases and prostaglandins, 20–1
  resorption by prostaglandins, 20, 21
Breast tumours, and prostaglandins, 19–22
Bretylium in arrhythmias, 109–110
Butyrophenones and causation of mania, 179

Carbamazepine
  in arrhythmias, 114
  in epilepsy, 147, 152–3, 159
    action, 152
    metabolism, 153
    pharmacokinetics, 148
Carcinogenesis, drug–induced, 195, 200
Cardiogenic shock, 132
Catecholamines
  in shock, 129–33
  urinary, in hypertension, 61–3
Cephaloridine nephrotoxicity, 200
Cephalothin nephrotoxicity, 200
Cerebral vessels, dilatation by dopamine, 131
Chlopromazine
  effect on dopamine action, 182
  plasma levels, dosage and clinical response, 170–2
    extrapyramidal side effects, 172
    metabolic pathway, 171
  and platelet aggregation, 174–5
Chlorthalidone in hypertension, 80
Cholecalciferol in epilepsy, 160
Clearance of drugs, kinetics, 2–7
  binding in blood, 4–5, 8, 9–10
  classification, 9–10
  hepatic, 3–5
    blood flow estimate, 6–7
    determinants, 4–5
  intrinsic, 2–3
    altered, 6
  oral, 5–7
  systemic, 5
  volume of distribution, 7–9
Clonazepam in epilepsy, 147, 155–6, 159
  action, 156
  clinical use, 156
  pharmacokinetics, 148

Clonidine, in hypertension, 65–6
  withdrawal syndrome, 65–6
Colloid solutions in shock, 127–8
Colloidal osmotic pressure in pulmonary oedema,
    126
Coronary vessels, effect of catecholamines in shock,
    129
Corticosteroids
  in epilepsy, 159, 160
  effect on prostaglandins, 26
  in shock, 137, 138
Crystalloid infusion in shock, 125
  burns, 125

Debrisoquine in hypertension, 71
Dextrans in shock, 127
Diarrhoea
  action of prostaglandins, 24–5
  and endocrine tumours, raised PG levels, 25
  nutmeg and prostaglandins, 25–6
  radiation, action of aspirin and prostaglandins, 25
Diazepam
  in epilepsy, 147
    pharmacokinetics, 148
  withdrawal symptoms, 196
Diazoxide in hypertension, 78–9
Digoxin in shock, 128–9
Diphenylhydantoin *see* Phenytoin
Disease causing adverse drug reactions, 192–4
Disopyramide in arrhythmias, 105–6
  adverse effects, 106
  pharmacokinetics, 106
Diuretics in hypertension, 80–1
  side effects, 81
Dobutamine, in shock, 129–130, 132
Dopamine
  in cardiogenic shock, 132
  hypothesis of causation of schizophrenia, 177,
    179–80
  neuropharmacology, 179–84
  in septic shock, 132–3
  in shock, 129–33
  vasodilation in shock, 130–1
Drugs
  dependence, 196
  fever following methyldopa, 67
  formulation errors, 197
  interaction, 196
    and lignocaine therapy, 102
    and quinidine therapy, 94–5
  levels, in body fluids, measuring, 13–14
    use of saliva, 14–15
    plasma, relation to pharmacological effects,
      11–15
  'mimicking' mental illness, 179
  reactions, adverse
    allergic and hypersensitivity, 192
    carcinogenesis, 194
    caused by additives or vehicle, 197
    changes in drug effects due to disease, 192–4
    classification, 191–7
    exaggerated therapeutic effect, 192

Drugs, *continued*
   genetically determined toxicity, 195
   hepatotoxicity, 198–200
   idiosyncrasy, 192
   incidence, 189–90
   inhibition of cell division, 194
   interference, with natural defence mechanisms
     and host resistance, 194, 200–1
     with growth, 194
     with nutrient absorption, 194
     with protein synthesis, 194
   mortality and cost, 190
   organ–specific toxicity, 192
   regulations, and reporting, 190
   secondary pharmacological actions, 192
   social effects, 196
   teratogenesis, 194
  toxicity, 189–204
   biochemical mechanisms, 197–201
   classification, 191–7
   epidemiology, 189
   recognition, 190–1
  withdrawal, 195
  with several pharmacological actions, monitoring,
    14
Ductus arteriosus, patent, closed by indomethacin,
  22

Electroconvulsive
  shocks, repeated, effects, 182–4
  treatment and causation of depression, 179, 180
Electrolytes, intracellular, in shock, 135
Endocrine tumours, diarrhoea and PG levels, 25
Endotoxin shock, 137
Enzymes
  drug metabolising, clearance, 2–3
  inhibition, caused by drugs, 197
Epilepsy, drugs, 147–62
  adverse effects, 159–60
  administration of vitamin D, 160
  corticosteroids given simultaneously, 160   diag-
    nosis, 157
  enzyme induction, 159
  folic acid deficiency, 160
  individual types, therapy, 156–8
  method of treatment, 158
  pharmacokinetics, 147–9
  quality control of drug measurements, 156
  of seizure, 157–8
  suitable drug, 158
  type, 157
Epinephrine, *see* Adrenaline
Essential hypertension, 58–63
  classification based on renin status, 58–60
  role of sympathetic nervous system, 60–3
Ethosuximide in epilepsy, 147, 155
  in children and young adults, 155
  pharmacokinetics, 148
External counterpulsation in shock, 134

Fluid therapy in shock, 125–8
Flupenthixol decanoate in schizophrenia, 175

Fluphenazine decanoate in schizophrenia, 175
Fluroxene, toxicity, 200
Fluspirilene, 175
Folic acid deficiency in epilepsy, 160
Frusemide hepatotoxicity, 199–200

Ganglionic blocking drugs in hypertension, 68
Gastric secretion, inhibition, 24
Gastrointestinal prostaglandins
  characteristics, 22–3
  role, 23
Genetic influence on drug metabolism, 13
Glucagon in shock, 128
Glucocorticoids in shock, 137, 138
Glucose solutions in shock, 125
Gold salts, and inhibition of prostaglandins, 27
Growth, drug interference, 194
Guanethidine in hypertension, 68–70
  and amphetamine, 69
  pharmacokinetics, 69–70
  protriptyline pretreatment, 69
  side–effects, 70
  venous reflex, 69

Haemorrhagic shock, 137
Halothane, toxicity, 200
Heart
  force, and catecholamines in shock, 129
  rate, and catecholamines in shock, 129
    control, 56–7
Hepatic clearance of drugs, 3–5
  determinants, 4–5
  drug binding in blood, 4–5
  hepatic blood flow estimate, 6–7
Hepatitis following methyldopa, 67
Hepatotoxicity, drug, 198–200
Hetastarch in shock, 127–8
Hydralazine in hypertension, 76–7
  side effects, 77
Hydroxyethyl starches in solution in shock, 127–8
5–Hydroxytryptamine
  blocking by beta adrenoceptors in hyperactivity
    syndrome, 176–7, 180
  induced platelet aggregation, 175
Hyperactivity syndrome
  effect of beta–adrenoceptors, 176–7, 180
  effect of drugs, 182
Hypercalcaemia, and prostaglandins, 21–2
Hypersensitivity, drug reaction, 192, 201
Hypertension
  drugs, 55–92
    individualisation, 82
    pharmacology, 65–81
    see also specific drugs and systems
   essential, 58–63
   see also Essential hypertension
   pathophysiology, 58–65
   renovascular, 63–5
Hypocalcaemia in epilepsy, 160
Hypoglycaemia in shock, 136
Hypoxia and shock, 135

Imipramine, 168–70
  plasma level and clinical response, 168–9
Immunological aspects of drug reaction, 194, 200–1
Indomethacin, to close patent ductus arteriosus, 22
Indoramin in hypertension, 72
Inflammation and prostaglandins, 26–7
Inotropic drugs in shock, 128–33
Intestinal fluid, stimulation by prostaglandins, 24–5
Intra–aortic balloon counter pulsation in shock, 134
Intrinsic clearance of drugs, 2–3
Isoetharine, properties, 42
Isoniazid hepatotoxicity, 199
Isoprenaline
  potency ratios, 40–1
  properties, 42
  in shock, 129–30
    cardiogenic, 132
    septic, 132–3
  sympathetic stimulation, 44–45
Isoproterenol *see* Isoprenaline

Kinetics of drug clearance, 2–7
  see also Clearance of drugs

Labetalol
  effect on hyperactivity syndrome, 177
  in hypertension, 76
Lactic acidosis in shock, 136
Lignocaine (Lidocaine) in arrhythmias, 99–102
  adverse effects upon conduction, 101–2
  clinical administration, 101
  drug interactions, 102
  haemodynamic effects, 101
  hepatic clearance, 3
  metabolism, 100–1
  pharmacokinetics, 100
  structure, 99, 103
Lithium and causation of mental illness, 179
LSD and 'mimicking' of mental illness, 179
Lysosomes in shock, 136–7

Mental illness
  causation, monoaminergic function, 178–180
  drugs mimicking, 179
Mesenteric vasodilation by dopamine, 131
Metabolic therapy in shock, 135–7
Methoxyflurane, toxicity, 200
Methyldopa, 66–8
  in hypertension, 66–7
  toxicity and side effects, 67–8
Metoprolol
  effect on hyperactivity syndrome, 177
  in hypertension, 75
  properties, 111
  selectivity, 48
Mexiletine in arrhythmias, 104
  structure, 103
Minoxidil in hypertension, 77–8
Monoamine oxidase inhibitors
  and causation of mental illness, 179, 181
  hypertension, 71–2
Monoaminergic function in causation of mental illness, 178–180

Mood and behaviour, cerebral mechanisms, neuropharmacology, 177–84
Myocardial infarction, beta–adrenoceptors in prophylaxis, 112

Neuroleptic drug therapy in schizophrenia
  depot, 175–7
  individualisation, 190–3
    metabolic pathway, 171
    plasma levels, dosage and clinical response, 170–2
Neuropharmacology, and mood and behaviour, 177–84
Nitrazepam, withdrawal symptoms, 195
Nitroprusside in hypertension, 79–80
Noradrenaline
  characteristics, 56
  levels in hypertension, 61–3
  in shock, 129–30
    cardiogenic, 132
    septic, 132–3
  synthesis, 55
Norepinephrine *see* Noradrenaline
Nortriptyline, 167–8, 169
  plasma concentration, 13
    and therapeutic effect, 167
Nutmeg, prostaglandins and diarrhoea, 25–6
Nutrient absorption, drug interference, 194

Obstructive lung disease, beta–adrenoceptor antagonists, 46–7
Oral drug clearance, 5–7
Orciprenaline, properties, 42
Oxprenolol
  effect on hyperactivity syndrome, 177
  in hypertension, 75
  properties, 111

Paracetamol hepatotoxicity, 198–9
Parasympathetic nervous system, 57
Penfluridol, in schizophrenia, 175
Peripheral vascular disease, effects of prostaglandins, 19
Peripheral vascular resistance, 57
Pharmacokinetics, 1–16
  see also Clearance of drugs
  development, 1–2
  plasma drug levels and pharmacological effects, 11–15
Phenacetin, hepatotoxicity, 199
Phenobarbitone in epilepsy, 147, 153–4
  metabolism, 153–4
  pharmacokinetics, 148
Phenothiazines and causation of schizophrenia, 179
Phenoxybenzamine in hypertension, 72
Phenytoin
  in arrhythmias, 102–3
  in epilepsy, 147, 149–152, 159
    action, 150
    characteristics, 149
    clinical effects, 150–2

Phenytoin–*continued*
  forms, 149–50
    pharmacokinetics, 148
    therapeutic range, 149, 151
Pimozide, 175
Pindolol
  effect on hyperactivity sydrome, 177
  in hypertension, 75
  properties, 111
  selectivity, 49–50
Plasma
  drug levels, relation to pharmacological effects,
    11–15
  renin activity in hypertension, 58–60
Platelet aggregation
  action of prostaglandins, 18–19
  and chlorpromazine therapy, 174–5
Polypeptides, effects on behaviour, 180–1
Postganglionic sympathetic nerve endings, drugs
    acting at, 68–72
Practolol, 44
  after acute myocardial infarction, 112, 113
  effect on hyperactivity syndrome, 177
  properties, 111
  selective antagonism, 47–8
  toxicity, 113–4
Prazosin in hypertension, 79
Primidone in epilepsy, 147, 154, 159
  metabolism, 154
  pharmacokinetics, 148
Prindolol *see* Pindolol
Procainamide in arrhythmias, 96–8
  accumulation, 97
  and lupus erythematosus, 96–7
  side effects, 96
  structure, 96
Propafenon in arrhythmias, 114–5
Propranolol
  after acute myocardial infarction, 112
  in arrhythmias, 98–9
  hepatic clearance, 3, 4
  in hypertension, 72–5
    side-effects, 74–5
  properties, 110–11
  in schizophrenia, 176–7
  structure, 98
  withdrawal phenomenon, 113
Prostacyclin *see* Prostaglandin PGI₂
Prostaglandins, 17–30
  and action of aspirin-like drugs in gastric bleed-
    ing, 24
  and Bartter's syndrome, 27
  and bone metastases, 20–21
  bone resorption, 20, 21
  and breast tumours, 19–22
  chemistry, 17–18
  in diarrhoea, 24–5
    of endocrine tumours, 25
    radiation, 25
  dilatation of ductus arteriosus, 22
  distribution in gut, role, 22–3
  and gastro-oesophageal reflux, 23

Prostaglandins–*continued*
  and hypercalcaemia, 21–2
  and inflammation, 26–7
    action of anti-inflammatory drugs, 26–7
  inhibition of gastric secretion, 24
  nutmeg and diarrhoea, 25–6
  and peripheral vascular disease, 19
  PGE, in shock, 133–4
  13, 14-dihydro-PGE₂ bone resorption, 20, 21
  PGI₂, structure, 18
    effect on vasodilation, 19
  6-oxo-PGF₂ bone resorption, 20
    structure, 18
Protriptyline in hypertension, 69
Psychopharmacology, clinical, 163–87
Psychotropic drug therapy, 163–6
  administration, 163
    compliance by patient, 163–4
  and causation of mental illness, 178, 179, 180
  cerebral mechanisms of mood and behaviour,
    177–84
  depot neuroleptics, 175–7
  monitoring techniques, 163–6
    sequence after administration, 163–6
      pharmacodynamic phase, 165–6
      therapeutic phase, 166
    see also specific drugs
  pharmacodynamic approaches, 173–5
Pulmonary
  blood flow, effect of dopamine, 131
  oedema, prevention, 126
Purified protein derivatives in solution in shock, 127

Quinethezone in hypertension, 80
Quinidine in arrhythmias, 93–6
  drug interactions, 94
  ECG tracings, 95
  side effects, 95–6
  structure, 93

Radiation diarrhoea, action of aspirin and prostag-
    landins, 25
Reductosis in shock, 135
Renal
  artery stenosis, diagnosis and management, 64–5
  vasodilatation by dopamine, 131
Renin-angiotensin-aldosterone system, role in blood
    pressure regulation, 57–8
Renin status of essential hypertension, 59–60
Renovascular hypertension, 63–5
Reserpine
  in hypertension, 71
  and 'mimicking' of mental illness, 179, 181
Resuscitation in shock, 124
Rimiterol
  potency ratios, 40–41
  properties, 42

Salbutamol
  potency ratios, 40–41
  properties, 42
Saliva, use in drug monitoring, 14–15

Salmefamol, properties, 42
Schizophrenia, neuroleptic drug therapy, 170–3
    depot, 175–7
    extra pyramidal side effects, 172
    plasma levels, dosage, clinical response, 170–1
    metabolic pathway, 171
    pharmacodynamic approaches, 173–5
        cellular biochemical pharmacology, 174–5
        neuroendocrine approach, 173–4
    and phenothiazines, 179–80
    propranolol, 176
    variation in clinical course, 170
Septic shock, 132–3
Shock
    adrenal corticosteroids in, 137, 138
    blood volume, 124
    cardiogenic, 132
    controlled clinical trials, 138
    drug therapy, 123–45
        catecholamines, 129–33
        constant re-evaluation, 123–4
        crystalloids, 125
        dobutamine, 132
        dopamine, 129–33
        inotropic drugs, 128–33
        resuscitation, 124
        vasodilators, 133–4
    endotoxin, 137
    fluid therapy, 125–8
        colloid solutions, 127–8
        crystalloids, 125
        heart filling pressures, 125–6
        plasma colloidal osmotic pressure, 126
    haemorrhagic, 137
    and hypoxia, 135
    mechanical circulatory support, 134
    metabolic therapy, 135–7
    prognostic factors, 138–9
    septic, 132–3
    stages of therapy, 123
Sinusoidal model, hepatic clearance, 4
Sodium valproate in epilepsy, 147, 154–5, 159
    metabolism, 154–5
    pharmacokinetics, 148
Sotalol
    effect on hyperactivity syndrome, 177
    in hypertension, 75
    properties, 111
Spironolactone in hypertension, 81
Sulphasalazine, effect on prostaglandin formation,
    27

Sympathetic nervous system
    central, drugs altering activity, 65–8
    role in blood pressure regulation, 55–8
    role in essential hypertension, 60–3
Systemic lupus erythematosus syndrome, induced
        by practolol, 113

Teratogenesis, drug causation, 194
Terbutaline properties, 42
Thiazide diuretics in hypertension, 80
Thioxanthenes and causation of mania, 179
Thromboxane A_2 (TXA_2) and B_2, structure, 18
Timolol
    effect on hyperactivity syndrome, 177
    in hypertension, 75
    properties, 111
Tocainide, in arrhythmias, 103–4
    structure, 103
Tolmalol
    properties, 111
    selectivity, 48
Toxicity *see* Drug toxicity
Triamterene in hypertension, 81
Tricyclic antidepressants
    and causation of mental illness, 179, 181
    individualisation, 166–70
    plasma concentrations and therapeutic effect, 166
Tumours, breast, and prostaglandins, 19–22
TXA_2 *see* Thromboxane A_2

Vascular
    effects of catecholamines in shock, 130
    selectivity of beta-adrenoceptor antagonists,
        47–50
Vasodilatation, dopaminergic, in shock, 130–1
Vasodilators
    in hypertension, 76–80
    in shock, 133–4
Vasopressin analogue in shock, 134
Venous
    capacitance, 57
    equilibration model, hepatic clearance, 4
Verapamil in arrhythmias, 107–8
    contraindications, 108
    structure, 107

Withdrawal symptoms, 195–6
    beta-adrenoceptors, 113
    diazepam, 196